TIMI Risk Score for UA/NSTEMI
Risk Score = Total Points (0–7)

Factor	Points	14-Day risk of cardiac events	
		SCORE	RISK (%)
Age ≥ 65	1	0/1	
≥ 3 CAD Risk factors	1		
Known coronary stenosis ≥ 50%			
ASA use in prior 7			
Recent severe ang			
Elevated cardiac bi			
ST deviation ≥ 0.5 r			

Antman et al. JAMA, 264:

CHADS 2 Score = sum of individual risk factors (0–6)		Score	Adjusted stroke rate (%/year)
Risk Factor	Points	0	1.9
Congestive Heart Failure	1	1	2.8
Hypertension	1	2	4
Age > 75 y	1	3	5.9
Diabetes mellitus	1	4	8.5
Prior stroke or TIA	2	5	12.5
		6	18.2

Gage et al. JAMA. 2001; 285:2854–2870

Duke Criteria for Infective Endocarditis

Definite endocarditis requires 2 major, 1 major and 3 minor, or 5 minor criteria

Major criteria	Positive blood culture
	Positive echocardiogram or new valve regurgitation
Minor criteria	Predisposing condition or IV drug use
	Fever >38° C
	Vascular phenomena: arterial emboli, septic pulmonary infarcts, mycotic aneurysm, intracranial and conjunctival hemorrhage, Janeway lesions
	Immunologic phenomena: glomerulonephritis, Osler's nodes, Roth spots, rheumatoid factor
	Positive blood cultures not meeting major criteria

Durack DT, Lukes AS, Bright DK. Am J Med. 96:200–209, 1994.

Framingham risk scoring system for men

Age

Years	Points
30–34	−1
35–39	0
40–44	1
45–49	2
50–54	3
55–59	4
60–64	5
65–69	6
70–74	7

Diabetes

	Points
No	0
Yes	2

Smoker

	Points
No	0
Yes	2

Coronary heart disease risk

Total points	10 yr risk (%)
< −3	1
−2	2
−1	2
0	3
1	4
2	5
3	6
4	7
5	9
6	11
7	14
8	18
9	22
10	27
11	33
12	40
13	47
14	56

LDL-C (mg/dL)

	Points
<100	−3
100–129	0
130–159	0
160–190	1
>190	2

HDL-C (mg/dL)

	Points
<35	2
35–44	1
45–49	0
50–54	0
>60	−1

SBP (mmHg) / DBP (mmHg)

SBP (mmHg)	< 80	80–84	85–89	90–99	≥100
<120	0	0	1	2	3
120–129	0	0	1	2	3
130–139	1	1	1	2	3
140–159	2	2	2	2	3
≥160	3	3	3	3	3

Oxford American Handbook of
Cardiology

About the Oxford American Handbooks in Medicine

The Oxford American Handbooks are pocket clinical books, providing practical guidance in quick reference, note form. Titles cover major medical specialties or cross-specialty topics and are aimed at students, residents, internists, family physicians, and practicing physicians within specific disciplines.

Their reputation is built on including the best clinical information, complemented by hints, tips, and advice from the authors. Each one is carefully reviewed by senior subject experts, residents, and students to ensure that content reflects the reality of day-to-day medical practice.

Key series features

- Written in short chunks, each topic is covered in a two-page spread to enable readers to find information quickly. They are also perfect for test preparation and gaining a quick overview of a subject without scanning through unnecessary pages.
- Content is evidence based and complemented by the expertise and judgment of experienced authors.
- The Handbooks provide a humanistic approach to medicine – it's more than just treatment by numbers.
- A "friend in your pocket," the Handbooks offer honest, reliable guidance about the difficulties of practicing medicine and provide coverage of both the practice and art of medicine.
- For quick reference, useful "everyday" information is included on the inside covers.

Published and Forthcoming Oxford American Handbooks

Oxford American Handbook of Clinical Medicine
Oxford American Handbook of Anesthesiology
Oxford American Handbook of Cardiology
Oxford American Handbook of Clinical Dentistry
Oxford American Handbook of Clinical Diagnosis
Oxford American Handbook of Clinical Pharmacy
Oxford American Handbook of Critical Care
Oxford American Handbook of Emergency Medicine
Oxford American Handbook of Geriatric Medicine
Oxford American Handbook of Nephrology and Hypertension
Oxford American Handbook of Neurology
Oxford American Handbook of Obstetrics and Gynecology
Oxford American Handbook of Oncology
Oxford American Handbook of Otolaryngology
Oxford American Handbook of Pediatrics
Oxford American Handbook of Physical Medicine and Rehabilitation
Oxford American Handbook of Psychiatry
Oxford American Handbook of Pulmonary Medicine
Oxford American Handbook of Rheumatology
Oxford American Handbook of Sports Medicine
Oxford American Handbook of Surgery
Oxford American Handbook of Urology

Oxford American Handbook of **Cardiology**

Edited by

Jeffrey R. Bender, MD

Robert I. Levy Professor of Preventive Cardiology
Associate Chief, Cardiovascular Medicine
Yale University School of Medicine
New Haven, Connecticut

Kerry S. Russell, MD, PhD

Associate Professor of Cardiovascular Medicine
Yale University School of Medicine
New Haven, Connecticut

Lynda E. Rosenfeld, MD

Associate Professor of Medicine and Pediatrics
Section of Cardiovascular Medicine
Yale University School of Medicine
New Haven, Connecticut

Sabeen Chaudry, MD

Fellow, Section of Cardiovascular Medicine
Yale University School of Medicine
New Haven, Connecticut

with

Punit Ramrakha

Jonathan Hill

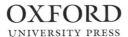

OXFORD
UNIVERSITY PRESS

OXFORD
UNIVERSITY PRESS

Oxford University Press, Inc. publishes works that further
Oxford University's objective of excellence
in research, scholarship and education.

Oxford New York

Auckland Cape Town Dar es Salaam Hong Kong Karachi
Kuala Lumpur Madrid Melbourne Mexico City Nairobi
New Delhi Shanghai Taipei Toronto

With offices in

Argentina Austria Brazil Chile Czech Republic France Greece
Guatemala Hungary Italy Japan Poland Portugal
Singapore South Korea Switzerland Thailand Turkey Ukraine Vietnam

Copyright © 2011 by Oxford University Press, Inc.

Published by Oxford University Press Inc.
198 Madison Avenue, New York, New York 10016

www.oup.com

Oxford is a registered trademark of Oxford University Press

First published 2011

Library of Congress Cataloging-in-Publication Data
Oxford American handbook of cardiology / edited by Jeffrey R. Bender ... [et al.].
p. ; cm.—Other title: American handbook of cardiology
Adapted from: Oxford handbook of neurology / Hadi Manji ... [et al.]. 2007.
Includes index.
ISBN 978-0-19-538969-2

1. Cardiovascular system—Diseases—Handbooks, manuals, etc. I. Bender, Jeffrey R.
II. Title: American handbook of cardiology.
[DNLM: Cardiovascular Diseases—Handbooks. WG 39 O98 2011]
RC669.15.O94 2011
616.1--dc22   2010003761

9 8 7 6 5 4 3 2 1
Printed in China
on acid-free paper

Preface

Despite major advances in prevention and treatment, cardiovascular disease remains the leading cause of death in the United States. There are greater than 1.4 million myocardial infarcts per year. Furthermore, the incidence of atrial fibrillation and of heart failure is rising, in part due to increased survival following acute coronary events, to our aging population, and to other undetermined factors. Management of cardiovascular disease spans a wide range, from acute care of the hemodynamically unstable patient, interventions directed at acute coronary obstructions and electrically unstable rhythms, to disease prevention and care of the chronically ill. In an era of genome-wide scans and growing lists of cardiovascular disease genes, we still require a careful and detailed understanding of disease pathophysiology and management.

In this Handbook, we attempt to represent this wide range of cardiovascular disease. We are fortunate to practice in this era of evidence-based medicine, in which care algorithms are developed and therapeutic approaches are carefully defined. The chapters of this Handbook provide the pathophysiological basis for many of these approaches, followed by delineation of management. Although these chapters will not replace the time dependent accumulation of experience in clinical care, we hope that this Handbook provides easy and rapid access to many major day-to-day management approaches to patients with cardiovascular problems. We hope it will appeal to a broad range of clinicians in many settings, including the coronary care unit, interventional laboratories, emergency departments, and medicine units, both inpatient and outpatient. It is designed to be a rapid reference guide for practicing cardiologists, internists, and relevant trainees.

There should still be sufficient space in white coat pockets for a handbook such as this one. It is our hope that pearls of cardiovascular care will be easily removed from these white pockets and extracted from our *Handbook of Cardiology*.

Acknowledgments

We, the four editors of the *Oxford American Handbook of Cardiology*, would like to express our gratitude to all contributors. This includes the chapter authors, who are all members of the Yale University Cardiovascular Medicine Division, either junior faculty or senior fellows. They carefully have reviewed the most recent data and recommendations for cardiovascular care, incorporating the latest large clinical trials and published recommendations of our largest cardiovascular organizations, the American Heart Association and the American College of Cardiology. Thus, this represents the most up-to-date guidelines and recommendations.

We also acknowledge all involved at Oxford University Press, most notably Andrea Seils, Senior Editor of Clinical Medicine. We are particularly grateful for Andrea's patience, as the coordination of this handbook production took longer than expected.

Most importantly, we want to formally and emphatically display our gratitude to Professors Ramrakha, Hill and all the authors of the original, U.K. version of the *Oxford Handbook of Cardiology*. They all did extraordinary work, assembling the original Handbook. Much of that work has been retained in the U.S. version. As noted, we have attempted to incorporate U.S. guidelines and recently published data into the new Handbook. However, many of the original chapters remain state-of-the-art, and required very little editing or conversion. The work done by the U.K. authors was more than the foundation for the U.S. version. If approval and commendations are forthcoming, as we hope they are, these must be directed to both the U.K. and U.S. authors.

Jeffrey Bender
Kerry Russell
Lynda Rosenfeld
Sabeen Chaudry

Contents

Detailed contents

6   **Preventive cardiology**   **245**

7   **Diseases of the myocardium and pericardium**   **285**

Myocardial diseases

Pericardial diseases

10   Heart disease in pregnancy   405

15   Major trials in cardiology   597

Contributors

Sarah Levin, MD
Fellow
Section of Cardiovascular Medicine
Yale University School of Medicine
New Haven, Connecticut

Brian J. Malm, MD
Assistant Professor
Section of Cardiovascular Medicine
Yale University School of Medicine
New Haven, Connecticut

Carlos Mena, MD
Clinical Instructor
Section of Cardiovascular Medicine
Yale University School of Medicine
New Haven, Connecticut

Rebecca Scandrett, MD
Clinical Instructor
Section of Cardiovascular Medicine
Yale University School of Medicine
New Haven, Connecticut

Symbols and Abbreviations

AAA	Abdominal aortic aneurysm
ABC	airway, breathing, circulation
ABG	arterial blood gas
ACC	American College of Cardiology
ACE	angiotensin-converting enzyme
ACLS	advanced cardiac life support
ACS	acute coronary syndrome; acute ST change
AD	after-depolarization
AED	automated external defibrillator
AF	atrial fibrillation
AFB	acid-fast bacillus
AFP	α-fetoprotein
AHA	American Heart Association
AICD	automatic implantable cardioverter defibrillator
AIH	aortic intramural hematoma
AMI	acute myocardial infarction
ANA	antinuclear antibody
ANP	atrial natriuretic peptide
AP	accessory pathway
APC	atrial premature complex
AR	aortic regurgitation
ARB	angiotensin II receptor blocker
ARDS	acute respiratory distress syndrome
ARVC	arrhythmogenic right ventricular cardiomyopathy
ARVD	arrhythmogenic right ventricular dysplasia
AS	aortic stenosis
ASA	acetylsalicylic acid
ASD	atrial septal defect
ASH	asymmetric septal hypertrophy
AST	aspartamine transferase
ATP	Adult Treatment Panel
AV	atrioventricular
AVN	atrioventricular node
AVNRT	Atrioventricular nodal reentry tachycardia
AVR	aortic valve replacement
AVRT	atrioventricular reentry tachycardia
BB	β-Blocker

bid	twice a day
BLS	basic life support
BMI	body mass index
BMS	bare metal stent
BNP	B-type natriuretic protein
BP	blood pressure
bpm	beats per minute
BUN	blood urea nitrogen
CABG	coronary artery bypass graft
CAC	coronary artery calcium
CAD	coronary artery disease
CAP	community-acquired pneumonia
CBC	complete blood count
CCB	calcium channel blocker
CCS	Canadian Cardiac Society
CCU	coronary care unit
CEA	carcinoembryonic antigen
CHB	complete heart block
CHF	congestive heart failure
CHD	congenital heart disease
CK	creatinine kinase
CMR	cardiac MRI
CMV	cytomegalovirus
CNS	central nervous system
COPD	chronic obstructive pulmonary disease
CPAP	continuous positive airway pressure
CPR	cardiopulmonary resuscitation
CRP	C-reactive protein
CRT	cardiac resynchronization therapy
CS	coronary sinus
CSNRT	corrected sinus node recovery time
CT	computerized tomography
CTO	chronic total occlusion
CVD	cardiovascular disease
CVP	central venous pressure
CW	continuous wave
CXR	chest radiograph
DBP	diastolic blood pressure
DCM	diluted cardiomyopathy
DES	drug-eluting stent
DFT	defibrillation threshold testing

DI	dimensionless index
DIC	disseminated intravascular coagulation
DM	diabetes mellitus
DT	deceleration time
DVT	deep vein thrombosis
EBCT	electron beam computed tomography
EBV	Epstein–Barr virus
ECG	electrocardiogram
ECHO	echocardiogram
EDD	end diastolic dimension
EF	ejection fraction
Egram	electrogram
EMD	electromechanical dissociation
EPS	electrophysiological study
ERNA	equilibrium nuclide angiography
EROA	effective regurgitant orifice area
ERP	effective refractory period
ERT	estrogen replacement therapy
ESD	end systolic dimension
ESR	erythrocyte sedimentation rate
ET	endotracheal
ETT	exercise treadmill testing
FDA	U.S. Food and Drug Administration
FFP	fresh frozen plasma
FFR	fractional flow response
GFR	glomerular filtration rate
GI	gastrointestinal
gp	glycoprotein
Hb	hemoglobin
HDL	high-density lipoprotein
HIS	His bundle
HOCM	hypertrophic obstructive cardiomyopathy
HR	heart rate
HRA	high right atrium
HRT	hormone replacement therapy
HSVPB	His synchronous ventricular premature beat
HTN	hypertension
IABD	intra-aortic balloon pump
ICD	implantable cardiac defibrillator
ICMP	ischemic cardiomyopathy
ICU	intensive care unit

IE	infective endocarditis
IGF	insulin-like growth factor
IHD	ischemic heart disease
IJV	internal jugular vein
IM	intramuscular
INR	International Normalized Ratio
IO	intraosseous
ISFC	International Society and Federation Cardiology
ISR	in-stent restenosis
IV	intravenous
IVC	inferior vena cava
IVP	intravenous push
IVRT	isovolumic relaxation time
IVUS	intravascular ultrasound
JVP	jugular venous pressure
LA	left atrium, atrial
LAD	left anterior descending (artery)
LAO	left anterior oblique
LBBB	left bundle branch block
LDH	lactate dehydrogenase
LDL	low-density lipoprotein
LFTs	liver function tests
LMS	left main stent
LMWH	low-molecular-weight heparin
LQTS	long QT syndrome
LV	left ventricular
LVAD	left ventricular assist device
LVEDP	left ventricular end diastolic pressure
LVF	left ventricular failure
LVH	left ventricular hypertrophy
LVOT	left ventricular outflow tract
MACE	major adverse cardiac event(s)
MDCT	multidetector computed tomography
MI	myocardial infarction
MPI	myocardial perfusion imaging
MR	mitral regurgitation; magnetic resonance
MRA	magnetic resonance angiography
MRI	magnetic resonance imaging
MVP	mitral valve prolapse
MVR	mitral valve replacement
NCEP	National Cholesterol Education Program

NCT	narrow complex tachycardia
NG	nasogastric
NO	nitric oxide
NPPE	negative pressure pulmonary edema
NPPV	noninvasive positive pressure ventilation
nREM	non-rapid eye movement sleep
NSAID	nonsteroidal anti-inflammatory drug
NSTEMI	non-ST elevation myocardial infarction
NYHA	New York Heart Association
OCP	oral contraceptive pill
OCT	optical coherence tomography
OM	obtuse marginal brach
OTC	over-the-counter (drugs)
OTW	over the wire
PA	pulmonary artery
PAD	peripheral arterial disease
PAN	polyarteritis nodosa
PCI	percutaneous coronary intervention
PCWP	pulmonary capillary wedge pressure
PDA	posterior descending artery
PDEI	phosphodiesterase inhibitor
PDGF	platelet-derived growth factor
PE	pulmonary embolus
PEA	pulseless electrical activity
PEEP	positive end expiratory pressure
PFFR	peak expiratory flow rate
PEG	percutaneous endoscopic gastrostomy
PET	positron emission tomography
PFO	patent foramen ovale
PHS	Physicians Health Study
PISA	proximal isovelocity surface area
PLAX	parasternal long axis
PMBV	percutaneous balloon mitral valuloplasty
PMT	pacemaker-mediated tachycardia
po	orally/by mouth
PR	pulmonary regurgitation
prn	as required
PS	pulmonary stenosis
PSAX	parasternal short axis
PTCA	percutaneous transluminal coronary intervention
PTFE	polytetrafluoroethylene

PV	pulmonary valve
PVE	prosthetic valve endocarditis
PVR	pulmonary vascular resistance
qid	four times a day
RA	rheumatoid arthritis; right atrium, atrial
RAS	renal artery stenosis
RBBB	right bundle branch block
RBC	red blood cells
RCA	right coronary artery
RF	radiofrequency; rheumatoid factor
RFA	radio frequency ablation
RHC	right heart catheterization
RIJ	right interior jugular
rtPA	recombinant tissue-type plasminogen activator
RV	right ventricular; regurgitant volume
RVA	right ventricular apex
RVAD	right ventricular assist device
RVF	right ventricular failure
RVH	right ventricular hypertrophy
RVOT	right ventricular outflow tract
RVSP	right ventricular systolic pressure
SACT	sinoatrial conduction time
SAH	subarachnoid hemorrhage
SAM	systolic anterior motion
SAN	sinoatrial node
SBE	subacute bacterial endocarditis
SBP	systolic blood pressure
SC	subcutaneous; subcostal
SCD	sudden cardiac death
SCM	sternocleidomastoid
SCV	subclavian vein
SK	streptokinase
SL	sublingual
SLE	systemic lupus erythematosus
SND	sinal node dysfunction
SNRT	sinus node reentrant tachycardia
SPECT	single photon electron computed tomography
SR	sinus rhythm
SS	suprasternal
STEMI	ST elevation myocardial infarction
SV	stroke volume

SVC	superior vena cava
SVG	saphenous vein graft
SVT	supraventricular tachycardia
TAA	thoracic aortic aneurysm
TB	tuberculosis
TCL	tachycardia cycle length
TDI	tissue Doppler imaging
TdP	torsades de pointes
TEE	transesophageal echocardiography
TFT	thyroid function test
TGF-β	transforming growth factor β
TIA	transient ischemic attack
tid	three times a day
TOF	tetralogy of Fallot
TR	tricuspid regurgitation
TS	tricuspid stenosis
TSH	thyroid-stimulating hormone
TST	tuberculin skin test
TTE	transthoracic echocardiogram
TV	tricuspid valve
TVI	time–velocity index
UA	unstable angina
UFH	unfractionated heparin
VF	ventricular fibrillation
VLDL	very low density lipoprotein
VMA	vanilmandelic acid
VPB	ventricular premature beats
VPC	ventricular premature complex
V/Q	ventilation–perfusion ratio
VSD	ventricular septal defect
VT	ventricular tachycardia
VVI	ventricular demand pacing
WBC	white blood cells
WCL	Wenckebach cycle length
WCT	wide complex tachycardia
WHO	World Health Organization
WMSI	wall motion score index
WPW	Wolff–Parkinson–White (syndrome)

Chapter 1

Cardiovascular emergencies and practical procedures

Cardiovascular emergencies

Adult basic life support

Basic life support (BLS) is the backbone of effective resuscitation following a cardiorespiratory arrest. The aim is to maintain adequate ventilation and circulation until the underlying cause for the arrest can be reversed. A period of 3–4 minutes without adequate perfusion (less if the patient is hypoxic) will lead to irreversible cerebral damage.

Occasionally you will be the first to discover the unresponsive patient, and it is important to rapidly assess the patient and begin cardiopulmonary resuscitation (CPR). The various stages in BLS are described here and summarized in Figure 1.1.

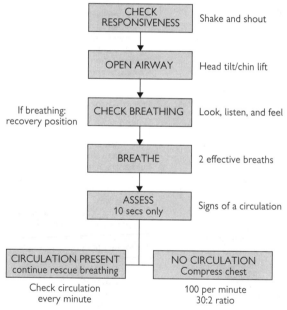

Send or go for help as soon as possible according to guidelines

Figure 1.1 Stages in basic life support. For further information, see BLS/ACLS AHA/ACC guidelines.

1. Assessment of the patient
- **Ensure safety of rescuer and victim.**
- **Check whether the patient is responsive.** Gently shake the victim and ask loudly, "Are you all right?"
  - If the victim responds, place them in recovery position and get help.
  - If the victim is unresponsive, shout for help and move on to assess airway (see below).

2. Airway assessment
- **Open the airway.** With two fingertips under the point of the chin, tilt the head up. If this fails, place your fingers behind the angles of the lower jaw and apply steady pressure upward and forward. Remove ill-fitting dentures and any obvious obstruction. If the patient starts breathing, roll patient over into the recovery position and try to keep the airway open until an orophyrangeal airway can be inserted. Use jaw thrust without head extension, if trauma is suspected (see Fig. 1.2).

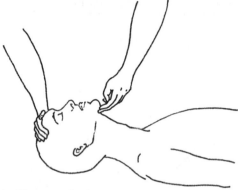

Jaw lift to open the airway

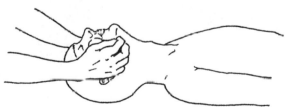

Jaw thrust (thrust the angle of the mandible upward)

Figure 1.2 Opening the airway. Reproduced with permission from Ramrakha PS, Moore KPK (2004). *Oxford Handbook of Acute Medicine*. Oxford, UK: Oxford University Press.

- **Keep the airway open; look, listen, and feel for breathing**. Look for chest movements, listen at the victim's mouth for breathing sounds, and feel for air on your cheek (for no more than 10 seconds).
  - If the patient is breathing, turn patient into the recovery position, check for continued breathing, and get help.
  - If the patient is not breathing or is making occasional gasps or weak attempts at breathing, send someone (or go for help if alone). (On return) Start rescue breaths by giving two slow effective breaths, each resulting in a visible rise and fall in the chest wall; a mouth-to-barrier device may be used.

3. Assessment of circulation

- Assess signs of circulation by feeling the carotid pulse for no more than 10 seconds.
  - If there are signs of circulation but no breathing, continue rescue breaths and check for signs of breathing every 10 breaths.
  - If there are no signs of circulation, start chest compression. Combine rescue breaths and compression at the rate of 30 compressions to two effective breaths, repeating this cycle 5 times in approximately 2 minutes.
- The ratio of compressions to lung inflation remains the same for resuscitation with two persons.

Adult advanced life support

It is unlikely that an effective spontaneous cardiac activity will be restored by BLS without more advanced techniques (intubation for effective ventilation, drugs, defibrillation, etc.). Do not waste time. As soon as help arrives, delegate CPR to someone less experienced in advanced cardiac life support (ACLS), so that you are able to continue.

- Attach the patient to an automated external defibrillator (AED) as soon as possible to determine if there is a shockable rhythm and treat appropriately (see p. 7 for the universal treatment algorithm).
- Oropharyngeal or nasopharyngeal airways help maintain the patency of the airway by keeping the tongue out of the way (see Fig. 1.3). Endotracheal (ET) intubation is the best method of securing the airway. *Do not attempt this if you are inexperienced.*
- Establish venous access. Central vein cannulation (internal jugular or subclavian) is ideal but requires more training and practice and is not for the inexperienced. If venous access fails, drugs may be given via an intraosseous (IO) route (more effective than an ET tube) or ET tube into the lungs (except for bicarbonate and calcium salts). Double the dose of drug if using this route, as absorption is less efficient than when given intravenously (IV).

Post resuscitation care

- *Try to establish the events* that precipitated the arrest from the history, staff, witnesses, and hospital notes of the patient. Is there an obvious cause (myocardial infarction [MI], hypoxia, hypoglycemia, stroke, drug overdose or interaction, electrolyte abnormality, etc.)? Record the duration of the arrest in the notes with the interventions, drugs (and doses) in chronological order.
- *Examine the patient* to check that both lung fields are being ventilated; check for ribs that may have broken during CPR. Listen for any cardiac murmurs. Check the neck veins. Examine the abdomen for an aneurysm or signs of peritoneal irritation. Insert urinary catheter. Consider a nasogastric (NG) tube if the patient remains unconscious. Record the Glasgow Coma Score and perform a brief neurological assessment.
- *Investigations:* **ECG** (electrocardiogram; looking for MI, ischemia, tall T-waves [suggesting hyperkalemia]); **ABG** (arterial blood gas; mixed metabolic and respiratory acidosis is common and usually responds to adequate oxygenation and ventilation once the circulation is restored); **CXR** (chest X-ray; check position of ET tube, look for pneumothorax); and glucose, **CBC** (complete blood count).
- After early and successful resuscitation from a primary cardiac arrest, the patient may rapidly recover completely. The patient must be transferred to an appropriate location (ICU) for monitoring and treatment.
- Change any venous lines that were inserted at the time of arrest for central lines inserted with sterile technique. Insert an arterial line and consider pulmonary artery (PA) catheter (Swan–Ganz) if requiring inotropes.

- Remember to talk to the relatives. Keep them informed of events and give a realistic picture of the arrest and possible outcomes.
- When appropriate, consider the possibility of organ donation and do not be frightened to discuss this with the relatives. Even if discussion with the relatives is delayed, remember that corneas and heart valves may be used up to 24 hours after death.
- Consider hypothermia for patients who do not immediately wake up, or who were "down" for a period of time.

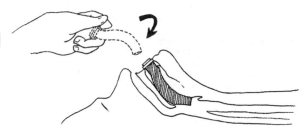

Insertion of oropharyngeal airway

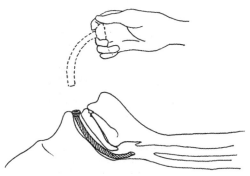

Insertion of nasopharyngeal airway

Figure 1.3 Insertion of nasopharyngeal airway. Reproduced with permission from Ramrakha PS, Moore KPK (2004). *Oxford Handbook of Acute Medicine*. Oxford, UK: Oxford University Press.

Universal treatment algorithm

Cardiac rhythms of cardiac arrest can be divided into two groups:
1. **Ventricular fibrillation/pulseless ventricular tachycardia (VF/VT).**
2. **Other cardiac rhythms,** which include **asystole** and **pulseless electrical activity (PEA).**

The principle difference in treatment of the two groups of arrhythmias is the need for attempted defibrillation in the VF/VT group of patients.

Figure 1.4 summarizes the algorithm for management of both groups of patients.

VF/VT

VF/VT are the most common rhythms at the time of cardiac arrest. Success in treatment of VF/VT is dependent on the delivery of prompt defibrillation. With each minute the chances of successful defibrillation declines by 7%–10%.

- Chest compressions and ventilation should be undertaken until the monitor and defibrillator are available. Typically, 120J to 200J for a biphasic defibrillator and 360J for a monophasic defibrillator is delivered in one shock. Continue CPR x 5 cycles then reassess. If there is persistent VF/VT a second shock is delivered, biphasic at an energy specific to the device and monophasic at 360J. At this time, epinephrine 1 mg IV/IO or vasopressin 40 U IV/IO can be given and repeated. Next, another shock is delivered and if there is persistent VF/VT, then antiarrhythmics (amiodarone 300 mg IV/IO once, then 150 mg IV/IO once, or lidocaine 1.0–1.5 mg/kg first dose and then 0.5–0.75 mg/kg IV/IO for a maximum of 3 mg/kg) should be considered
- After each shock CPR is resumed immediately for 5 cycles, after which the carotid pulse should be palpated only if the waveform changes to one usually capable of providing a cardiac output.
- Shock cycle is repeated every minute if VF/VT persists.
- Myocardial and cerebral viability must be maintained after each shock cycle with chest compressions and ventilation.
- In between cycles of defibrillation, reversible factors must be identified and corrected, the patient intubated (if possible), and venous access obtained.

Non-VF/VT rhythms

The outcome from these rhythms is generally worse than that with VF/VT unless a reversible cause can be identified and treated promptly.

- Chest compressions and ventilation should be undertaken for 3 minutes with each loop of the algorithm (1 minute if directly after a shock).
- With each cycle, attempts must be made to intubate the patient, gain IV access, and give adrenaline.

Asystole

- Atropine 3 mg IV should be given to block all vagal output.
- In the presence of p waves on the ECG strip/monitor, pacing (external or transvenous) must be considered.

Pulseless electrical activity (PEA)

- Identification of the underlying cause and its correction are both vital for successful resuscitation. Resuscitation must be continued while reversible causes are being sought.

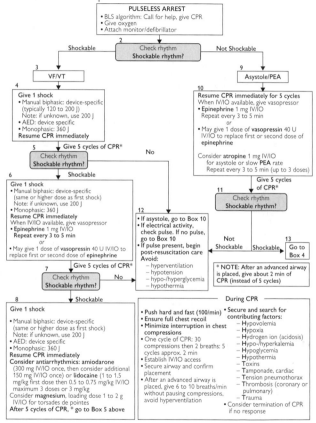

Figure 1.4 Advanced cardiac life support pulseless arrest algorithm. Reprinted with permission from 2005 American Heart Association Guidelines for Cardiopulmonary Resuscitation and Emergency Cardiovascular Care Part 7.2: Management of Cardiac Arrest. *Circulation* 2005; 112(Suppl IV):IV58–IV66. ©2005, American Heart Association, Inc.

Acute pulmonary edema: assessment

Presentation

- Acute breathlessness, cough, frothy blood-stained (pink) sputum
- Collapse, cardiac arrest, or shock
- Associated features may reflect underlying cause:
  - Chest pain or palpitations—? ischemic cardiomyopathy (ICMP)/MI, arrhythmia
  - Preceding history of dyspnea on exertion—? ICMP, poor left ventricular (LV) function
  - Oliguria, hematuria—? acute renal failure
  - Seizures, signs of intracranial bleed

Causes

A diagnosis of pulmonary edema or "heart failure" is not adequate. Underlying causes must be sought in order to direct treatment appropriately. These may be divided into the following:

- Increased pulmonary capillary pressure (hydrostatic)
- Increased pulmonary capillary permeability
- Decreased intravascular oncotic pressure

Often a combination of factors is involved (e.g., pneumonia, hypoxia, cardiac ischemia). See Table 1.1.

The main differential diagnosis is acute exacerbation of chronic obstructive pulmonary disease (COPD) (previous history, quiet breath sounds ± wheeze, fewer crackles). It may be difficult to differentiate the two clinically.

Principles of management

1 Stabilize the patient—relieve distress and begin definitive treatment.
2 Look for an underlying cause.
3 Address hemodynamic and respiratory issues.
4 Optimize and introduce long-term therapy.

Initial rapid assessment

- If the patient is unstable (e.g., unable to speak, hypoxic, systolic blood pressure [SBP] <100 mmHg), introduce stabilizing measures and begin treatment immediately before detailed examination and investigations (see p. 12).
- If the patient is stable and/or if there is doubt as to the diagnosis, give oxygen and diuretic, but await the outcome of clinical examination, CXR, and blood tests such as B-type natriuretic peptide (BNP) level before deciding on definitive treatment.

Urgent investigations for all patients

- ECG   Sinus tachycardia most common.
               ? Any cardiac arrhythmia (SVT, VT).
               ? Evidence of acute ST change (ACS).
               ? Evidence of underlying heart disease (LVH, P mitrale).

- CXR   To confirm diagnosis, looking for interstitial shadowing,
               enlarged hila, prominent upper lobe vessels, pleural
               effusion, and Kerley B lines. Cardiomegaly may or may
               not be present. Also exclude pneumothorax, pulmon-
               ary embolus (oligemic lung fields), and consolidation.

- Laboratory   ? Pre-existing renal impairment. Regular K^+ and Mg
               measurements (once on IV diuretics). Anemia. Signs of
               infection.

- ECHO   As soon as practical to assess LV function, valve abnor-
               malities, ventricular septal defect (VSD), or pericardial
               effusion.

- ABG   Typically low PaO_2, PCO_2 levels may be low (hyper-
               ventilation) or increased depending on severity. Pulse
               oximetry may be inadequate if peripheral vasoconstric-
               tion is present.

Pulmonary edema: causes

Table 1.1 Look for an underlying cause for pulmonary edema

Increased pulmonary capillary pressure (hydrostatic)	
↑ Left atrial (LA) pressure	• Mitral valve disease • Arrhythmia (e.g., AF) with pre-existing mitral valve disease • Left atrial myxoma
↑ Left ventricular end diastolic pressure (LVEDP)	• Ischemia • Arrhythmia • Aortic valve disease • Cardiomyopathy • Uncontrolled hypertension • Pericardial constriction • Fluid overload • High-output states (anemia, thyrotoxicosis, Paget's, atrioventricular (AV) fistula, beri-beri) • Renovascular disease
↑ Pulmonary venous pressure Neurogenic High-altitude pulmonary edema	• L → R shunt (e.g., VSD) • Veno-occlusive disease • Intracranial hemorrhage • Cerebral edema • Postictal
Increased pulmonary capillary permeability	
Acute lung injury	Acute respiratory distress syndrome (ARDS)
Decreased intravascular oncotic pressure	
Hypoalbuminemia	• ↑ Losses (e.g., nephrotic syndrome, liver failure) • ↓ Production (e.g., sepsis) • Dilution (e.g., crystalloid transfusion).

Note: the critical LA pressure for hydrostatic edema = serum albumin (g/L) × 0.57.

Pulmonary edema: management

Stabilize the patient

Patients with acute pulmonary edema should initially be continuously monitored and managed where full resuscitation facilities are available.

- Sit the patient up in bed.
- Give 100% oxygen by facemask, unless contraindicated, i.e., COPD.
- If the patient is severely distressed, the patient may require continuous positive airway pressure (CPAP) or mechanical ventilation.
- Treat any hemodynamically unstable arrhythmia (urgent synchronized DC shock may be required, (p. 78).
- Give
  - Morphine 2.5–5 mg IV (caution: abnormal ABGs)
  - Frusemide 40–120 mg slow IV injection
- Secure venous access and send blood for urgent blood work.
- Unless thrombolysis is indicated, take ABG.
- If SBP ≥90 mmHg and the patient does not have aortic stenosis:
  - Give sublingual nitroglycerin spray (2 puffs).
  - Start IV nitroglycerin infusion 1–10 mg/hr; increase the infusion rate every 15–20 minutes, titrating against blood pressure (aiming to keep SBP ~100 mmHg).
- If SBP <90 mmHg, treat patient as cardiogenic shock.
- Insert a urinary catheter to monitor urine output.
- Repeat ABG and K^+ if the clinical condition deteriorates or fails to improve, or after 2 hours if there is improvement and the original sample was abnormal.
- Monitor pulse, BP, respiratory rate, O_2 saturation with a pulse oximeter (if an accurate reading can be obtained), and urine output.

Further management

The subsequent management of the patient is aimed at ensuring adequate ventilation/gas exchange, ensuring hemodynamic stability, and correcting any reversible precipitants of acute pulmonary edema. If the patient stabilizes, begin investigations looking for a cause.

If the patient remains unstable and/or deteriorates conduct the assessments listed next.

Assess patient's respiratory function

Wheeze may be caused by interstitial pulmonary edema. If there is a history of asthma, give nebulized salbutamol (2.5–5 mg), nebulized ipratropium bromide (500 µg), and hydrocortisone (200 mg) IV.

Indications for further respiratory support

- Patient exhaustion or continuing severe breathlessness
- Persistent hypoxemia
- Rising P_aCO_2
- Persistent or worsening acidosis (pH < 7.2)

Continuous positive airway pressure (CPAP)
This may be tried for cooperative patients who can protect their airway, have adequate respiratory muscle strength, and who are not hypotensive. The positive pressure reduces venous return to the heart and may compromise BP.

Endotracheal intubation and mechanical ventilation
This may be required, and some positive end expiratory pressure (PEEP) should be used. PEEP may also lower SBP.

Discuss the patient with the on-call anesthesiologist and ICU team early.

Assess patient's hemodynamic status

It is important to distinguish between cardiogenic and noncardiogenic pulmonary edema, as further treatment is different for the two groups. Making this distinction may be difficult clinically. A central venous or PA (Swan–Ganz) catheter must be inserted if the patient's condition will allow this procedure.

Management

The general approach involves a combination of diuretics, vasodilators, ⊥ inotropes. Patients may be divided into two groups:
• Patients in shock (with SBP <90 mmHg)
• Hemodynamically stable patients with SBP >90 mmHg

Patients with SBP <90 mmHg

The choice of inotropic agent depends on the clinical condition of the patient and, to some extent, the underlying diagnosis:

SBP <90 mmHg give:
• **Dopamine** at doses of >2.5 μg/kg/min has a pressor action in addition to direct and indirect inotropic effects and may be used at higher doses (10–20 μg/kg/min) if the blood pressure remains low. However, it tends to raise the pulmonary capillary filling pressure further and should be combined with vasodilators (e.g., nitroprusside or hydralazine) once the blood pressure is restored (see below). Beware of arrhythmias at these dosages.
• **Epinephrine** infusion may be preferred to high-dose dopamine as an alternative inotrope. Once the blood pressure is restored (>100 mmHg), vasodilators such as nitroprusside/hydralazine or nitroglycerin infusion should be added to counteract the pressor effects. Epinephrine can be combined with dobutamine and/or a phosphodiesterase inhibitor, especially in the context of a poor ventricle.
• **Dobutamine** infusion at 5 μg/kg/min, increasing by 2.5 μg/kg/min every 10–15 minutes to a maximum of 20 μg/kg/min until BP >100 mmHg. This may be combined with dopamine (2.5–5 μg/kg/min). However, tachycardia and/or hypotension secondary to peripheral vasodilation may limit its effectiveness.
• **Phosphodiesterase inhibitors** (milrinone) should be considered where dobutamine fails.

- **Intra-aortic balloon counterpulsation** should also be used with or without inotropes in the context of a potentially reversible cause for the pulmonary edema and shock (e.g., ongoing myocardial ischemia, VSD, acute mitral regurgitation [MR]).
- Further doses of diuretic may be given.

Patients with SBP ≥90 mmHg
- Further doses of diuretic may be given (furosemide 40–80 mg IV q3–4h or as a continuous infusion [10–80 mg/hr]).
- Continue the nitroglycerin infusion, increasing the infusion rate every 15–20 minutes up to 10 mg/hr, titrating against blood pressure (aiming to keep SBP ~100 mmHg).

Long-term management
- Unless a contraindication exists, start an angiotensin-converting enzyme (ACE) inhibitor, increasing the dose to as near the recommended maximum dose as possible. In the context of LV impairment, ACE inhibitors have significant prognostic benefit.
- If ACE inhibitors are contraindicated or not tolerated, consider use of hydralazine and long-acting oral nitrate in combination.
- If the patient is already on high doses of diuretics and ACE inhibitors, consider addition of spironolactone (25–50 mg) (monitor renal function and serum potassium).
- In the context of stable patients (no clinical features of failure) and poor LV function, β-blockers have significant mortality and some symptomatic benefit (start with very small dose and increase gradually every 2 weeks with regular monitoring). Bisoprolol, carvedilol, and metoprolol can all be used.
- Ensure that all arrhythmias are treated.
- Digoxin can be used for symptomatic improvement.
- Consider cardiac resynchronization therapy (biventricular pacing) in the context of severe LV dysfunction, broad QRS complex ± MR on ECHO.
- Patients in atrial fibrillation (AF) or with poor LV function should be considered for long-term anticoagulation.
- Patients <60 years with severe irreversible LV dysfunction and debilitating symptoms must be considered for cardiac transplantation.

Pulmonary edema: specific conditions

Diastolic LV dysfunction

This typically occurs in elderly hypertensive patients with left ventricular hypertrophy (LVH), where there is impaired relaxation of the ventricle in diastole. There is marked hypertension, pulmonary edema, and normal, or only mild, systolic LV impairment.

With tachycardia, diastolic filling time shortens. As the ventricle is "stiff" in diastole, LA pressure is increased and pulmonary edema occurs (exacerbated by AF as filling by atrial systole is lost).

Treatment involves control of hypertension with IV nitrates (and/or nitroprusside), calcium blockers (verapamil or nifedipine), and even certain β-blockers (e.g., carvedilol, bisoprolol) and, if appropriate, restoration of sinus rhythm.

Fluid overload

Standard measures are usually effective.
- Check that the patient is not anemic (Hb ≥10 g/dL). Remove 500 mL blood via cannula in a large vein and repeat if necessary.
- If anemic (e.g., renal failure) and acutely unwell, consider dialysis.

Known (or unknown) renal failure

- Unless the patient is permanently anuric, large doses of IV furosemide may be required in addition to standard treatment.
- If this fails or the patient is known to be anuric, dialysis will be required.
- In patients not known to have renal failure an underlying cause should be sought.

Anemia

- Cardiac failure may be worsened or precipitated by the presence of significant anemia. Symptoms may be improved in the long term by correcting this anemia.
- If the anemia is thought to be exacerbating pulmonary edema, ensure that an adequate diuresis is obtained prior to transfusion. Give slow transfusion (3–4 hours per unit) of packed cells, with IV furosemide 20–40 mg before each transfusion.

Hypoproteinemia

- Treatment involves diuretics, cautious albumin replacement, spironolactone (if there is secondary hyperaldosteronism), and treatment of the underlying cause for hypoproteinemia.

Acute aortic regurgitation

Presentation
- Sudden, severe aortic regurgitation (AR) presents as cardiogenic shock and acute pulmonary edema.
- The hemodynamic changes are markedly different from those seen in chronic AR. The previous normal-sized LV results in a smaller effective forward flow and higher LVEDP for the same degree of AR.
- Patients are often extremely unstable, tachycardic, and peripherally vasoconstricted and often have pulmonary edema. Unlike chronic AR, pulse pressure may be near normal.
- If available, ask about history of previous valvular heart disease, hypertension, features of Marfan's syndrome (family history), and risk factors for infective endocarditis.
- Physical signs of severe AR include a quiet aortic closure sound (S2); an ejection systolic murmur over the aortic valve (turbulent flow); high-pitched and short, early diastolic murmur (AR); quiet S1 (premature closure of the mitral valve).
- Examine specifically for signs of an underlying cause.
- Where there is no obvious underlying cause (e.g., acute MI), assume infective endocarditis until proven otherwise.

Causes
- Infective endocarditis
- Ascending aortic dissection
- Collagen vascular disorders (e.g., Marfan's)
- Connective tissue diseases (large- and medium-vessel arteritis)
- Trauma
- Dehiscence of a prosthetic valve

Diagnosis
Diagnosis is based on a combination of clinical features and transthoracic and/or transesophageal ECHO.

Management
Acute AR is a surgical emergency and all other management measures are only aimed at stabilizing the patient until urgent aortic valve replacement (AVR) can take place. The patient's clinical condition will determine the urgency of surgery (and risk of mortality).

General measures
- Admit the patient to intensive care unit (ICU).
- Give oxygen and begin treating any pulmonary edema with diuretics.
- Monitor blood gases; mechanical ventilation may be necessary.
- Blood cultures × 3 are essential.
- Serial ECG: watch for developing atrioventricular (AV) block or conduction defects in endocarditis.

Specific measures
- Every patient must be discussed with a cardiothoracic surgeon.
- In the context of good systemic BP, vasodilators such as sodium nitroprusside or hydralazine may temporarily improve forward flow and relieve pulmonary edema.
- Inotropic support may be necessary if the patient is hypotensive. However, inotropes are best avoided as any increase in systemic pressures and peripheral vasoconstriction may worsen AR.
- All patients with hemodynamic compromise should have immediate or urgent AVR.
- *Infective endocarditis*: indications for surgery are given on p. 208.
- Intra-aortic balloon pump (IABP) must be avoided, as it will worsen AR.

Acute mitral regurgitation

Presentation

- Patients most commonly present with acute shortness of breath and severe pulmonary edema. Symptoms may be less severe, or spontaneously improve as left atrial compliance increases. There may be a history of previous murmur, angina, or myocardial infarction.
- The signs are different from those seen in chronic MR because of the presence of a nondilated and relatively noncompliant LA. Acute MR results in a large LA systolic pressure wave (v wave) and hence pulmonary edema.
- Patients may be acutely ill with tachycardia, hypotension, peripheral vasoconstriction, and pulmonary edema, and a pan-systolic murmur of MR.
- Later in the illness, probably because of sustained high left atrial and pulmonary venous pressures, right heart failure develops.
- Examine for signs of any underlying conditions.
- When there is no obvious underlying cause (e.g., acute MI; see Box 1.1), assume the patient has infective endocarditis until proven otherwise.

Diagnosis

Diagnosis is based on a combination of clinical features and ECHO. Transthoracic echocardiography (TTE) can be used to readily diagnose and quantify MR. It also provides information on LV status (in particular regional wall motion abnormalities that can give rise to MR).

TEE can provide specific information about etiology of valve dysfunction, including papillary muscle rupture and MV leaflet (anterior and posterior) structural abnormalities. This information will be vital for a decision regarding definitive management. The important differential diagnosis is a VSD.

TTE and Doppler studies can readily differentiate between the two conditions. Alternatively, if ECHO is not available, pulmonary artery catheterization in acute MR will exclude the presence of a left-to-right shunt and the pulmonary capillary wedge pressure (PCWP) trace will demonstrate a large v-wave.

General measures

- Admit patient to ICU.
- Give oxygen and begin treating any pulmonary edema with diuretics.
- Monitor blood gases; mechanical ventilation may be necessary.
- Blood cultures × 3 are essential.
- If present, MI should be treated in the standard manner.

Specific measures

Pulmonary edema may be very resistant to treatment.

- In the presence of good BP, reduction in preload (nitroglycerin infusion) and afterload, especially with ACE inhibitors, is important. Systemic vasodilators such as hydralazine (12.5–100 mg tid) can also be added.

- An IABP will help decrease LVEDP and increase coronary blood flow.
- *Patients may require inotropic support.* There are multiple combinations and etiologies of MR and hemodynamic status, and local policy and expertise should dictate choice of agent.
- CPAP and intubation and positive-pressure ventilation are extremely useful and must be considered in all severe and/or resistant cases.
- Hemodynamic disturbance and severe pulmonary edema in the context of acute MR is a surgical emergency.
- *Infective endocarditis:* indications for surgery are given on p. 208.
- *Post-infarct MR:* management depends on the patient's condition following resuscitation. Patients who are stabilized may have mitral valve replacement (MVR) deferred because of risks of surgery in the post-infarct patient. Preoperative management should consist of diuretics and vasodilators, including ACE inhibitors, if tolerated. Opening the infarct-related artery (angioplasty) may improve acute MR.

Box 1.1 Causes of acute mitral regurgitation

- Infective endocarditis
- Papillary muscle dysfunction or rupture (post-MI).
- Rupture of chordae tendinae (e.g., infection, myxomatous degeneration, systemic lupus erythematosus [SLE])
- Trauma (to leaflets, papillary muscle, or chordae)
- Prosthetic valve malfunction (e.g., secondary to infection)
- Left atrial myxoma
- Acute rheumatic fever
- Collagen vascular disorders (e.g., Marfan's)
- Connective tissue diseases (large- and medium-vessel arteritis)

Deep vein thrombosis: assessment

Presentation

- Deep vein thrombosis (DVT) is most commonly asymptomatic. Minor leg discomfort or isolated swelling (>65%) in the affected limb are the most common clinical features. Breathlessness or chest pain may be secondary to pulmonary embolism (PE).
- Signs include erythema and swelling of the leg, dilated superficial veins, and calf discomfort on dorsiflexion of the foot (Homan's sign). The thrombus may be palpable as a fibrous cord in the popliteal fossa. Confirm the presence of swelling (>2 cm) by measuring the limb circumference 15 cm above and 10 cm below the tibial tuberosity.
- In all cases of leg swelling, abdominal and rectal (and pelvic in women) examination must be carried out to exclude an abdominal cause.

See Table 1.2 for risk factors for DVT.

Investigations

- *Real-time B-mode venous compression ultrasonography* of leg veins is largely replacing venography as the initial investigation of choice. It is quick and noninvasive, with sensitivity and specificity of over 90%, and does not carry the risk of contrast allergy or phlebitis. It can simultaneously assess extent of proximal progression of the thrombus, in particular, extension into pelvic vessels.
- *D-dimers* have a high negative predictive value for DVT. A low clinical probability of DVT and a negative D-dimer does not require further investigation. A positive D-dimer result should be followed by ultrasonography.
- *Venography:* use if results are uncertain and clinical suspicion is high.
- Consider baseline-investigation blood work.
- If appropriate, look for an underlying cause.
- *Procoagulant screen*: refer to local screening policy and get hematology advice (e.g., prothrombin time [INR] and partial thromboplastin time, C-reactive protein [CRP], erythrocyte sedimentation rate (ESR), proteins C and S, antithrombin III levels, factor V_{Leiden} mutation, auto-Ab screen, immunoglobulins and immunoelectrophoretic strip, anticardiolipin antibody, Ham test, etc.)
- *Screen for malignancy*: ultrasound ± computed tomography (CT) (abdomen and pelvis), CXR, liver function tests (LFTs), prostate-specific antigen (PSA), carcinoembryonic antigen (CEA), CA-125, CA-19.9, β-HCG, etc.

Table 1.2 Risk factors for DVT

Procoagulant states

Congenital	Acquired
Factor V$_{Leiden}$	Malignant disease (~5%)
Antithrombin III deficiency	Antiphospholipid syndrome
Protein C deficiency	Myeloproliferative disorders
Protein S deficiency	Oral contraceptive pill (especially with Factor V$_{Leiden}$ mutation)
	Nephrotic syndrome (via renal AT III losses)
	Homocystinuria
	Paroxysmal nocturnal hemoglobinuria

Venous stasis

Immobility (e.g., long journeys)	Recent surgery
Pelvic mass	Pregnancy or recent childbirth
	Severe obesity

Miscellaneous

Hyperviscosity syndromes
Previous DVT or PE
Family history of DVT/PE

Deep vein thrombosis: management

If there is high clinical suspicion of DVT (the presence of risk factors and absence of an alternative diagnosis), start empiric anticoagulation with low-molecular-weight heparin (LMWH). This may be stopped if subsequent investigations are negative.

Below-knee DVT

Thrombi limited to the calf have a lower risk of embolization and may be treated with compression stockings and subcutaneous (SC) prophylactic doses of LMWH until the patient is mobile, to deter proximal propagation of thrombus. A brief period of systemic anticoagulation with LMWH may lessen the pain from below-knee DVT.

Above-knee DVT

Thrombi within the thigh veins warrant full anticoagulation with LMWH/ unfractionated heparin (UFH) and subsequently with warfarin.

Anticoagulation

Heparin

- LMWHs have now superceded UFH for management of both DVT and PE. They require no monitoring on a daily basis and allow outpatient treatment.
- There must be a period of overlap between LMWH/UFH therapy and anticoagulation with warfarin until the INR is within therapeutic range and stable.
- LMWH are administered primarily as a once-daily subcutaneous (SC) injection, and dosage is determined by patient weight. It may require adjustment for renal dysfunction.

Warfarin

- Always anticoagulate with LMWH/UFH before starting warfarin. Protein C (a vitamin K–dependent anticoagulant) has a shorter half-life than that of the other coagulation factors and levels fall sooner, resulting in a transient procoagulant tendency.
- If DVT is confirmed, begin warfarin and maintain on LMWH/UFH until INR >2.
- Anticoagulate (INR 2–2.5) for 3 months.
- If there is recurrent DVT or the patient is at high risk of recurrence, consider lifelong anticoagulation.

Thrombolysis

This should be considered for recurrent, extensive, proximal venous thrombosis (e.g., femoral or iliac veins), as it is more effective than anticoagulation alone in promoting clot dissolution and produces a better clinical outcome.

Catheter-directed thrombolytic therapy (rt-PA or SK) is superior to systemic thrombolysis.

One approach is streptokinase (SK) 250,000 U over 30 minutes then 100,000 U every hour for 24–72 hours. See p. 100 for contraindications to thrombolysis.

Further management

Women taking the combined oral contraceptive pill (OCP) should be advised to stop this.

If there are contraindications to anticoagulation, consider the insertion of a caval filter to prevent PE.

All patients should be treated with thigh-high compression stockings to try to reduce symptomatic venous distension when mobilizing.

Pulmonary embolism (PE): assessment

Symptoms

- Classically presents with sudden-onset, pleuritic chest pain, associated with breathlessness and hemoptysis. Additional symptoms include postural dizziness or syncope.
- Massive PE may present as cardiac arrest (particularly with electromechanical dissociation) or shock.
- Presentation may be atypical, i.e., unexplained breathlessness or unexplained hypotension or syncope only.
- Pulmonary emboli should be suspected in all breathless patients with risk factors for DVT or with clinically proven DVT.
- Recurrent PEs may present with chronic pulmonary hypertension and progressive right heart failure.

Signs

- Examination may reveal tachycardia and tachypnea only. Look for postural hypotension (in the presence of raised jugular venous pressure [JVP]).
- Look for signs of raised right heart pressures and cor pulmonale (raised JVP with prominent a-wave, tricuspid regurgitation, parasternal heave, right ventricular S3, loud pulmonary closure sound with wide splitting of S2, pulmonary regurgitation).
- Cyanosis suggests a large PE.
- Examine for a pleural rub (may be transient) or effusion.
- Examine lower limbs for obvious thrombophlebitis.
- Mild fever (>37.5°C) may be present. There may be signs of coexisting COPD.

Causes

Most frequently PE is secondary to DVT (leg >> arm).

Other causes

- Rarely secondary to right ventricular thrombus (post-MI)
- Septic emboli (e.g., tricuspid endocarditis)
- Fat embolism (post-fracture)
- Air embolism (venous lines, diving)
- Amniotic fluid
- Parasites
- Neoplastic cells
- Foreign materials (e.g., venous catheters)

Prognostic features

The prognosis in patients with pulmonary emboli varies greatly and is associated in part with any underlying condition. Generally worse prognosis is associated with larger PE; poor prognostic indicators include the following:

- Hypotension
- Hypoxia
- ECG changes (other than nonspecific T-wave changes)

Pulmonary embolism: investigations

General investigations

- ABG

  Normal ABG does not exclude a PE.
  $\downarrow P_aO_2$ is invariable with larger PEs. Other changes include mild respiratory alkalosis and $\downarrow P_aCO_2$ (due to tachypnea) and metabolic acidosis (secondary to shock).

- ECG

  Commonly shows sinus tachycardia $\pm$ nonspecific ST- and T-wave changes in the anterior chest leads. The classical changes of acute cor pulmonale such as $S_1Q_3T_3$, right axis deviation, or right bundle branch block (RBBB) are only seen with massive PE. Less common findings include AF.

- CXR

  May be normal; a near-normal chest film in the context of severe respiratory compromise is highly suggestive of a PE. Less commonly may show focal pulmonary oligemia (*Westermark's sign*), a raised hemidiaphragm, small pleural effusion, wedge-shaped pleural shadow, subsegmental atelectasis, or dilated proximal pulmonary arteries.

- Blood tests

  There is no specific test. Mildly elevated CK, troponin, BNP may be seen.

- ECHO

  Insensitive for diagnosis but can exclude other causes of hypotension and raised right-sided pressures (e.g., tamponade, RV infarction). In PE may show RV dilatation and global hypokinesia (with sparing of apex [*McConnell's sign*]) and pulmonary artery dilation, and Doppler may show tricuspid/pulmonary regurgitation, allowing estimation of RV systolic pressure. Rarely, the thrombus in the pulmonary artery may be visible.

Specific investigations

D-dimer

- A highly sensitive but nonspecific test.
- Useful in ruling out PE in patients with low probability.
- Results can be affected by advancing age, pregnancy, trauma, surgery, malignancy, and inflammatory states.

Ventilation/perfusion (V/Q) lung scanning

A perfusion lung scan (with IV technetium-99-labeled albumin) can be considered in suspected cases of PE, especially if there is a contraindication to giving contrast. A ventilation scan (inhaled xenon-133) in conjunction increases the specificity by assessing whether the defects in the ventilation and perfusion scans "match" or "mismatch." Pre-existing lung disease makes interpretation difficult.

A normal perfusion scan rules out significant-sized PE.

Abnormal scans are reported as low, medium, or high probability:

- A high-probability scan is strongly associated with a PE, but there is a significant minority of false positives.
- A low-probability scan with a low clinical suspicion of PE should prompt a search for another cause for the patient's symptoms.

Box 1.2 Investigations for an underlying cause for PE

- Ultrasound of deep veins of legs
- Ultrasound of abdomen and pelvis (? occult malignancy, pelvic mass, lymphadenopathy)
- CT of abdomen/pelvis
- Screen for inherited procoagulant tendency (e.g., proteins C, S, anti thrombin III, factor V_{Leiden}, etc.)
- Autoimmune screen (anticardiolipin antibody, antinuclear antibody [ANA])
- Biopsy of suspicious lymph nodes or masses

If clinical suspicion of PE is high and the scan is of low or medium probability, alternative investigations are required.

CT pulmonary angiography (CTPA)

This is the recommended initial lung imaging modality in patients with PE as long as there are no contraindications.

- It allows direct visualization of emboli as well as other potential parenchymal disease, which may provide alternative explanation for symptoms.
- Sensitivity and specificity are high (>90%) for lobar pulmonary arteries but not so high for segmental and subsegmental pulmonary arteries.
- A patient with a positive CTPA does not require further investigation.
- A patient with a negative CTPA in the context of a high or intermediate probability of a PE should undergo further investigation.

Evaluation of leg veins with ultrasound

This is not very reliable. Almost half of patients with PE do not have evidence of a DVT and thus a negative result cannot rule out a PE.

Ultrasound is a useful second-line investigation as an adjunct to a CTPA/VQ scan.

Outcome studies have demonstrated that it would be safe not to anticoagulate patients with a negative CTPA and lower limb ultrasound who have an intermediate or low probability of a PE.

Pulmonary angiography

This is the gold-standard investigation. It is indicated in patients in whom diagnosis of embolism cannot be established by noninvasive means. Look for sharp cutoff of vessels or obvious filling defects. It is an invasive investigation and can be associated with 0.5% mortality.

If there is an obvious filling defect, the catheter or a guide wire passed through the catheter may be used to disrupt the thrombus.

After angiography, the catheter may be used to give thrombolytics directly into the affected pulmonary artery (see below).

The contrast can cause systemic vasodilatation and hemodynamic collapse in hypotensive patients.

MR pulmonary angiography

Results are comparable to those of pulmonary angiography in preliminary studies. It can simultaneously assess ventricular function.

Pulmonary embolism: management

1. Stabilize the patient

- Unless an alternative diagnosis is made, the patient should be treated as for a pulmonary embolus until this can be excluded.
- Monitor cardiac rhythm, pulse, BP, and respiration rate every 15 minutes with continuous pulse oximetry and cardiac monitor. Ensure full resuscitation facilities are available.
- Obtain venous access and start IV fluids (crystalloid or colloid).
- Give maximal inspired oxygen via facemask to correct hypoxia. Mechanical ventilation may be necessary if the patient is tiring (beware of cardiovascular collapse when sedation is given for ET intubation).
- **Give LMWH or UFH to all patients with high or intermediate risk of PE until diagnosis is confirmed.** Meta-analysis of multiple trials has shown LMWH to be superior to UFH with a reduction in mortality and bleeding complications. For doses, consult local formulary.
- If there is evidence of hemodynamic instability (systemic hypotension, features of right heart failure) or cardiac arrest, patients will benefit from thrombolysis with recombinant tissue plasminogen activator (rtPA) or streptokinase (see Table 1.3; same doses used for treatment of STEMI [see p. 100]). Local delivery of thrombolytics to the site of thrombus via a PA catheter may also be considered.

2. Analgesia

- Patients may respond to oral nonsteroidal anti-inflammatory drugs.
- Opiate analgesia should be used with caution. The vasodilatation caused by these drugs may precipitate or worsen hypotension. Give small doses (1–2 mg morphine IV) slowly. Hypotension should respond to IV colloid.
- Avoid IM injections (anticoagulation and possible thrombolysis).

3. Anticoagulation

Patients with a positive diagnosis must undergo anticoagulation with warfarin. There should be a period of overlap with LMWH/UFH until INR values are therapeutic. Target INR is 2–3 for most cases.

Standard duration of anticoagulation is as follows:

- 3 months for temporary risk factor
- 3 months for first idiopathic cases
- At least 6 months for other cases
- With recurrent events and underlying predisposition to thromboembolic events (e.g., antiphospholipid antibody syndrome) lifelong anticoagulation may be needed (as well as higher target INR >3).

Table 1.3 Dosage of thrombolytic agents for pulmonary embolus	
rtPA	100 mg over 2 hours or 0.6 mg/kg over 15 minutes (maximum of 50 mg) followed by heparin
Streptokinase	250,000 U over 30 minutes followed by 100,000 U/hr infusion for 24 hours

Contraindications for thrombolysis are identical to those for STEMI (p. 100).

Cardiac arrest (also see p. 5)

Massive PE may present as cardiac arrest with electromechanical dissociation (EMD). Exclude the other causes of EMD.

Hypotension

The acute increase in pulmonary vascular resistance results in right ventricular dilatation and pressure overload, which mechanically impairs LV filling and function. Patients require a higher than normal right-sided filling pressure but may be worsened by fluid overload.

- Insert an internal jugular sheath prior to anticoagulation. This can be used for access later if necessary.
- Give thrombolysis if there are no contraindications.
- If hypotensive give IV fluids.
- If hypotension persists, invasive monitoring and/or inotropic support is required. The JVP is a poor indicator of the left-sided filling pressures in such cases. Adrenaline is the inotrope of choice.
- Femorofemoral cardiopulmonary bypass may be used to support the circulation until thrombolysis or surgical embolectomy can be performed.
- Pulmonary angiography in a hypotensive patient is hazardous as the contrast may cause systemic vasodilatation and cardiovascular collapse.

Pulmonary embolectomy

In patients who have contraindications to thrombolysis and are in shock requiring inotropic support, there may be a role for embolectomy if appropriate skills are on site.

This can be performed percutaneously in the catheterization laboratory using a number of devices or surgically on cardiopulmonary bypass Percutaneous procedures may be combined with peripheral or central thrombolysis.

Seek specialist advice early. Best results are obtained before onset of cardiogenic shock.

Radiological confirmation of the extent and site of embolism is preferable before thoracotomy.

Mortality is ~25%–30%.

Inferior vena cava (IVC) filter

There is little evidence that use of an IVC filter improves short- or long-term mortality rates.

Filters are positioned percutaneously and, if possible, patients must remain anticoagulated to prevent further thrombus formation. Most IVC filters are positioned infrarenally (bird's nest filter) but can also be suprarenal (Greenfield filter).

Indications for IVC filter use include the following:

- Anticoagulation contraindicated—e.g., active bleeding, heparin-induced thrombocytopenia, planned intensive chemotherapy.
- Anticoagulation failure despite adequate therapy.
- Prophylaxis in high-risk patients—e.g., progressive venous thrombosis, severe pulmonary hypertension, extensive trauma.

Fat embolism

This is commonly seen in patients with major trauma. There is embolization of fat and microaggregates of platelets, red blood cells (RBCs), and fibrin in systemic and pulmonary circulation. Pulmonary damage may result directly from the emboli (infarction) or from chemical pneumonitis and ARDS.

Clinical features

There may be a history of fractures followed (24–48 hours later) by breathlessness, cough, hemoptysis, confusion, and rash.

Examination reveals fever (38–39°C), widespread petechial rash (25%–50%), cyanosis, and tachypnea. There may be scattered rales in the chest, although examination may be normal. Changes in mental state may be the first sign with confusion, drowsiness, seizures, and coma. Examine the eyes for conjunctival and retinal hemorrhages; occasionally fat globules may be seen in the retinal vessels.

Severe fat embolism may present as shock.

Investigations

- ABG
  Hypoxia and a respiratory alkalosis (with low P_aCO_2) as for thromboembolic PE

- CBC
  Thrombocytopenia, acute intravascular hemolysis

- Coagulation
  Disseminated intravascular coagulation

- Chemistries and glucose
  Renal failure, hypoglycemia

- Ca^{2+}
  May be low

- Urine
  Microscopy for fat and dipstick for hemoglobin.

- ECG
  Usually nonspecific (sinus tachycardia; occasionally signs of right heart strain)

- CXR
  Usually lags behind the clinical course. There may be patchy, bilateral, air space opacification. Effusions are rare

- CT head
  Consider if there is a possibility of head injury with expanding subdural or epidural bleed

Differential diagnosis

This includes pulmonary thromboembolism, other causes of ARDS, septic shock, hypovolemia, cardiac or pulmonary contusion, head injury, aspiration pneumonia, and transfusion reaction.

Management

- Treat respiratory failure. Give oxygen (maximal via face mask, CPAP and mechanical ventilation if necessary).
- Ensure adequate circulating volume and cardiac output. Central venous pressure (CVP) is not a good guide to left-sided filling pressures, and a PA catheter (Swan–Ganz) may be used to guide fluid replacement. Try to keep PCWP 15–18 mmHg and give diuretics if necessary. Use inotropes to support circulation as required.

- Aspirin, heparin, and Dextran 40 (500 mL over 4–6 hours) are of some benefit in the acute stages but may exacerbate bleeding from sites of trauma.
- High-dose steroids (methylprednisolone 30 mg/kg q8h for 3 doses) have been shown to improve hypoxemia,[1] but steroids are probably most effective if given prophylactically.

1 Lindeque BG, Schoeman HS, Dommisse GF, Boeyens MC, Vlok AL (1987). Fat embolism and the fat embolism syndrome. A double-blind therapeutic study. *J Bone Joint Surg*, 69:128–131.

Hypertensive emergencies

Hypertensive crisis

Hypertensive crisis is defined as a severe elevation in BP (SBP >200 mmHg, DBP >120 mmHg). Rate of change in BP is important. A rapid rise is poorly tolerated and leads to end-organ damage, whereas a gradual rise in a patient with existent poor BP control is better tolerated. Hypertensive crises are classified as follows:

1. **Hypertensive emergency**, where a high BP is complicated by acute target organ dysfunction (see Box 1.3) and includes
- *Hypertensive emergency with retinopathy*—there is marked elevation in BP (classically DBP >140 mmHg) with retinal hemorrhages and exudates (previously called accelerated hypertension), and
- *Hypertensive emergency with papilledema* with a similarly high BP and papilledema (previously called malignant hypertension).
2. **Hypertensive urgency**, where there is a similar rise in BP but without target organ damage.

Conditions presenting as hypertensive emergency

- Essential hypertension.
- Renovascular hypertension: atheroma, fibromuscular dysplasia, acute renal artery occlusion.
- Renal parenchymal disease: acute glomerulonephritis, vasculitis, scleroderma.
- Endocrine disorders: pheochromocytoma, Cushing's syndrome, primary hyperaldosteronism, thyrotoxicosis, heperparathyroidism, acromegaly, adrenal carcinoma.
- Eclampsia and pre-eclampsia.
- Vasculitis.
- Drugs: presence of cocaine, amphetamines, MAOI interactions, or cyclosporine, or withdrawal of β-blocker or clonidine.
- Autonomic hyperactivity in the presence of spinal cord injury.
- Coarctation of the aorta.

Presentation

Occasionally there are minimal nonspecific symptoms such as mild headache and nosebleed.

A small group of patients present with symptoms resulting from BP-induced microvascular damage:
- Neurological symptoms: severe headache, nausea, vomiting, visual loss, focal neurological deficits, seizures, confusion, intracerebral hemorrhage, coma (see below)
- Chest pain (hypertensive heart disease, MI, or aortic dissection) and congestive cardiac failure
- Symptoms of renal failure: renal impairment may be chronic (secondary to long-standing hypertension) or acute (from the necrotizing vasculitis of malignant hypertension)

Patients may present with hypertension as one manifestation of an underlying "disease" (renovascular hypertension, chronic renal failure, CREST syndrome, pheochromocytoma, pregnancy).

Examination should be directed at looking for evidence of end-organ damage even if the patient is asymptomatic (heart or renal failure, retinopathy, papilledema, focal neurological symptoms).

Box 1.3 Hypertensive emergencies

- Hypertensive emergency with retinopathy/papilledema
- Hypertensive encephalopathy
- Hypertension-induced intracranial hemorrhage/stroke
- Hypertension with cardiovascular complications:
  - Aortic dissection
  - MI
  - Pulmonary edema
- Pheochromocytoma
- Pregnancy-associated hypertensive complications
  - Eclampsia and pre-eclampsia
- Acute renal insufficiency
- Hypertensive emergency secondary to acute withdrawal syndromes (e.g., β-blockers, centrally acting antihypertensives)

Hypertensive emergencies: management

Priorities in management are as follows:
1. Confirm the diagnosis and assess the severity.
2. Identify those patients needing specific emergency treatment.
3. Plan long-term treatment.

Diagnosis and severity

- Ask about previous BP recordings, previous and current treatment, sympathomimetics, antidepressants, nonprescription drugs, and recreational drugs.
- Check the blood pressure yourself, in both arms, after a period of rest and, if possible, on standing.
- Examine carefully for clinical evidence of cardiac enlargement or heart failure, peripheral pulses, renal masses, or focal neurological deficit. Always examine the fundi—dilate if necessary.

All patients should have the following tests:

• CBC	Microangiopathic hemolytic anemia with malignant hypertension
• Chemistries	Renal impairment and/or $\downarrow K^+$ (diffuse intrarenal ischemia and secondary hyperaldosteronism)
• Coagulation screen	Disseminated intravascular coagulation (DIC) with malignant hypertension
• CXR	Cardiac enlargement Aortic contour (dissection?) Pulmonary edema
• Urinalysis	Protein and red cells ± casts

Other investigations depending on clinical picture and possible etiology include the following:

• 24-hour urine collection	Creatinine clearance Free catecholamines, metanephrines or vanilmandellic acid (VMA)
• ECHO	LVH, aortic dissection
• Renal US and Doppler	Size of kidneys and renal artery stenosis
• MR renal angiogram	Renal artery stenosis
• CT/MR brain	Intracranial bleed
• Drug screen	Cocaine, amphetamine, others

Indications for admission

- Diastolic blood pressure persistently ≥120 mmHg
- Retinal hemorrhages, exudates or papilledema
- Renal impairment

Treatment principles

- **Rapid reduction in BP is unnecessary, must be avoided, and can be very dangerous**. This can result in cerebral and cardiac hypoperfusion (abrupt change of >25% in BP will exceed cerebral BP autoregulation).
- Initial BP reduction (of 25%) should be achieved over 1–4 hours with a less rapid reduction over 24 hours to a diastolic blood pressure (DBP) of 100 mmHg.
- The only two situations where BP must be lowered rapidly are in the context of aortic dissection and MI.

Treatment

Most patients who are alert and otherwise well may be treated with oral therapy to lower BP gradually.

First-line treatment should be with a β-blocker (unless contraindicated) with a thiazide diuretic, or a low-dose calcium antagonist.

Urgent invasive monitoring (arterial line) prior to drug therapy is indicated for patients with the following:

- Evidence of hypertensive encephalopathy
- Complications of hypertension (e.g., aortic dissection, acute pulmonary edema or renal failure)
- Treatment of underlying condition (e.g., glomerulonephritis, pheochromocytoma, CREST crisis)
- Patients with persistent diastolic BP ≥140 mmHg
- Eclampsia

Sublingual nifedipine must be avoided.

Conditions requiring specific treatment

See Box 1.4.

Long-term management

- Investigate as appropriate for an underlying cause.
- Select a treatment regime that is tolerated and effective. Tell the patient why long-term therapy is important.
- Try to reduce all cardiovascular risk factors by advising the patient to stop smoking (if applicable), giving appropriate dietary advice (cholesterol), and aiming for optimal diabetic control.
- Monitor long-term control and look for end-organ damage (regular fundoscopy, ECG, blood work). Even poor control is better than no control.

Box 1.4 Conditions requiring specific treatment

- Accelerated and malignant hypertension
- Hypertensive encephalopathy
- Eclampsia
- Pheochromocytoma
- Hypertensive patients undergoing anesthesia

Drugs for hypertensive emergencies

Table 1.4 Drugs for treatment of hypertensive emergencies: IV therapy

Drug	Dosage	Onset of action	Comments
Labetalol	20–80 mg IV bolus q10min 20–200 mg/min by IV infusion, increasing every 15 minutes	2–5 minutes	Drug of choice in suspected pheochromocytoma or aortic dissection. Avoid if there is LVF. May be continued orally (see below)
Nitroprusside	0.25–10 µg/kg/min IV infusion	Seconds	Drug of choice in LVF and/or encephalopathy
Nitroglycerine	1–10 mg/hr IV infusion	2–5 minutes	Mainly venodilatation. Useful in patients with LVF or angina
Hydralazine	5–10 mg IV over 20 minutes 50–300 µg/min IV infusion	10–15 minutes	May provoke angina
Esmolol HCl	500 µg/kg/min IV loading dose 50–200 µg/kg/min IV infusion	Seconds	Short-acting β-blocker also used for SVTs
Phentolamine	2–5 mg IV over 2–5 minutes prn	Seconds	

NB: It is dangerous to reduce the blood pressure quickly. Aim to reduce DBP to 100–110 mmHg within 2–4 hours. Unless there are good reasons to commence IV therapy, always use oral medicines.

Table 1.5 Drugs for treatment of hypertensive emergencies: oral therapy

Drug	Dosage	Onset of action	Comment
Atenolol	50–100 mg po daily	30–60 minutes	There are numerous alternative β-blockers
Nimodipine	10–20 mg po q8h (q12h if slow release)	15–20 minutes	Avoid sublingual use, as the fall in BP is very rapid
Labetalol	100–400 mg po q12h	30–60 minutes	Use if pheochromocytoma suspected. Safe in pregnancy
Hydralazine	10–50 mg po q8h	20–40 minutes	Safe in pregnancy
Minoxidil	5–10 mg po od	30–60 minutes	May cause marked salt and water retention Combine with a loop diuretic (e.g. furosemice 40–240 mg daily)
Clonidine	0.2 mg po followed by 0.1 mg hourly max. 30–60 minutes 0.8 mg total for urgent therapy, or 0.05–0.1 mg po q8h increasing every 2 days	30–60 minutes	Sedation is common. Do not stop abruptly as here is a high incidence of rebound hypertensive crisis

Note: Aim to reduce DBP to 100–110 mmHg in 2–4 hours and normalize BP in 2–3 days.

Hypertensive emergency with retinopathy (accelerated and malignant hypertension)

This is part of a continuum of disorders (see Box 1.5) characterized by hypertension (DBP often >120 mmHg) and acute microvascular damage (seen best in the retina but present in all organs). It may be difficult to decide whether the damage in some vascular beds is the cause or effect of hypertension (e.g., an acute glomerulonephritis).

Accelerated hypertension (grade 3 retinopathy) may progress to malignant hypertension, with widespread necrotizing vasculitis of the arterioles (and papilledema).

Presentation is commonly with headache or visual loss and varying degrees of confusion. More severe cases present with renal failure, heart failure, microangiopathic hemolytic anemia, and DIC.

Management

- Transfer the patient to the ICU.
- Insert an arterial line and consider central venous line if there is evidence of necrotizing vasculitis and DIC. Catheterize the bladder.
- Monitor neurological state, ECG, fluid balance.
- Aim to lower the DBP to 100 mmHg or by 15–20 mmHg, whichever is higher, over the first 24 hours.
- Those patients with early features may be treated successfully with oral therapy (β-blockers, calcium channel blockers—see Table 1.5).
- Patients with late symptoms or who deteriorate should be given parenteral therapy aiming for more rapid lowering of BP.
  - If there is evidence of pulmonary edema or encephalopathy, give furosemide 40–80 mg IV.
  - If there is no left ventricular failure (LVF), give a bolus of labetalol followed by an infusion. For patients with LVF, nitroprusside or hydralazine is preferable.
- Consult renal team for patients with acute renal failure or evidence of acute glomerulonephritis (>2+ proteinuria, red cell casts). Dopamine should be avoided as it may worsen hypertension.
- Consider giving an ACE inhibitor. High circulating renin levels may not allow control of hypertension, which in turn causes progressive renal failure. ACE inhibitors will block this vicious circle. There may be marked first-dose hypotension, so start cautiously.
- Hemolysis and DIC should recover with control of BP.

Hypertension in the context of acute stroke or intracranial bleed

Stroke or bleed may be the result of hypertension or vice versa. In the acute setting there is impaired autoregulation of cerebral blood flow and autonomic function. Small changes in systemic BP may result in catastrophic falls in cerebral blood flow.

Systemic BP should not be treated unless DBP >130 mmHg and/or there is severe cerebral edema (with clinical manifestations).

In most cases, BP tends to settle over 24–36 hours. If treatment is indicated, BP reduction principles must be adhered to and a combination of nitroprusside, labetalol, and calcium channel blockers can be used.

Centrally acting agents must be avoided as they cause sedation.

In patients with subarachnoid hemorrhage (SAH), a cerebroselective calcium channel blocker, such as nimodipine, is used to decrease cerebral vasospasm.

Systemic BP must also be treated if it qualifies by principles and/or if it remains elevated after 24 hours. There is no evidence that this reduces further events in the acute phase.

Box 1.5 Hypertensive retinopathy

Grade 1	Tortuous retinal arteries, silver wiring
Grade 2	Atrioventricular (AV) nicking
Grade 3	Flame shaped hemorrhages and cotton wool exudates
Grade 4	Papilledema

Hypertensive encephalopathy

This condition is caused by cerebral edema secondary to loss of cerebral autoregulatory function.

It is usually gradual in onset and may occur in previously normotensive patients at blood pressures as low as 150/100 mmHg. It is rare in patients with chronic hypertension and pressures are also much higher.

Symptoms

- Headache, nausea and vomiting, confusion, grade III and IV hypertensive retinopathy.
- Late features consist of focal neurological signs, seizures, and coma.

Diagnosis

This is a diagnosis of exclusion and other diagnoses must be ruled out (e.g., stroke, encephalitis, tumors, bleeding, vasculitis).

History is helpful, particularly of previous seizures, SAH usually being sudden in onset and strokes being associated with focal neurological deficit. Always exclude hypoglycemia.

Starting hypotensive treatment for hypertension associated with a stroke can cause extension of the stroke.

An urgent MRI or CT brain must be obtained to rule out some of the other diagnoses.

Management

The primary principle of blood pressure control is to reduce DBP by 25% or reduce DBP to 100 mmHg, whichever is higher, over a period of 1–2 hours.

- Transfer the patient to the ICU for invasive monitoring
- Monitor neurological state, ECG, fluid balance.
- Correct electrolyte abnormalities (K^+, Mg^{2+}, Ca^{2+}).
- Give furosemide 40–80 mg IV.
- Nitroprusside is the first-line agent as it is easy to control BP changes, despite its tendency to increase cerebral blood flow.
- Labetalol and calcium channel blockers such as nicardipine are second-line agents and should be added in if necessary.
- It is vital to avoid agents with potential sedative action such as β-blockers, clonidine, and methyldopa.
- In selected patients who are stable, oral therapy with a combination of β-blockers and calcium blockers may be sufficient.

Aortic dissection: assessment

Aortic dissection is a surgical and medical emergency; untreated it has a >90% 1-year mortality rate. Dissection begins with formation of a tear in the intima and the force of the blood cleaves the media longitudinally to various lengths. Predisposing factors are summarized in Box 1.6.

Classification

There are three classifications, illustrated in Figure 1.5—DeBakey, Stanford, and descriptive. Dissections involving the ascending aorta and/or aortic arch are surgical emergencies and ones limited to the descending aorta are treated medically.

Presentation

• **Chest pain** classically has abrupt onset, is very severe in nature, and most commonly is anterior chest pain radiating to the interscapular region. Usually it is tearing in nature and, unlike the pain of myocardial infarction, most severe at its onset. Pain felt maximally in the anterior chest is associated with ascending aortic dissection, whereas interscapular pain suggests dissection of the descending aorta. Patients often use adjectives such as *tearing, ripping, sharp,* and *stabbing* to describe the pain.
• **Sudden death** or **shock:** is usually due to aortic rupture or cardiac tamponade.
• **Congestive cardiac failure** is due to acute aortic incompetence and/or myocardial infarction.

Box 1.6 Conditions associated with aortic dissection

• Hypertension	Smoking, dyslipidemia, cocaine/crack
• Connective tissue disorders	Marfan's syndrome* Ehlers–Danlos syndrome
• Hereditary vascular disorders	Bicuspid aortic valve Coarctaion
• Vascular inflammation	Giant cell arteritis Takayasu arteritis Behçet's disease Syphilis
• Deceleration trauma	Car accident Falls
• Chest trauma	
• Pregnancy	
• Iatrogenic	Catheterization Cardiac surgery

*Marfan's syndrome: arm span > height, pubis to sole > pubis to vertex, depressed sternum, scoliosis, high arched palate, upward lens dislocation, thoracic aortic dilation/aortic regurgitation, increased urinary hydroxyprolene.

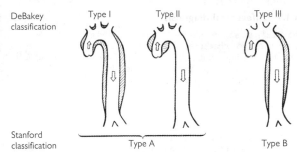

Figure 1.5 Classification of aortic dissection.

Patients may also present with symptoms and signs of occlusion of one of the branches of the aorta. Examples include:
- Stroke or acute limb ischemia—due to compression or dissection
- Paraplegia with sensory deficits—spinal artery occlusion
- Myocardial infarction—usually the right coronary artery
- Renal failure and renovascular hypertension
- Abdominal pain—celiac axis or mesenteric artery occlusion

Aortic dissection may be painless.

Ask specifically about history of hypertension, previous heart murmurs, or aortic valve disease and previous CXR that may be useful for comparison.

Examination

This may be normal. Most patients are hypertensive on presentation. Hypotension is more common in dissections of the ascending aorta (20%–25%) and may be due to blood loss, acute aortic incompetence (which may be accompanied by heart failure), or tamponade (distended neck veins, tachycardia, pulsus paradoxus).

Pseudohypotension may be seen if flow to either or both subclavian arteries is compromised. Look for unequal blood pressure in the arms and document the presence of peripheral pulses carefully. Absent or changing pulses suggest extension of the dissection.

Auscultation may reveal aortic valve regurgitation and occasionally a pericardial friction rub. Descending aortic dissections may rupture or leak into the left pleural space, and the effusion results in dullness in the left base.

Neurological deficits may be due to carotid artery dissection or compression (hemiplegia) or spinal artery occlusion (paraplegia with sensory loss).

Box 1.7 Differential diagnosis

- The chest pain may be mistaken for acute MI, and acute MI may complicate aortic dissection. Always look for other signs of dissection (see Presentation, p. 40), as thrombolysis will be fatal.
- Severe chest pain and collapse may also be due to pulmonary embolism, spontaneous pneumothorax, acute pancreatitis, and penetrating duodenal ulcer.
- Pulse deficits without backache should suggest other diagnoses: atherosclerotic peripheral vascular disease, arterial embolism, Takayasu's arteritis, etc.
- Acute cardiac tamponade with chest pain is also seen in acute viral or idiopathic pericarditis and acute myocardial infarction with external rupture.

Aortic dissection: investigations

General

ECG may be normal or nonspecific (LVH, ST/T abnormalities). Look specifically for evidence of acute MI (inferior MI is seen if the dissection compromises the right coronary artery ostium).

CXR may appear normal. Look for widened upper mediastinum, haziness or enlargement of the aortic knuckle, irregular aortic contour, separation (>5 mm) of intimal calcium from outer aortic contour, displacement of trachea to the right, enlarged cardiac silhouette (pericardial effusion), pleural effusion (usually on left). Compare with previous films if available.

Bloods: Base-line CBC, chemistries, cardiac enzymes as well as crossmatch. A novel monoclonal antibody assay to smooth muscle myosin heavy chains can accurately differentiate an acute dissection from an MI.

Diagnostic

Echocardiography

Transthoracic echocardiogram (TTE) may be useful in diagnosing aortic root dilatation, aortic regurgitation, and pericardial effusion/tamponade.

Transesophageal echocardiogram (TEE) is the investigation of choice, as it allows better evaluation of both ascending aorta and descending aorta, may identify the origin of intimal tear, allows evaluation of the origins of the coronary arteries in relation to the dissection flap, and provides information on aortic insufficiency. It is not good at imaging the distal ascending aorta and proximal arch.

MRI angiography

This is the gold standard for diagnosing aortic dissection. It has all the positive features of TEE and in particular also provides accurate information on all segments of ascending/arch/descending aorta, entry/exit sites and branch vessels. Images can be displayed in multiple views as well as reconstructed in three dimensions.

However, there are a number of disadvantages: 1) availability of service after hours and cost; 2) presence of metallic valves or pacemakers may preclude patients from having an MRI; 3) monitoring of unstable patients in the scanner can be difficult and unsafe.

Spiral (helical) CT with contrast

This allows three-dimensional display of all segments of the aorta and adjacent structures. True and false lumen are identified by differential contrast flow, and entry and exit sites of intimal flap can be seen as well as pleural and pericardial fluid.

However, it cannot demonstrate disruption of the aortic valve, which may be associated with ascending aortic dissection. It requires the use of iodinate contrast

Angiography
Angiography using the femoral or axillary approach may demonstrate altered flow in the two lumens, aortic valve incompetence, and involvement of the branches and the site of the intimal tear. It is invasive and associated with a higher risk of complications in an already high-risk patient. It has largely been superseded by CT/MRI and TEE.

Selecting a diagnostic modality (see Box 1.8)

- Confirm or refute a diagnosis of dissection.
- Is the dissection confined to the descending aorta or does it involve the ascending/arch?
- Identify the extent, sites of entry and exit, and presence and absence of thrombus.
- See whether there is aortic regurgitation, coronary involvement, or pericardial effusions.
- Rule out other causes of symptoms.

Box 1.8 Selecting a diagnostic modality

- Where available, TEE should be the first-line investigation. It is safe and can provide all the information necessary to take the patient to the operating room.
- If TEE is not available or if it fails to provide the necessary information, a spiral contrast CT should be performed.
- MRI should generally be reserved for follow-up images.
- Angiography is rarely used but is of value if other modalities have failed to provide a diagnosis and/or extensive information is needed on branch vessels.

Aortic dissection: management

Stabilize the patient

- If the diagnosis is suspected, transfer the patient to an area where full resuscitation facilities are readily available.
- Secure **venous access** with large-bore cannulas.
- **Take blood** for CBC, chemistries, and cross-match (10 units).
- When the diagnosis is confirmed or in cases with cardiovascular complications, **transfer to ICU**, insert an **arterial line** (radial unless the subclavian artery is compromised when a femoral line is preferred), **central venous line,** and **urinary catheter**.
- Immediate measures should be taken to correct blood pressure (see below).
- Give adequate analgesia (morphine 2.5–10 mg IV and metoclopramide 10 mg IV).

Plan definitive treatment

This depends on the type of dissection (see Fig. 1.5) and its effects on the patient. General principles are as follows:

- Patients with involvement of the ascending aorta should have **emergency surgical repair and BP control**.
- Patients with dissection limited to the descending aorta are managed initially medically with aggressive blood pressure control.

However, this may change in the near future with emerging encouraging data from deployment of endovascular stent-grafts.

Indications and principles for surgery

- Involvement of the ascending aorta
- External rupture (hemopericardium, hemothorax, effusions)
- Arterial compromise (limb ischemia, renal failure, stroke)
- Contraindications to medical therapy (AR, CHF)
- Progression (continued pain, expansion of hematoma on further imaging, loss of pulses, pericardial rub, or aortic insufficiency)

The aim of surgical therapy is to replace the ascending aorta, thereby preventing retrograde dissection and cardiac tamponade (the main cause of death). The aortic valve may need reconstruction and resuspension unless it is structurally abnormal (bicuspid or Marfan's), when it is replaced.

Indications and principles for medical management

Medical therapy is the treatment of choice for the following:

- Uncomplicated type B dissection.
- Stable isolated arch dissection.
- Chronic (>2 weeks duration) stable type B dissection.

In all but those patients who are hypotensive, initial management is aimed at reducing systemic blood pressure and myocardial contractility. The goal is to stop spread of the intramural hematoma and to prevent rupture. The best guide is control of pain. Strict bed rest in a quiet room is essential.

Control blood pressure

Reduce systolic BP to 100–120 mmHg.

- Start on IV β-blocker (if no contraindications) aiming to reduce the heart rate to 60–70/min (see Table 1.6).
- Once this is achieved, if blood pressure remains high, add a vasodilator such as sodium nitroprusside (see Table 1.6). Vasodilators in the absence of β-blockade may increase myocardial contractility and the rate of rise of pressure (dP/dt). Theoretically this may promote extension of the dissection.
- Further antihypertensive therapy may be necessary and other conventional agents such as calcium channel blockers, β-blockers, and ACE inhibitors can be used.
- In patients with aortic regurgitation and congestive cardiac failure, myocardial depressants should not be given. Aim to control blood pressure with vasodilators only.

Hypotension

This may be due to hemorrhage or cardiac tamponade.

- Resuscitate with rapid IV volume (ideally colloid or blood, but crystalloid may be used also). A central venous or pulmonary artery wedge catheter (Swan–Ganz) may be used to monitor the wedge pressure and guide fluid replacement.
- If there are signs of aortic regurgitation or tamponade, arrange for an urgent ECHO and discuss with the surgeons.

Table 1.6 Medical therapy of aortic dissection

β-Blockade (aim for HR <60–70/min)	
Labetalol	20–80 mg slow IV injection over 10 minutes, then 20–200 mg/hr IV, increasing every 15 minutes 100–400 mg po q12h
Atenolol	5–10 mg slow IV injection then 50 mg po after 15 minutes and at 12 hours, then 100 mg po daily
Propranolol	0.5 mg IV (test dose), then 1 mg every 2–5 minutes up to max 10 mg; repeat every 2–3 hours 10–40 mg po 3–4 times daily
When HR 60–70 /min (or if β-Blocker contraindicated), add	
Nitroprusside	0.25–10 µg/kg/min IV infusion
Hydralazine	5–10 mg IV over 20 minutes 50–300 µg/min IV infusion 25–50 mg po q8h
Nitroglycerin	1–10 mg/hr IV infusion
Amlodipine	5–10 mg po qd

Emerging indications and principles for interventional therapy

There are increasing reports and short case series demonstrating favorable outcome (prognostic as well as symptomatic) data for use of endovascular stent-grafts in management of primarily type B and, to a lesser extent, type A aortic dissections.

On the basis of the current evidence, endovascular stent-grafts should be considered to seal entry to false lumen and to enlarge compressed true lumen in the following situations:

- Unstable type B dissection
- Malperfusion syndrome (proximal aortic stent-graft and/or distal fenestration/stenting of branch arteries)
- Patients with high-risk type B dissections who represent high surgical risk
- Routine management of type B dissection (under evaluation)

Cardiac tamponade: if the patient is relatively stable, pericardiocentesis may precipitate hemodynamic collapse and should be avoided. The patient should be transferred to the operating room for direct repair as urgently as possible. In the context of tamponade and EMD or marked hypotension, pericardiocentesis is warranted.

Long-term treatment must involve strict blood pressure control.

Prognosis

The mortality rate for untreated aortic dissection is roughly 20%–30% at 24 hours and 65%–75% at 2 weeks.

For dissections confined to the descending aorta, short-term survival is better (up to 80%) but ~30%–50% will have progression of dissection despite aggressive medical therapy and will require surgery.

Operative mortality is of the order of 10%–25% and depends on the condition of the patient preoperatively. Postoperative 5-year actuarial survival of up to 75% may be expected.

Acute pericarditis: assessment

Presentation

- Typically presents as central chest pain—often pleuritic—relieved by sitting forward and can be associated with breathlessness.
- Other symptoms (e.g., fever, cough, arthralgia, rash, faintness or dizziness secondary to pain/↑HR) may reflect the underlying disease.
- A pericardial friction rub is pathognomonic. This may be positional and transient and may be confused with the murmur of TR or MR.
- Venous pressure rises if an effusion develops. Look for signs of cardiac tamponade (p. 51).

Causes of acute pericarditis are listed in Box 1.9.

Investigations

ECG

- May be normal in up to 10%.
- *Saddle-shaped ST-segment elevation* (concave upward), with variable T inversion (usually late stages) and
- *PR-segment depression* (opposite to p-wave polarity). Minimal lead involvement considered typical includes I, II, aVL, aVF, and V3–V6.
- ST segment is always depressed in aVR, frequently depressed or isoelectric in V1, and sometimes depressed in V2.
- It may be difficult to distinguish from acute MI. Features suggesting pericarditis are the following:
  - Concave ST elevation (vs. convex)
  - All leads involved (vs. a territory, e.g., inferior)
  - Failure of usual ST evolution and no Q waves
  - No AV block, bundle branch block (BBB), or QT prolongation
- Early repolarization (a normal variant) may be mistaken for pericarditis. In the former; ST elevation occurs in precordial and rarely in V6 or the limb leads and is unlikely to show ST depression in V1 or PR segment depression.

Box 1.9 Causes of acute pericarditis

- Idiopathic
- Infection (viral, bacterial, tuberculosis [TB], and fungal)
- Acute MI
- Dressler's syndrome, postcardiotomy syndrome
- Malignancy (e.g., breast, bronchus, lymphoma)
- Uremia
- Autoimmune disease (e.g., SLE, rheumatoid arthritis [RA], Wegner's, scleroderma, polyarteritis nodosa [PAN])
- Granulomatous diseases (e.g., sarcoid)
- Hypothyroidism
- Drugs (hydralazine, procainamide, isoniazid)
- Trauma (chest trauma, iatrogenic)
- Radiotherapy

- ECG is usually not helpful in diagnosing pericarditis post-MI.
- The voltage drops as an effusion develops and in tamponade there is electrical alternans best seen in QRS complexes.

ECHO
- May demonstrate a pericardial collection
- Useful to monitor LV function in case of deterioration due to associated myopericarditis
- We recommend that every patient have an ECHO prior to discharge to assess LV function.

Other
Other investigations depend on the suspected etiology.

All patients should have
- CBC and biochemical profile
- ESR and CRP (levels rise proportionate to intensity of disease)
- Serial cardiac enzymes (CK, CK-MB, troponin)—elevations indicate subpericardial myocarditis
- CXR (heart size, pulmonary edema, infection)
- Echocardiogram: evaluate size, hemodynamic consequences of any effusion

Where appropriate
- Viral titers (acute +2 weeks later) and obtain infectious disease opinion
- Blood cultures
- Autoantibody screen (RF, ANA, anti-DNA, complement levels)
- Thyroid function tests
- Fungal precipitins (if immunosuppressed), ↑PPD
- Sputum culture and cytology
- Diagnostic pericardial tap (culture, cytology)

Acute pericarditis: management

General measures

- **Admit?** This depends on the clinical picture. We recommend admission of most patients for observation for complications, especially effusions, tamponade, and myocarditis. Patients should be discharged when pain free.
- **Bed rest**
- **Analgesia:** NSAIDs are the mainstay. Ibuprofen is well tolerated and increases coronary flow (200–800 mg qid). Aspirin is an alternative (650 mg q6h po). Indomethacin should be avoided in adults as it reduces coronary flow and has marked side effects. Use proton pump inhibitor (PPI) (lansoprazole 30 mg od) to minimize gastrointestinal (GI) side effects. Opioid analgesia may be required. Colchicine used as monotherapy or in addition to NSAIDs may help reduce pain acutely and prevent recurrence.
- **Steroids** may be used if the pain does not decrease within 48 hours (e.g., prednisolone 40–60 mg po qd for up to 2 weeks, tapering down when pain decreases). Use in conjunction with NSAID and taper steroids first before stopping NSAID. It is also of value if pericarditis is secondary to autoimmune disorders.
- **Colchicine:** There is evidence to support that either used as monotherpay or in conjunction with NSAIDs it may help to reduce pain acutely and prevent relapses (1 mg/day divided doses). Stop if patient develops diarrhea, nausea (1 mg stat, 500 µg q6h for 48 hours).
- **Pericardiocentesis** should be considered for significant effusion or if there are signs of tamponade (p. 75), diagnostically if persistent or recurrent effusion.
- **Antibiotics** should be given only if bacterial infection is suspected.
- **Oral anticoagulants** should be discontinued (risk of hemopericardium). Patients should be given IV UFH if absolutely necessary, which is easier to reverse (IV protamine) if complications arise.

Cardiac tamponade: presentation

Cardiac tamponade occurs when a pericardial effusion causes hemo-dynamically significant cardiac compression. The presentation depends on the speed with which fluid accumulates within the pericardium.

Acute tamponade may occur with 100–200 mL in a relatively restricted pericardial sac.

Chronic pericardial collections may contain up to 1000 mL of fluid without clinical tamponade.

Causes

Acute tamponade

- Cardiac trauma
- Iatrogenic
  - Post-cardiac surgery
  - Post-cardiac catheterization
  - Post-pacing/EP study
- Aortic dissection
- Spontaneous bleed
  - Anticoagulation
  - Uremia
  - Thrombocytopenia
- Cardiac rupture post-MI

Subacute tamponade

- Malignant disease
- Idiopathic pericarditis
- Uremia
- Infections
- Bacterial
  - Tuberculosis
- Radiation
- Hypothyroidism
- Postpericardiotomy
- SLE
- Other autoimmune disease

Presentation

Patients commonly present with either cardiac arrest (commonly electrical mechanical dissociation) or hypotension, confusion, stupor, and shock.

Patients who develop cardiac tamponade slowly are usually acutely unwell, but not in extremis. Their main symptoms include the following:
- Shortness of breath, leading to air hunger at rest.
- There may be a preceding history of chest discomfort.
- Symptoms resulting from compression of adjacent structures by a large effusion (i.e., dysphagia, cough, hoarseness, or hiccough).
- There may be symptoms due to the underlying cause.
- Insidious development may present with complications of tamponade, including renal failure, liver and/or mesenteric ischemia, and abdominal plethora.

Important physical signs

Most physical findings are nonspecific and include the following:
- Tachycardia (except in hypothyroidism and uremia).
- Hypotension (+ shock) with postural hypotension.
- Raised JVP (often >10 cm) with a prominent systolic x descent and absent diastolic y descent (see Box 1.10). If the JVP is visible and either remains static or rises with inspiration, it indicates concomitant pericardial constriction (Kussmaul's sign).
- Auscultation may reveal diminished heart sounds. Pericardial rub may be present and suggests a small pericardial collection.

- Look for pulsus paradoxus (a decrease in the palpable pulse and SBP of >10 mmHg on inspiration). This may be so marked that the pulse and Korotkoff sounds may be completely lost during inspiration. This can be measured using a BP cuff[1] or arterial catheter if in situ already. Other conditions that can cause a pulsus paradoxus include acute hypotension, obstructive airways disease, and pulmonary embolus.

Other physical signs include cool extremities (ears, nose), tachypnea, hepatomegaly, and signs of underlying cause of the pericardial effusion.

Box 1.10 Causes of hypotension with a raised JVP

- Cardiac tamponade
- Constrictive pericarditis
- Restrictive cardiomyopathy
- Severe biventricular failure
- Right ventricular infarction
- Pulmonary embolism
- Tension pneumothorax
- Acute severe asthma
- Malignant superior vena cava (SVC) obstruction and sepsis (e.g., lymphoma)

---

1 Teaching **point:** To establish presence of pulsus paradoxus noninvasively, inflate BP cuff to 15 mmHg above highest systolic pressure. Deflate cuff gradually until first beats are heard and hold pressure at that level concentrating on disappearance and reappearance of sounds with respiration (bump-bump, silence-silence, bump-bump, where noise reflects expiration). Continue to deflate slowly, paying attention to the same pattern until all beats are audible. The difference between the initial and final pressure should be >10 mmHg when paradox is present.

Cardiac tamponade: management

Tamponade should be suspected in patients with hypotension, elevated venous pressure, falling BP, ↑HR and ↑RR (with clear chest), and pulsus paradoxus, especially if predisposing factors are present.

Investigations

- **CXR:** the heart size may be normal (e.g., in acute hemopericardium following cardiac trauma). With slower accumulation of pericardial fluid (>250 mL) the cardiac silhouette will enlarge with a globular appearance. The size of the effusion is unrelated to its hemodynamic significance. Look for signs of pulmonary edema.
- **ECG** usually shows a sinus tachycardia, with low-voltage complexes and variable ST-segment changes. With large effusions, electrical alternans may be present with beat-to-beat variation in the QRS morphology possibly resulting form the movement of the heart within the pericardial effusion.
- **Echocardiography** confirms presence of a pericardial effusion. The diagnosis of tamponade is a clinical one. ECHO signs highly suggestive of tamponade include 1) chamber collapse during diastole (RA, RV, RV outflow tract), 2) marked variation in transvalvular flow, and 3) dilated IVC with little or no diameter change on respiration.

If available, examine the central venous pressure trace for the characteristic exaggerated x descent and absent y descent.

Management

Following confirmation of the diagnosis:

- While preparing for drainage of the pericardial fluid, the patient's circulation may temporarily be supported by loading with IV colloid (500–1000 mL stat) and starting inotropes (i.e., adrenaline).
- The effusion should be urgently drained (see p. 75 for pericardiocentesis), guided by ECHO or fluoroscopy. **In the event of circulatory collapse, drainage must happen immediately without imaging.**
- Surgical drainage is indicated if the effusion is secondary to trauma.
- Avoid intubation and positive pressure ventilation as this reduces CO.
- In patients with cardiac arrest, chest compression has little or no value, as there is no room for additional filling.
- Uremic patients will also need dialysis.
- The cause of the effusion should be established (see p. 309). Pericardial fluid should be sent for cytology, microbiology including TB, virology, and, if appropriate, Hb, glucose, and amylase.

Further management is of the underlying cause.

Special cases

Recurrent pericardial effusion

In some cases, pericardial effusion recurs. This requires either a change in the treatment of the underlying cause or a formal surgical drainage procedure such as a surgical pericardial window or pericardiectomy.

Low-pressure tamponade

This is seen in the setting of dehydration. The JVP is not raised, right atrial pressure is normal, and tamponade occurs even with small volumes of pericardial fluid.

- The patient may respond well to IV fluids.
- If there is a significant pericardial collection, this should be drained.

Practical procedures

Central line insertion

Check list of required materials
- Sterile dressing pack and gloves
- 10 mL and 5 mL syringe (21G) and (25G) needles
- Local anesthetic (e.g., 2% lidocaine)
- Central line (e.g., 16G long Abbocath® or Seldinger catheter)
- Saline flush
- Silk suture and needle
- No 11 scalpel blade
- Sterile occlusive dressing (e.g., Tegaderm®)

Risks
- Arterial puncture (remove and apply local pressure)
- Pneumothorax (insert chest drain or aspirate if required)
- Hemothorax
- Chylothorax (mainly left subclavian lines)
- Infection (local, septicemia, bacterial endocarditis)
- Brachial plexus or cervical root damage (over infiltration with local anesthetic)
- Arrhythmias

General procedure
The basic technique is the same regardless of the type of vein being cannulated (see Fig. 1.6).
- Lay the patient supine (± head-down tilt).
- Turn the patient's head away from the side you wish to cannulate.
- Clean the skin with chlorhexidine—from the angle of the jaw to the clavicle for internal jugular vein (IJV) cannulation and from the midline to axilla for the subclavian approach.
- Use the full drapes to isolate the sterile field.
- Flush the lumen of the central line with saline.
- Identify your landmarks.
- Infiltrate skin and subcutaneous tissue with local anesthetic.
- Have the introducer needle and Seldinger guide wire within easy reach so that you can reach them with one hand without having to release your other hand. Your fingers may be distorting the anatomy slightly, making access to the vein easier, and if released it may prove difficult to relocate the vein.
- With the introducer needle in the vein, check that you can aspirate blood freely. Use the hand that was marking the landmarks to immobilize the needle relative to the skin and mandible or clavicle.
- Remove the syringe and pass the guide wire into the vein; it should pass freely. If there is resistance, remove the wire, check that the needle is still within the lumen, and try again.
- Remove the needle, leaving the wire within the vein, and observe for any arrhythmia from the wire "tickling" the atrium or ventricle.

- With a No.11 blade, make a nick in the skin where the wire enters to facilitate dilatation of the subcutaneous tissues. Pass the dilator over the wire and remove, leaving the wire in situ.
- Pass the central line over the wire into the vein. Remove the guide wire, flush the lumen with fresh saline, and close off to air.
- Suture the line in place and cover the skin penetration site with a sterile occlusive dressing.

Box 1.11 Measuring the CVP—tips and pitfalls

- When asked to see a patient at night with an abnormal CVP reading, it is good to always recheck the zero and the reading yourself.
- Always do measurements with the mid-axillary point as the zero reference. Sitting the patient up will drop the central filling pressure (pooling in the veins).
- Look at the rate and character of the venous pressure tracing. It should fall to its value quickly and swing with respiration.
- If it fails to fall quickly, consider whether the line is open (i.e., saline running in), blocked with blood clot, positional (up against vessel wall; ask patient to take some deep breaths), arterial blood (blood tracks back up the line). Raise the whole dripstand (if you are strong), and make sure that the level falls. If it falls when the whole stand is elevated, it may be that the CVP is very high.
- It is easier, and safer, to cannulate a central vein with the patient supine or head down. There is an increased risk of air embolus if the patient is semi-recumbent.

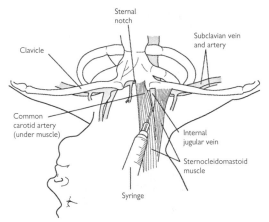

Figure 1.6 Technique for catheterization at the internal jugular and subclavian sites. Reproduced with permission from McGee DC, Gould MK (2003). *N Engl J Med* 348(12):1123–1133. Copyright © 2003 Massachusetts Medical Society. All rights reserved.

Internal jugular vein cannulation

The IJV runs just posterolateral to the carotid artery within the carotid sheath and lies medial to the sternocleidomastoid (SCM) in the upper part of the neck, between the two heads of SCM in its medial portion, and enters the subclavian vein near the medial border of the anterior scalene muscle (see Fig. 1.7).

There are three basic approaches to IJV cannulation: medial to (SCM), between the two heads of SCM, or lateral to SCM. The approach used varies and depends on the experience of the operator and the institution.

- Locate the carotid artery between the sternal and clavicular heads of the SCM at the level of the thyroid cartilage; the IJV lies just lateral and parallel to it.
- Keeping the fingers of one hand on the carotid pulsation, infiltrate the skin with LA thoroughly, aiming just lateral to this and ensuring that you are not in a vein.
- Ideally, first locate the vein with a 21G needle. Advance the needle at 45° to the skin, with gentle negative suction on the syringe, aiming for the ipsilateral nipple, lateral to the pulse.
- If you fail to find the vein, withdraw the needle slowly, maintaining negative suction on the syringe (you may have inadvertently have transfixed the vein). Aim slightly more medially and try again.
- Once you have identified the position of the vein, change to the syringe with the introducer needle, cannulate the vein, and pass the guide wire into the vein.

Tips and pitfalls

Venous blood is dark, and arterial blood is pulsatile and bright red!

Once you locate the vein, change to the syringe with the introducer needle, taking care not to release your fingers from the pulse; they may be distorting the anatomy slightly, making access to the vein easier, and if released it may prove difficult to relocate the vein.

The guide wire should pass freely down the needle and into the vein. With the left IJV approach, there are several acute bends that need to be negotiated. If the guide wire keeps passing down the wrong route, ask your assistant to hold the patient's arms out at 90° to the bed, or even above the patient's head, to coax the guide wire down the correct path.

For patients who are intubated or require respiratory support, it may be difficult to access the head of the bed. The anterior approach may be easier (see Fig. 1.7) and may be done from the side of the bed (the left side of the bed for right-handed operators, using the left hand to locate the pulse and the right to cannulate the vein)

The IJV may also be readily cannulated with a long Abbocath®. No guide wire is necessary, but as a result, misplacement is more common than with the Seldinger technique.

When using an Abbocath®, on cannulating the vein, remember to advance the sheath and needle a few millimeters to allow the tip of the plastic sheath (~1 mm behind the tip of the beveled needle) to enter the vein. Holding the needle stationary, advance the sheath over it into the vein.

Arrange for a CXR to confirm the position of the line and rule out pneumothorax.

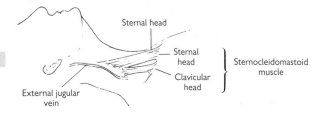

(a) Surface anatomy of external and internal jugular veins

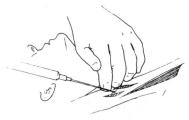

(b) Anterior approach: the chin is in the midline and the skin puncture is over the sternal head of SCM muscle

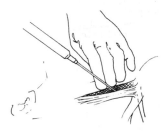

(c) Central approach: the chin is turned away and the skin puncture is between the two heads of SCM muscle

Figure 1.7 Internal jugular vein cannulation.

Subclavian vein cannulation

The axillary vein becomes the subclavian vein (SCV) at the lateral border of the first rib and extends for 3–4 cm just deep to the clavicle. It is joined by the ipsilateral IJV to become the brachiocephalic vein behind the sternoclavicular joint.

The subclavian artery and brachial plexus lie posteriorly separated from the vein by the scalenus anterior muscle (see Fig. 1.8). The phrenic nerve and the internal mammary artery lie behind the medial portion of the SCV, and on the left lies the thoracic duct.

Checklist

- The patient should be in the Trendelenberg position. Select the point 1 cm below the junction of the medial third and middle third of the clavicle. If possible, place a bag of saline between the scapulae to extend the spine.
- Clean the skin with iodine or chlorhexidine.
- Infiltrate skin and subcutaneous tissue and periosteum of the inferior border of the clavicle with local anesthetic up to the hilt of the green (21G) needle, ensuring that it is not in a vein.
- Insert the introducer needle with a 10 mL syringe, guiding gently under the clavicle. It is safest to initially hit the clavicle and "walk" the needle under it until the inferior border is just cleared. In this way you keep the needle as superficial to the dome of the pleura as possible. Once it has just skimmed underneath the clavicle, advance it slowly toward the contralateral sternoclavicular joint, aspirating as you advance. Using this technique, the risk of pneumothorax is small, and success is high.
- Once the venous blood is obtained, rotate the bevel of the needle toward the heart. This encourages the guide wire to pass down the brachiocephalic rather than up the IJV.
- The wire should pass easily into the vein. If there is difficulty, try advancing during the inspiratory and expiratory phases of the respiratory cycle; do not force the wire. Observe for arrhythmia.
- Once the guide wire is in place, nick the skin with a blade, remove the introducer needle, and pass the dilator over the wire. When removing the dilator, note the direction that it faces; it should be slightly curved downward. If it is slightly curved upward, then it is likely that the wire has passed up into the IJV. The wire may be manipulated into the brachiocephalic vein under fluoroscopic control. If this is not available it is safer to remove the wire and start again.
- After removing the dilator, pass the central venous catheter over the guide wire, remove the guide wire, and secure as above.
- A CXR is mandatory after subclavian-line insertion to exclude a pneumothorax and to confirm satisfactory placement of the line, especially if fluoroscopy was not employed.

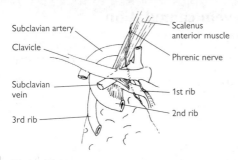

Figure 1.8 The subclavian vein and surrounding structures.

Pulmonary artery catheterization

Indications

Pulmonary artery (PA) catheters (Swan–Ganz catheters) allow direct measurement of a number of hemodynamic parameters that aid clinical decision-making in critically ill patients (evaluate right and left ventricular function, guide treatment, and provide prognostic information). Consider inserting a PA catheter in any critically ill patient, after discussion with an experienced physician, if the measurements will influence decisions on therapy (and not just to reassure yourself).

Careful and frequent clinical assessment of the patient should always accompany measurements, and PA catheterization should not delay treatment of the patient.

General indications (not a comprehensive list) include the following:

- Management of complicated myocardial infarction
- Assessment and management of shock
- Assessment and management of respiratory distress (cardiogenic vs. noncardiogenic pulmonary edema)
- Evaluating effects of treatment in unstable patients (e.g., inotropes, vasodilators, mechanical ventilation, etc.)
- Delivering therapy (e.g., thrombolysis for pulmonary embolism, prostacyclin for pulmonary hypertension, etc.)
- Assessment of fluid requirements in critically ill patients

Equipment required

Full resuscitation facilities should be available and the patient's ECG should be continuously monitored.

- Bag of saline for flushing the catheter and transducer set for pressure monitoring. (Check that your assistant is experienced in setting up the transducer system BEFORE you start.)
- 8F introducer kit (prepackaged kits contain the introducer sheath and all the equipment required for central venous cannulation)
- PA catheter: commonly a triple lumen catheter, which allows simultaneous measurement of RA pressure (proximal port) and PA pressure (distal port) and incorporates a thermistor for measurement of cardiac output by thermodilution; and a balloon to facilitate flotation of the catheter. Check your catheter before you start.
- Fluoroscopy is preferable, though not essential.

General technique

Do not attempt this without supervision if you are inexperienced.

- Observe strict aseptic technique using sterile drapes, etc.
- Insert the introducer sheath (at least 8F in size) into either the internal jugular or subclavian vein in the standard way. Flush the sheath with saline and secure to the skin with sutures (see Fig. 1.9).
- Do not attach the plastic sterile expandable sheath to the introducer yet, but keep it sterile for use later once the catheter is in position (the catheter is easier to manipulate without the plastic covering).

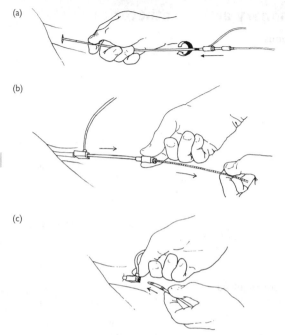

(a)

(b)

(c)

Figure 1.9 Pulmonary artery catheterization. (a) The sheath and dilator are advanced into the vein over the guide wire. A twisting motion makes insertion easier. (b) The guide wire and dilator are then removed. The sheath has a hemostatic valve at the end preventing leakage of blood. (c) The PA catheter is then inserted through the introducer sheath into the vein.

Thread it onto the catheter and have it ready for use when the catheter is positioned.
• Flush all the lumens of the PA catheter and attach the distal lumen to the pressure transducer. Check that the transducer is zeroed (conventionally to the mid-axillary point). Check the integrity of the balloon by inflating it with the syringe provided (1–2 mL air) and then deflate the balloon.

Insertion technique
• Flush all the lumens of the PA catheter and attach the distal lumen to the pressure transducer. Check that the transducer is zeroed (conventionally to the mid-axillary point). Check the integrity of the balloon by inflating it with the syringe provided and then deflate the balloon. Lock the valve.

- Pass the tip of the PA catheter through the plastic sheath, keeping the sheath compressed. The catheter is easier to manipulate without the sheath over it; once in position, extend the sheath over the catheter to keep it sterile and lock in place.
- With the balloon deflated, advance the tip of the catheter to approximately 10–15 cm from the right IJV or SCV, 15–20 cm from the left (the markings on the side of the catheter are at 10 cm intervals: 2 lines = 20 cm). Check that the pressure tracing is typical of the RA pressure (see Table 1.7 and Fig. 1.10).
- Inflate the balloon and advance the catheter gently. The flow of blood will carry the balloon (and catheter) across the tricuspid valve, through the right ventricle and into the pulmonary artery (see Fig. 1.10).
- Watch the ECG tracing closely while the catheter is advanced. The catheter commonly triggers runs of VT when crossing the tricuspid valve and through the RV. The VT is usually self-limiting but should not be ignored. Deflate the balloon, pull back, and try again.
- If more than 15 cm of catheter is advanced into the RV without the tip entering the PA, this suggests the catheter is coiling in the RV. Deflate the balloon, withdraw the catheter into the RA, reinflate the balloon, and try again using clockwise torque while advancing in the ventricle, or flushing the catheter with cold saline to stiffen the plastic. If this fails repeatedly, try under fluoroscopic guidance.
- As the tip passes into a distal branch of the PA, the balloon will impact and not pass further—the wedge position—and the pressure tracing will change (see Fig. 1.10).
- Deflate the balloon and check that a typical PA tracing is obtained. If not, try flushing the catheter lumen, and if that fails, withdraw the catheter until the tip is within the PA and begin again.
- Reinflate the balloon slowly. If the pulmonary capillary wedge (PCW) pressure is seen before the balloon is fully inflated, it suggests that the tip has migrated further into the artery. Deflate the balloon, withdraw the catheter 1–2 cm, and try again.
- If the pressure tracing flattens and then continues to rise, you have "overwedged." Immediately deflate the balloon, pull back the catheter 1–2 cm, and start again.
- When a stable position has been achieved, extend the plastic sheath over the catheter and secure it to the introducer sheath. Clean any blood from the skin insertion site with antiseptic and secure a coil of the PA catheter to the patient's chest to avoid inadvertent removal. Dress the catheter sterilely.
- Obtain a CXR to check the position of the catheter and rule out pneumothorax. The tip of the catheter should ideally be no more than 3–5 cm from the midline.

Tips and pitfalls

- Never withdraw the catheter with the balloon inflated.
- Never advance the catheter with the balloon deflated.
- Never inject liquid into the balloon.
- Never leave the catheter with the balloon inflated, as pulmonary infarction may occur.

Table 1.7 Normal values of right heart pressures and flows

Right atrial pressure	0–8 mmHg
Right ventricle	
Systolic	15–30 mmHg
End diastolic	0–8 mmHg
Pulmonary artery	
Systolic/diastolic	15–30/4–12 mmHg
Mean	9–16 mmHg
Pulmonary capillary wedge pressure	2–10 mmHg
Cardiac index	2.8–4.2 L/min/m^2

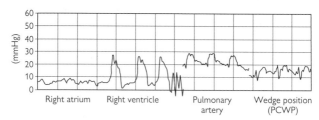

Figure 1.10 Pressure tracings during pulmonary artery catheterization.

- The plastic of the catheter softens with time at body temperature and the tip of the catheter may migrate further into the PA branch. If the pressure tracing with the balloon deflated is "partially wedged" (and flushing the catheter does not improve this), withdraw the catheter 1–2 cm and reposition.
- Sometimes it is impossible to obtain a wedged trace. In this situation one has to use the PA diastolic pressure as a guide. In health there is ~2–4 mmHg difference between PA diastolic pressure and PCWP. Any condition that causes pulmonary hypertension (e.g., severe lung disease, ARDS, long-standing valvular disease) will alter this relationship.
- *Valvular lesions, VSDs, prosthetic valves, and pacemakers:* If these are present seek advice from a cardiologist. The risk of subacute bacterial endocarditis (SBE) may be sufficiently great that the placement of a PA catheter may be more detrimental than beneficial.
- *Positive end-expiratory pressure (PEEP):* Measurement and interpretation if PCWP in patients on PEEP depends on the position of the catheter. Ensure that the catheter is below the level of the left atrium on lateral CXR. Removing PEEP during measurement causes marked fluctuations in hemodynamics and oxygenation, and the pressures do not reflect the state once back on the ventilator.

Complications

Arrhythmias

Watch the ECG tracing closely while the catheter is advanced. The catheter commonly triggers runs of VT when crossing the tricuspid valve and through the RV. If this happens, deflate the balloon, pull back, and try again. The VT is usually self-limiting, but should not be ignored.

Pulmonary artery rupture

Occurrence of PA rupture was ~0.2% in one series. Damage may occur if the balloon is overinflated in a small branch.

Risk factors include mitral valve disease (large v wave confused with poor wedging), pulmonary hypertension, and multiple inflations or hyperinflations of balloon. Hemoptysis is an early sign. It is safer to follow PA diastolic pressures if these correlate with the PCWP.

Pulmonary infarction

Knots

These usually occur at the time of initial placement in patients where there has been difficulty in traversing the RV. Signs include loss of pressure tracing, persistent ectopy, and resistance to catheter manipulation. If this is suspected, stop manipulation and seek expert help.

Infection

Risks increase with length of time the catheter is left in situ. Pressure transducer may occasionally be a source of infection, so keep in place for the shortest possible time. Remove the catheter and introducer and replace only if necessary.

Other complications

Other complications are those associated with central line insertion, thrombosis and embolism, balloon rupture, and intracardiac damage.

Indications for temporary pacing

1. Following acute myocardial infarction

- Asystole
- Symptomatic complete heart block (CHB) (any territory)
- Symptomatic secondary heart block (any territory)
- Trifascicular block (currently often managed with Zoll defibrillator)
  - Alternating LBBB and RBBB
  - First-degree AV block + RBBB + LAD
  - New RBBB and left posterior hemiblock
  - LBBB and long PR interval
- After anterior MI
  - Asymptomatic CHB
  - Asymptomatic second-degree (Mobitz II) block
- Symptomatic sinus bradycardia unresponsive to atropine
- Recurrent VT for atrial or ventricular overdrive pacing

2. Unrelated to myocardial infarction

- Symptomatic sinus or junctional bradycardia unresponsive to atropine (e.g., carotid sinus hypersensitivity)
- Symptomatic second-degree heart block or sinus arrest
- Symptomatic CHB
- Torsades de pointes tachycardia due to bradycardia
- Recurrent VT for atrial or ventricular overdrive pacing
- Bradycardia-dependent tachycardia
- Drug overdose (e.g., verapamil, β-blockers, digoxin)
- Permanent pacemaker box change in a pacing-dependent patient (not usually done)

3. Before general anesthesia

- Use the same principles as for acute MI
- Sinus node disease and second-degree (Wenckebach) heart block need prophylactic pacing only if there are symptoms of syncope or presyncope.
- CHB.

Transvenous temporary pacing

The technique of temporary wire insertion is described on p. 68.

The most commonly used pacing mode and the mode of choice for life-threatening bradyarrhythmias is ventricular demand pacing (VVI) with a single bipolar wire positioned in the right ventricle.

In critically ill patients with impaired cardiac pump function and symptomatic bradycardia (especially with right ventricular infarction), cardiac output may be increased by up to 20% by maintaining atrioventricular (AV) synchrony. This requires two pacing leads, one atrial and one ventricular, and a dual pacing box.

Indications for temporary transvenous cardiac pacing are listed in Table 1.8.

Epicardial temporary pacing

Following cardiac surgery, patients may have epicardial wires (attached to the pericardial surface of the heart) left in for up to 1 week in case of postoperative bradyarrhythmia. These are used in the same way as trans-venous pacing wires, but the threshold may be higher. They are removed prior to discharge.

Table 1.8 Indications for temporary transvenous cardiac pacing

Emergency/acute

Acute myocardial infarction (class I: ACC/AHA)*

- Asystole
- Symptomatic bradycardia (sinus bradycardia with hypotension and type I second-degree AV block with hypotension not responsive to atropine)
- Bilateral bundle branch block (alternating BBB or RBBB with alternating LAHB/LPHB)
- New or indeterminate age bifascicular block with first-degree AV block
- Mobitz type II second-degree AV block

Bradycardia not associated with acute myocardial infarction

- Asystole
- Second- or third-degree AV block with hemodynamic compromise or syncope at rest
- Ventricular tachyarrhythmias secondary to bradycardia

Elective

- Support for procedures that may promote bradycardia
- General anesthesia with:
  - Second- or third-degree AV block
  - Intermittent AV block
  - First degree AV block with bifascicular block
  - First degree AV block and LBBB
- Cardiac surgery (not usual)
  - Aortic surgery
  - Tricuspid surgery
  - Ventricular septal defect closure
  - Ostium primum repair

Rarely considered for coronary angioplasty (usually to right coronary artery)

Overdrive suppression of tachyarrhythmias

* Ryan TJ, et al. (1996), ACC/AHA guidelines for the management of patients with acute myocardial infarction. *J Am Coll Cardiol* 28:1328–1428.

Reproduced with permission from Gammage MD (2000). Temporary cardiac pacing. *Heart* 83:715–720.

Temporary ventricular pacing

For a checklist for inserting a pacing wire, see Box 1.12.

- *Cannulate a central vein:* The wire is easiest to manipulate via the right interior jugular (RIJ) approach but is more comfortable for the patient via the right subclavian (SC) vein. The LIJ approach is best avoided as there are many acute bends to negotiate and a stable position is difficult to achieve. Avoid the left subclavicular area as this is the preferred area for permanent pacemaker insertion and should be kept "virgin" if possible. The femoral vein may be used (incidence of DVT and infection is high).
- *Insert a sheath* (similar to that for PA catheterization) through which the pacing wire can be fed. Pacing wires are commonly 5F or 6F and a sheath at least one size larger is necessary. Most commercially available pacing wires are prepacked with an introducer needle and plastic cannula similar to an Abbocath®, which may be used to position the pacing wire. However, the cannula does not have a hemostatic seal. The plastic cannula may be removed from the vein, leaving the bare wire entering the skin, once a stable position has been achieved. This reduces the risk of wire displacement but also makes repositioning of the wire more difficult should this be necessary, and infection risk is higher.
- *Pass the wire* through the sterile plastic cover that accompanies the introducer sheath and advance into the upper right atrium (see Fig. 1.11) but do not unfurl the cover yet. The wire is much easier to manipulate with gloved hands without the hindrance of the plastic cover.
- *Advance the wire* with the tip pointing toward the right ventricle; it may cross the tricuspid valve easily. If it fails to cross, point the tip to the lateral wall of the atrium and form a loop. Rotate the wire and the loop should fall across the tricuspid valve into the ventricle.

Advance and rotate the wire so that the tip points inferiorly as close to the apex of the right ventricle (laterally) as possible.

Box 1.12 Checklist for pacing wire insertion

- Check that the fluoroscopy and monitoring equipment and defibrillator are working.
- Check the type of pacing wire: atrial wires have a preformed "J" that allows easy placement in the atrium or appendage and are very difficult to manipulate into a satisfactory position in the ventricle. Ventricular pacing wires have a more open, gentle "J."
- Check the pacing box (single vs. dual or sequential pacing box) and leads to attach to the wire(s). Familiarize yourself with the controls on the box; you may need to connect up in a hurry if the patient's intrinsic rhythm slows further.
- Remember to put on the lead apron before wearing the sterile gown, mask, and gloves.

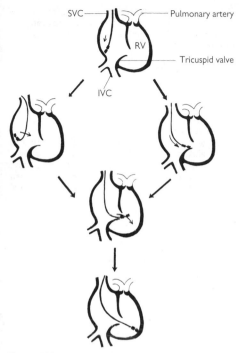

Figure 1.11 Insertion of a ventricular pacing wire (see text for details). Reproduced with permission from Ramrakha P, Moore K (2004). *Oxford Handbook of Acute Medicine*, 2nd ed. Oxford, UK: Oxford University Press.

If the wire does not rotate down to the apex easily, it may be because you are in the coronary sinus rather than in the right ventricle. (The tip of the wire points to the left shoulder).

- *Withdraw the wire* and re-cross the tricuspid valve. Leave some slack in the wire; the final appearance should be like the outline of a sock with the "heel" in the right atrium, the "arch" over the tricuspid valve and the "big toe" at the tip of the right ventricle.
- *Connect the wire* to the pacing box and check the threshold. Ventricular pacing thresholds should be <1.0 V, but threshold up to 1.5 V is acceptable if another stable position cannot be achieved.
- *Check for positional stability.* With the box pacing at a rate higher than the intrinsic heart rate, ask the patient to take some deep breaths, cough forcefully, and sniff. Watch for failure of capture; if this happens, reposition the wire.

- *Set the output* to 5 V and the box on "demand." If the patient is in sinus rhythm and has an adequate blood pressure, set the box rate to just below the patient's rate. If there is complete heart block or bradycardia, set the rate at 70–80/min.
- *Dress sterilely.* Cover the wire with the plastic sheath and suture sheath and wire securely to the skin. Loop the rest of the wire and fix to the patient's skin with adhesive dressing.
- When the patient returns to the ward, obtain a CXR to confirm satisfactory positioning of the wire and to exclude a pneumothorax.

Temporary pacemaker placement can be done with ECG guidance (clip lead V1 to end of pacing wire) but fluoroscopy guidance is preferred.

If it is anticipated that a temporary pacer will be needed for more than a short period of time (infected or hemodynamically unstable patient), a permanent screw-in pacemaker lead may be placed, externalized, and connected to a nonsterile permanent pacemaker generator which is then secured to the patient's skin. This is especially useful if "temporary" atrial or dual chamber pacing is needed.

Temporary atrial pacing

The technique of inserting an atrial temporary wire is similar to that of ventricular pacing.
- Advance the atrial wire until the "J" is re-formed in the right atrium.
- Rotate the wire and withdraw slightly to position the tip in the right atrial appendage. Aim for a threshold of <1.5 V.

If atrial wires are not available, a ventricular pacing wire may be manipulated into a similar position or passed into the coronary sinus for left atrial pacing. Alternatively, a screw-in permanent lead may be used as described on p. 398.

AV sequential pacing

In critically ill patients with impaired cardiac pump function and symptomatic bradycardia (especially with right ventricular infarction), cardiac output may be increased by up to 20% by maintaining atrioventricular synchrony. This requires two pacing leads, one atrial and one ventricular, and a dual pacing box.

Patients most likely to benefit from AV sequential pacing

- Acute MI (especially RV infarction)
- "Stiff" left ventricle: aortic stenosis, hypertrophic cardiomyopathy (HCM), hypertensive heart disease, amyloidosis
- Low cardiac output states (cardiomyopathy)
- Recurrent atrial arrhythmias

Temporary pacing: complications

1. Ventricular ectopy or tachycardia

Nonsustained ventricular tachycardia (VT) is common as the guide or pacing wire crosses the tricuspid valve (especially in patients receiving a catecholamine infusion) and does not require treatment.

Try to avoid long runs of VT and, if necessary, withdraw the wire into the atrium and wait until the rhythm has settled.

If ectopy persists after the wire is positioned, try adjusting the amount of slack in the wire in the region of the tricuspid valve (either more or less).

Pacing the right ventricular outflow tract can provoke runs of VT.

2. Failure to pace and/or sense

It is difficult to get low pacing thresholds (<1.0 V) in patients with extensive myocardial infarction (especially of the inferior wall) or cardiomyopathy or who have received class I antiarrhythmic drugs. Accept a slightly higher value if the position is otherwise stable and satisfactory.

If the position of the wire appears satisfactory and yet the pacing thresholds are high, the wire may be in a left hepatic vein or may have perforated. Pull the wire back into the atrium and try again, looking specifically for the ventricular ectopy as the wire crosses the tricuspid valve. Monitor closely for signs of hemodynamic compromise.

- The pacing threshold commonly doubles in the first few days due to endocardial edema.
- If the pacemaker suddenly fails, the most common reason is usually wire displacement.
- Increase the pacing output of the box.
- Check all the connections of the wire and the battery of the box.
- Try moving the patient to the left lateral position until arrangements can be made to reposition the wire.

3. Perforation

A pericardial rub may be present in the absence of perforation (especially post-MI).

Presentation

Watch for pericardial chest pain, increasing breathlessness, falling blood pressure, enlarged cardiac silhouette on CXR, signs of cardiac tamponade, left diaphragmatic pacing at low output, increased threshold.

Management

If there are signs of cardiac tamponade, arrange for urgent ECHO, drainage of fluid, and repositioning of the wire.

Monitor the patient carefully over the next few days with repeat ECHOs to detect incipient cardiac tamponade.

4. Diaphragmatic pacing

High-output pacing (10 V), even with satisfactory position of the ventricular lead, may cause pacing of the left hemidiaphragm. At low voltages this suggests perforation (see above).

Right hemidiaphragm pacing may be seen with atrial pacing and stimulation of the right phrenic nerve.

Reposition the wire if symptomatic (painful twitching, dyspnea).

Box 1.13 Complications of temporary pacing

- Complications associated with central line insertion
- Ventricular ectopy
- Nonsustained VT
- Perforation
- Pericarditis
- Diaphragmatic pacing
- Infection
- Pneumothorax

Pericardiocentesis

Equipment

Establish peripheral venous access and check that full facilities for resuscitation are available. Pre-prepared pericardiocentesis sets may be available. You will need the following:

- Table for central line insertion with chlorhexidine for skin, dressing pack, sterile drapes, local anesthetic (lidocaine 2%), syringes (including a 50 mL), needles (25G and 22G), No 11 blade, and silk sutures
- Pericardiocentesis needle (15 cm, 18G) or similar Wallace cannula
- J-guide wire (≥80 cm, 0.035 diameter)
- Dilators (up to 7 French)
- Pigtail catheter (≥60 cm with catheter with multiple side holes)
- Drainage bag and connectors
- Facilities for fluoroscopy or echocardiographic screening
- Often done with a pulmonary artery catheter in place to document initial filling pressures and improvement

Technique

- Position the patient at ~30°. This allows the effusion to pool inferiorly and anteriorly within the pericardium.
- Sedate the patient lightly with midazolam (2.5–7.5 mg IV) and fentanyl 50–200 µg IV) if necessary. Use with caution, as this may drop the BP in patients already compromised by the effusion.
- Wearing a sterile gown and gloves, clean the skin from mid-chest to mid-abdomen and put the sterile drapes on the patient.
- Infiltrate the skin and subcutaneous tissues with local anesthetic starting 1–1.5 cm below the xiphoid and just to the left of midline, aiming for the left shoulder and staying as close as possible to the inferior border of the rib cartilages.
- The pericardiocentesis needle is introduced into the angle between the xiphoid and the left costal margin angled at ~30°. Advance slowly, aspirating gently and then injecting more lidocaine every few millimeters, aiming for the left shoulder.
- As the parietal pericardium is pierced, you may feel a "give" and fluid will be aspirated. Remove the syringe and introduce the guide wire through the needle (see Fig. 1.12).
- Check the position of the guide wire by screening. It should loop within the cardiac silhouette only and not advance into the SVC or pulmonary artery.
- Remove the needle, leaving the wire in place. Enlarge the skin incision slightly using the blade and dilate the track.
- Insert the side-hole catheter over the wire into the pericardial space and remove the wire. Measure intrapericardial pressure.
- Take specimens for microscopy, culture (and inoculate a sample into blood culture bottles), cytology, and hematocrit if blood stained (a CBC tube; ask the hematologists to run on the Coulter counter for rapid estimation of Hb).

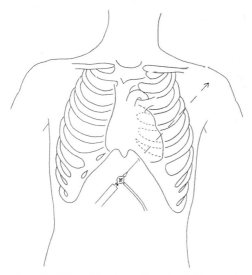

Figure 1.12 Pericardial aspiration. Reproduced with permission from Ramrakha P, Moore K (2004). *Oxford Handbook of Acute Medicine*, 2nd ed. Oxford, UK: Oxford University Press.

- Aspirate to dryness, watching the patient carefully. Symptoms and hemodynamics (tachycardia) often start to improve with removal of as little as 100 mL of pericardial fluid.
- If the fluid is heavily blood stained, withdraw fluid cautiously—if the pigtail is in the right ventricle, withdrawal of blood may cause cardiovascular collapse. Arrange for urgent Hb/hematocrit.
- Leave on free drainage and attached to the drainage bag.
- Suture the pigtail to the skin securely and cover with a sterile occlusive dressing.

Aftercare
- Closely observe the patient for recurrent tamponade (obstruction of drain) and follow repeat ECHO studies.
- Discontinue anticoagulants.
- Remove the drain after 24 hours or when the drainage stops.
- Consider the need for surgery (drainage, biopsy, or pericardial window) or specific therapy (chemotherapy if malignant effusion, antimicrobials if bacterial, dialysis if renal failure, etc.).

Tips and pitfalls

A summary of complications of pericardiocentesis is provided in Box 1.14.

1. If the needle touches the heart's epicardial surface, you may feel a "ticking" sensation transmitted down the needle: withdraw the needle a few millimeters, angulate the needle more superficially, and try cautiously again, aspirating as you advance.

2. If you do not enter the effusion, and the heart is not encountered:
- Withdraw the needle slightly and advance again, aiming slightly deeper, but still toward the left shoulder.
- If this fails, try again, aiming more medially (mid-clavicular point or even suprasternal notch).
- Consider trying the apical approach (starting laterally at cardiac apex and aiming for right shoulder), if echo confirms sufficient fluid at the cardiac apex.

3. If available, *intrathoracic ECG* can be monitored by a lead attached to the needle as it is advanced. This is seldom clinically useful in our experience. Penetration of the myocardium results in ST elevation, suggesting that the needle has been advanced too far.

4. If there is difficulty with inserting the side-hole catheter:
- This may be due to insufficient dilatation of the tract (use a larger dilator).
- Holding the wire taught (by gentle traction) while pushing the catheter may help; take care not to pull the wire out of the pericardium.

5. With hemorrhagic effusion vs. blood
- Compare the Hb of the pericardial fluid with the venous blood Hb.
- Place some of the fluid in a clean container; blood will clot, whereas hemorrhagic effusion will not, as the "whipping" action of the heart tends to defibrinate it.
- Confirm the position of the needle by first withdrawing some fluid and then injecting 10–20 mL of contrast; using fluoroscopy, see if the contrast stays within the cardiac silhouette.
- Alternatively, if using ECHO guidance, inject 5–10 mL saline into the needle, looking for "microbubble contrast" in the cavity containing the needle tip. Injecting 20 mL saline rapidly into a peripheral vein will produce "contrast" in the right atrium and ventricle and may allow them to be distinguished from the pericardial space.
- Connect a pressure line to the needle; a characteristic waveform will confirm penetration of the right ventricle.

Box 1.14 Complications of pericardiocentesis

- Penetration of a cardiac chamber (usually right ventricle)
- Laceration of an epicardial vessel
- Arrhythmia (atrial arrhythmias as the wire is advanced, ventricular arrhythmias if the RV is penetrated)
- Pneumothorax
- Perforation of abdominal viscus (liver, stomach, colon)
- Ascending infection

DC cardioversion

Relative contraindications

- Digoxin toxicity
- Electrolyte disturbance ($\downarrow$Na$^+$, $\downarrow$K$^+$, $\uparrow$K, $\downarrow$Ca^{2+}, $\downarrow$Mg^{2+}, acidosis)
- Fever and ongoing metabolic abnormalities

Checklist for DC cardioversion

• Defibrillator	Check that this is functioning, with a fully equipped crash cart on hand in case of arrest.
• Informed consent	Unless life-threatening emergency
• 12 lead ECG	AF, flutter, SVT, VT, signs of ischemia or digoxin. If ventricular rate is slow, have an external (transcutaneous) pacing system nearby in case of asystole.
• Nothing by mouth	For at least 6 hours
• Anticoagulation	Does the patient require anticoagulants? Is the INR > 2.0? (Has it been so for >3 weeks?)
• Potassium	Check that this is >3.5 mmol/L.
• Digoxin	Check that there are no features of digoxin toxicity. If taking ≥250 µg/day, check that renal function and recent digoxin level are normal. If there is frequent ventricular ectopy, give IV Mg^{2+} 2 g.
• Thyroid function	Treat thyrotoxicosis or myxedema first, if patient is stable.
• IV access	Peripheral venous cannula
• Sedation	Short general anesthesia (propofol) is preferable to sedation with benzodiazepine and fentanyl. Bag the patient with 100% oxygen.
• Select energy	See Box 1.16.
• Synchronization	Check that this is selected on the defibrillator for all shocks (unless the patient is in VF or hemodynamically unstable). Adjust the ECG gain so that the machine is only sensing QRS complexes and not P or T waves.
• Paddle placement	Conductive gel pads should be placed between the paddles and the skin or, preferably, self-adhesive patches should be used. Place one anteriorly just left of the sternum, and one posteriorly to the left of midline. Alternatively, position one just to the right of the sternum and the other to the left of the left nipple (anterior–mid-axillary line).
• Cardioversion	Check that no one is in contact with the patient or with the metal bed. Ensure your own legs are clear of the bed! Apply firm pressure on the paddles if they are used.

• Successful	Repeat ECG. Place patient in recovery position until awake. Monitor for 2–4 hours and ensure that effects of sedation have passed.
	If being discharged, patients should be accompanied home by a friend or relative. In addition, they should not drive or operate heavy equipment for 24 hours.

Special situations

Pregnancy

DC shock during pregnancy appears to be safe. Auscultate the fetal heart before and after cardioversion and, if possible, fetal ECG should be monitored. Because of the increased risk of gastric reflux, airway protection (intubation) is usually necessary.

Pacemakers/AICDs

There is a danger of damage to the pacemaker generator box or the junction at the tip of the pacing wire(s) and endocardium. Position the paddles away from the generator, and not in the same vector as the device.

Facilities for backup pacing (external or transvenous) should be available. Check the pacemaker/ICD post-cardioversion—both early and late problems have been reported. These problems are very rare with newer devices and are minimized by not delivering a shock over the generator.

The presence of a defibrillator is not a contraindication to an external shock if this is needed.

Box 1.15 Complications of DC cardioversion

- Asystole/bradycardia
- Ventricular fibrillation
- Thromboembolism
- Transient hypotension
- Skin burns
- Aspiration pneumonitis.

Box 1.16 Suggested initial energies for DC shock for elective cardioversion

• Sustained monomorphic VT	200 J biphasic	Synchronized
• Atrial fibrillation	50–200 J	Synchronized
• Atrial flutter	50 J	Synchronized
• Other SVTs	50 J	Synchronized

- If the initial shock is unsuccessful, increase the energy (50, 100, 200, 360 J) and repeat.
- If still unsuccessful, consider changing paddle position and try 200 J again.

Intra-aortic balloon counterpulsation

Indications

- Cardiogenic shock post-MI
- Acute severe mitral regurgitation
- Acute ventricular septal defect
- Preoperative (LM disease, triple-vessel disease with severely depressed EF with high filling pressures)
- Weaning from cardiopulmonary bypass

Rarely

- Treatment of ventricular arrhythmias post-MI.
- Unstable angina (as a bridge to CABG)
- Hemodynamic support as a bridge to transplant or assist device placement

Contraindications

- Aortic regurgitation
- Aortic dissection
- Severe aortoiliac atheroma.

- Bleeding diathesis
- Dilated cardiomyopathy (if patient is not a candidate for transplantation)

Complications

- Aortic dissection
- Arterial perforation
- Limb ischemia
- Infection

- Trombocytopenia
- Peripheral embolism/stroke
- Balloon rupture

Principle

The device consists of a catheter with a balloon (34 mL up to 40 mL size) at its tip, which is positioned in the descending thoracic aorta.

The balloon inflation and deflation is synchronized to the ECG. The balloon should inflate just after the dicrotic notch (in diastole), thereby increasing pressure in the aortic root and increasing coronary perfusion. The balloon deflates just before ventricular systole, thereby decreasing afterload and improving left ventricular performance (see Fig. 1.13).

Counterpulsation has a number of beneficial effects on the circulation:

- Increased in coronary perfusion in diastole
- Reduced LV end-diastolic pressure
- Reduced myocardial oxygen consumption
- Increased cerebral and peripheral blood flow

The IAB cannot assist the patient in asystole or VF. It is often less effective in the setting of severe tachycardia (rapid atrial fibrillation or atrial flutter). It requires a minimum cardiac index of 1.2–1.4 L/min/m^2, often necessitating additional inotropes.

Technique

Balloon insertion

Previous experience is essential. Formerly, a cut-down to the femoral artery was required, but newer balloons come equipped with a sheath that may be introduced percutaneously.

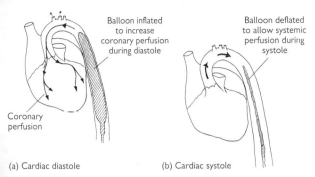

Figure 1.13 Operation of intra-aortic balloon pump. Reproduced with permission from Ramrakha P, Moore K (2004). *Oxford Handbook of Acute Medicine*, 2nd ed. Oxford, UK: Oxford University Press.

Using fluoroscopy, the balloon is positioned in the descending thoracic aorta with the tip just below the origin of the left subclavian artery. Fully anticoagulate the patient with IV heparin.

Some units routinely give IV antibiotics (vancomycin) to cover against *Staph*. infection.

Triggering and timing

The balloon pump may be triggered either from the patient's ECG (R wave) or from the arterial pressure waveform. Slide switches on the pump console allow precise timing of inflation and deflation during the cardiac cycle. Set the pump to 1:2 to allow you to see the effects of augmentation on alternate beats (see Fig. 1.14).

Troubleshooting

Seek help from an expert! There is usually an on-call cardiac perfusionist or technician or senior cardiac physician or surgeon.

Counterpulsation is inefficient with heart rates over 130/min. Consider antiarrhythmics or 1:2 augmentation instead.

Triggering and timing

For ECG triggering, select a lead with most pronounced R wave; ensure that the pump is set to trigger from ECG, not pressure. Permanent pacemakers may interfere with triggering—select a lead with a negative and the smallest pacing artifact. Alternatively, set the pump to be triggered from the external pacing device.

A good arterial waveform is required for pressure triggering; the timing will vary slightly depending on the location of the arterial line (slightly earlier for radial artery line than femoral artery line). Be guided by the hemodynamic effects of balloon inflation and deflation rather than precise value of delay. See Figure 1.15 for timing errors.

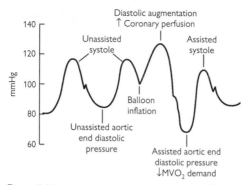

Figure 1.14 Arterial waveform variations during 1:2 IABP therapy.

Limb ischemia is exacerbated by poor cardiac output, adrenaline, nor-adrenaline, and peripheral vascular disease. Wean patient off and remove the balloon.

Thrombocytopenia is commonly seen; it does not require transfusion unless there is overt bleeding and returns to normal once the balloon is removed.

IABP removal

The patient may be progressively weaned by gradually reducing the counterpulsation ratio (1:2, 1:4, 1:8, etc.) and checking that the patient remains hemodynamically stable.

• Stop the heparin infusion and wait for the ACT (activated clotting time) to fall <150 seconds (APTT <1.5 normal).
• Using a 50 mL syringe, have an assistant apply negative pressure to the balloon.
• Pull the balloon down until it abuts the sheath; do not attempt to pull the balloon into the sheath.
• Withdraw both balloon and sheath and apply firm pressure on the femoral puncture site for at least 30 minutes or until the bleeding is controlled.

(a) Inflation of the IAB prior
to aortic valve closure

Waveform characteristics:
- Inflation of IAB prior to dicrotic notch
- Diastolic augmentation encroaches onto systole (may be unable to distinguish)

Physiologic effects:
- Potential premature closure of aortic valve
- Potential increase in LVEDV and LVEDP or PCWP
- Increased left ventricular wall stress or afterload
- Aortic regurgitation
- Increased MVO_2 demand

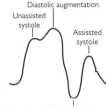

(b) Inflation of the IAB markedly after
closure of the aortic valve

Waveform characteristics:
- Inflation of the IAB after the dicrotic notch
- Absence of sharp V
- Sub-optimal diastolic augmentation

Physiologic effects:
- Sub-optimal coronary artery perfusion

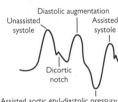

(c) Premature deflation of the IAB during
the diastolic phase

Waveform characteristics:
- Deflation of IAB is seen as a sharp drop following diastolic augmentation
- Sub-optimal diastolic augmentation
- Assisted aortic end-diastolic pressure may be equal to or less than the unassisted aortic end-diastolic pressure
- Assisted systolic pressure may rise

Physiologic effects:
- Sub-optimal coronary perfusion
- Potential for retrograde coronary and carotid blood flow
- Angina may occur as a result of retrograde coronary blood flow
- Sub-optimal afterload reduction
- Increased MVO_2 demand

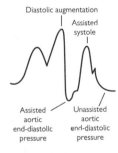

(d) Deflation of the IAB as the aortic valve
is beginning to open

Waveform characteristics:
- Assisted aortic end-diastolic pressure may be equal to the unassisted aortic end-diastolic pressure
- Rate of rise of assisted systole is prolonged
- Diastolic augmentation may appear widened

Physiologic effects:
- Afterload reduction is essentially absent
- Increased MVO_2 consumption due to the left ventricle ejecting against a greater resistance and a prolonged isovolumetric contraction phase
- IAB may impede left ventricular ejection and increase the afterload

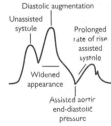

Figure 1.15 Timing errors. (a) Early inflation; (b) late inflation; (c) early deflation; (d) late deflation.

Coronary artery disease

Angina pectoris

Angina pectoris refers to the pain caused by myocardial ischemia. Ischemia is usually caused by mismatched oxygen demand (tachycardia, anemia, aortic stenosis, left ventricular hypertrophy of other etiologies) and delivery in the setting of a hemodynamically significant coronary stenosis due to atheroma, but it may have other causes such as coronary artery spasm (Prinzmetal's variant angina).

In more unusual cases the etiology is not completely understood—e.g., syndrome X (chest pain with normal coronary arteries). Alternatively, these conditions may coexist and be exacerbated by emotional stress.

History and examination

Angina pectoris is characterized by a deep and diffusely distributed central chest discomfort. Certain features of pain are of discriminative value. Patients will not be able to point to where the pain is coming from with one finger but will use an open palm or fist over the center or left parasternal aspect of their chest.

- The pain is not sharp (some patients confuse "sharp" with "severe").
- Pain lasts longer than a few seconds and rarely exceeds an hour without varying in severity. Most episodes will last 1–5 minutes.
- The response to nitroglycerin, if any, will be almost immediate. Generally, responses taking more than 5 minutes are unlikely to be related to the drug.

Chest wall tenderness suggests musculoskeletal pain and does not accompany angina.

Dyspnea, fatigue, nausea, and recurrent belching may also represent underlying ischemia and can occur in the absence of the classical central chest pain. The clue to underlying ischemic heart disease (IHD) lies in their precipitation by exertion or emotional stress.

Angina is often classified according to its temporal pattern and its relation to exertion because this loosely reflects prognosis.

- *Stable angina* is characterized by pain occurring after a relatively constant level of exertion.
- *Unstable angina* is characterized by pain on minor exertion or at rest, which is either new onset or a dramatic worsening of existing angina. Also, it can present as pain on ever-diminishing levels of exertion, usually over a period of days.

The Canadian Cardiovascular Society (CCS) system provides a quantitative means to describe exertional capacity and is divided into four classes:

I. Minimal limitation of ordinary activity. Angina occurs with strenuous, rapid, or prolonged exertion at work or recreation.
II. Slight limitation of ordinary activity; angina occurs on walking or climbing stairs rapidly; walking in cold, in wind, or under emotional stress.
III. Marked limitation of ordinary physical activity; angina occurs on walking 50–100 m on level ground or climbing 1 flight of stairs at a normal pace in normal conditions.
IV. Inability to perform any physical activity without discomfort; angina symptoms may be present at rest.

Physical examination

- Measure the pulse rate. This may be slowed by inferior ischemia due to atrioventricular (AV) node ischemia. A resting tachycardia, if present, usually represents activation of the sympathetic nervous system but may be due to an arrhythmia precipitated by ischemia.
- Blood pressure measurement is essential to look for evidence of hypertension (predisposing to atheroma) or hypotension (may reflect cardiac dysfunction or overmedication).
- Precordial examination should include palpation for left ventricular hypertrophy (LVH), cardiac enlargement, or dyskinesis, and auscultation for added heart sounds (heart failure or acute ischemia), aortic stenosis, or mitral regurgitation (due to papillary muscle dysfunction).
- Examine for signs of heart failure by listening for fine, late-inspiratory crackles at the lung bases and looking for dependent pitting edema (typically bilateral ankle ± leg edema, but sacral edema may be the only manifestation if the patient has been recumbent for some time).
- Look for evidence of peripheral vascular disease by palpating for aortic aneurysm; feeling the carotid and limb pulses; listening for carotid, renal, or femoral artery bruits; and assessing tissue integrity and capillary refill of the legs and feet.
- Examine for signs of hypercholesterolemia: the eyes for xanthelasmata and corneal arcus, and the skin and tendons (especially the Achilles) for xanthomata.

Differential diagnosis

The differential diagnosis of anginal chest pain is wide and includes
- Anxiety and hyperventilation
- Musculoskeletal chest wall pain
- Cervical or thoracic root pain
- Pneumothorax, pneumonia, or pulmonary embolus
- Esophageal problem (inflammation/spasm)
- Other upper gastrointestinal (GI) problem (gastritis, peptic ulcer, pancreatitis, cholecystitis)
- Pericarditis
- Aortic dissection
- Mitral valve prolapse
- Coronary emboli (LV mural thrombus, atrial myxoma)

Investigations

Further risk stratification will add to the diagnostic certainty achieved by history and examination. Measure complete blood count (CBC), chemistries, a full fasting lipid profile (total, LDL and HDL cholesterol and triglyceride levels), and blood glucose.

Chest X-ray (CXR) is not mandatory but should be performed if there is suspicion of heart failure, aortic dissection, a pulmonary condition or an abnormality of the bony structures of the chest wall.

12 Lead ECG

A resting electrocardiogram (ECG) may not confirm the diagnosis but can point toward ischemic heart disease. The presence of Q waves suggests previous myocardial injury. The presence of ST depression and, to a lesser extent, T-wave inversion during pain is a marker of ischemia and patients with these signs should be further investigated. If ST-segment deviation is observed at rest, an acute coronary syndrome must be excluded.

A 12-lead ECG can also help identify other causes of chest pain (LVH, arrhythmia, pericarditis).

Tests for inducible ischemia

Tests such as exercise ECG, stress echocardiogram (ECHO), or myocardial perfusion scanning are useful adjuncts to confirm the diagnosis and aid management.

Management

Lifestyle

Smoking cessation is of paramount importance. Encourage daily aerobic exercise within limits of exercise capacity. Look at the patient's occupational needs and advise adjustment if symptom level is not compatible. Advise a healthy diet, collaborating with dieticians if required.

Aspirin

Provide aspirin in all cases unless there is active peptic ulcer disease, allergy (desensitizing may be required), or bleeding diathesis. Those with past peptic ulcer disease may take a gastroprotective agent such as an H2 antagonist or proton pump inhibitor.

Anti-anginals

- *β-Blockers:* First line (e.g., atenolol 25–100 mg qd or metoprolol 25–50 mg bid). Start on suspicion of ischemic heart disease. Avoid only if contraindicated (asthma with confirmed β-agonist response (mortality improved in patients with angina and concomitant COPD if they can tolerate bronchospasm), uncontrolled severe LV dysfunction, bradycardia, coronary artery spasm).
- *Calcium antagonists* (e.g., amlodipine or diltiazem): If β-blocker contraindicated or concern for vasospasm, calcium antagonists become the drug of choice.
- *Nitrates* (e.g., nitroglycerin): Used for control of breakthrough angina. Long-acting nitrates (e.g., isosorbide mononitrate 60–120 mg qd) are a useful addition to β-blockers for prevention of attacks.

Statins

Statins (HMG-CoA reductase inhibitors) reduce mortality by approximately one-third in all risk groups. However, the underlying risk of events must be taken into account when considering starting the drug, because absolute risk reduction in young patients with low-risk IHD may be very small, with possible harm of myositis, hepatic failure, and reduced compliance with other medications.

Acute coronary syndromes

Acute coronary syndrome (ACS) is a term used to describe a constellation of symptoms resulting from acute myocardial ischemia. An ACS resulting in myocardial injury is termed *myocardial infarction* (MI). ACS includes the diagnosis of unstable angina (UA), non-ST elevation myocardial infarction (NSTEMI), and ST elevation myocardial infarction (STEMI).

Definition

The current nomenclature divides ACS into two major groups on the basis of delivered treatment modalities (see Fig. 2.1).

ST elevation myocardial infarction (STEMI)—an ACS in which patients present with chest discomfort and ST-segment elevation on ECG. This group of patients must undergo reperfusion therapy on presentation.

Non-ST elevation myocardial infarction (NSTEMI) and unstable angina (UA)—ACS in which patients present with ischemic chest discomfort associated with transient or permanent non-ST-elevation ischemic ECG changes. If there is biochemical evidence of myocardial injury, the condition is termed NSTEMI, and in the absence of biochemical myocardial injury the condition is termed UA. This group of patients is not treated with thrombolysis.

Initial management of ACS

- All patients with suspected ACS should have continuous ECG monitoring and access to a defibrillator.
- Rapid assessment and stabilization is imperative.

Immediate assessment should include

- **Rapid examination** to exclude hypotension, note the presence of murmurs, and identify and treat acute pulmonary edema.
- Secure IV access.
- 12 Lead ECG should be obtained and reported within 10 minutes of presentation.
- Give the following:
  - Oxygen (initially only 28% if history of COPD)
  - Morphine 2.5–10 mg IV prn for pain relief
  - Aspirin 325 mg po
  - Nitroglycerin, unless hypotensive
  - Heparin IV and/or Integrilin
  - Consider addition of Plavix
- Take blood for the following:

• CBC/chemistries	Supplement K+ to keep it at 4–5 mmol/L
• Glucose	May be ↑ acutely post MI, even in nondiabetics, reflecting a stress-catecholamine response and may resolve without treatment

  - Biochemical markers of cardiac injury
  - Lipid profile   Total cholesterol, LDL, HDL, triglycerides
  - Serum cholesterol and HDL remain close to baseline for 24–48 hours but fall thereafter and take ≥8 weeks to return to baseline.

- Portable CXR to assess cardiac size and pulmonary edema and to exclude mediastinal enlargement.
- General examination should include peripheral pulses, fundoscopy, and abdominal examination for organomegaly and aortic aneurysm.

Box 2.1 Conditions mimicking pain in ACS

- Pericarditis
- Dissecting aortic aneurysm
- Pulmonary embolism
- Esophageal reflux, spasm, or rupture
- Biliary tract disease
- Perforated peptic ulcer
- Pancreatitis

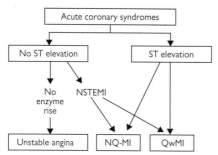

Figure 2.1 Nomenclature of ACS. Patients with ACS may present with or without ST elevation on the ECG. Most patients with ST elevation (large arrows) ultimately develop Q-wave MI (QwMI), whereas a minority (small arrow) develop a non-Q-wave MI (NQ-MI). Patients without ST elevation are experiencing either unstable angina or an NSTEMI depending on the absence or presence of cardiac enzymes (e.g., troponin) detected in the blood. This figure was published in Libby et al., *Braunwald's Heart Disease*, 8th edition. Copyright Elsevier 2007.

ST elevation myocardial infarction (STEMI)

Patients with ACS who have ST-segment elevation or new left bundle branch block (LBBB) on their presenting ECG benefit significantly from immediate reperfusion and are treated as one group under the term *ST elevation myocardial infarction* (STEMI).

Presentation

• **Chest pain** is usually similar in nature to angina, but of greater severity and longer duration and is not relieved by sublingual (SL) nitroglycerin. Associated features are nausea and vomiting, sweating, breathlessness, and extreme distress.
• The pain may be **atypical** (e.g., epigastric) or radiate to the back.
• Diabetics and elderly or hypertensive patients may suffer painless (**"silent" infarcts**) and/or **atypical infarction.** Presenting features include breathlessness from acute pulmonary edema, syncope or coma from arrhythmias, acute confusional states (mania/psychosis), diabetic hyperglycemic crises, hypotension or cardiogenic shock, central nervous system (CNS) manifestations resembling stroke secondary to sudden reduction in cardiac output, and peripheral embolization.

Management

Diagnosis is normally made on presentation followed by rapid stabilization to ensure institution of reperfusion therapy without delay. This is in contrast to NSTEMI/UA, where diagnosis may evolve over a period of 24–72 hours. Management principles of the various stages are outlined below and expanded subsequently (see also Box 2.2).

Stabilizing measures are generally similar for all ACS patients.
• All patients with suspected STEMI should have continuous ECG monitoring in an area with full resuscitation facilities.
• Patients should receive immediate aspirin 325 mg po (if no contraindications), analgesia, and oxygen. Secure IV access.
• Conduct rapid examination to exclude hypotension, note the presence of murmurs, and identify and treat acute pulmonary edema. Right ventricular failure (RVF) out of proportion to left ventricular failure (LVF) suggests RV infarction.

Diagnosis must be made on the basis of history, ECG (ST elevation/new LBBB), and biochemical markers of myocardial injury. (Reperfusion must not be delayed to wait for biochemical markers.)
• Blood for CBC, biochemical profile, markers of cardiac injury, lipid profile, and glucose, and portable CXR

Treatment
• General medical measures (p. 96)
• Reperfusion (p. 98).

All patients with STEMI should be admitted to an intensive care unit (ICU), e.g., coronary ICU (CICU).

Discharge and risk prevention

Box 2.2 Factors associated with a poor prognosis

- Age >70 years
- Previous MI or chronic stable angina
- Anterior MI or right ventricular infarction
- Left ventricular failure at presentation
- Hypotension (and sinus tachycardia) at presentation
- Diabetes mellitus
- Mitral regurgitation (acute)
- Ventricular septal defect

STEMI: diagnosis

STEMI diagnosis is based on a **combination of history, ECG, and biochemical markers of cardiac injury.** In practice, history and ECG changes are normally diagnostic, resulting in immediate reperfusion and medical treatment. Biochemical markers of cardiac injury usually become available later and help reconfirm the diagnosis and provide prognostic information (magnitude of rise).

ECG changes

- **ST-segment elevation** occurs within minutes and may last for up to 2 weeks. ST elevation of ≥2 mm in adjacent chest leads and ≥1 mm in adjacent limb leads is necessary to fulfill thrombolysis criteria. Persisting ST elevation after 1 month suggests formation of LV aneurysm. Infarction site can be localized from ECG changes as indicated in Table 2.1.
- **Pathological Q waves** indicate significant abnormal electrical conduction but are not synonymous with irreversible myocardial damage. In the context of a "transmural infarction" the Q waves may take hours or days to develop and usually remain indefinitely. In the standard leads, the Q wave should be ≥25% of the R wave, 0.04 s in duration, with negative T waves. In the precordial leads, Q waves in V4 should be >0.4 mV (4 small sq) and in V6 >0.2 mV (2 small sq), in the absence of LBBB (QRS width <0.1 s or 3 small sq).
- **ST-segment depression** in a second territory (in patients with ST-segment elevation) is secondary to ischemia in a territory other than the area of infarction (often indicative of multivessel disease) or reciprocal electrical phenomena. Overall, it implies a poorer prognosis.

Table 2.1 Localization of infarcts from ECG changes

Anterior	ST elevation and/or Q waves in V1–V4/V5
Anteroseptal	ST elevation and/or Q waves in V1–V3
Anterolateral	ST elevation and/or Q waves in V1–V6 and I and aVL
Lateral	ST elevation and/or Q waves in V5–V6 and T-wave inversion/ST elevation/Q waves in I and aVL
Inferolateral	ST elevation and/or Q waves in II, III, aVF, and 5–V6 (sometimes I and aVL)
Inferior	ST elevation and/or Q waves in II, III, and aVF
Inferoseptal	ST elevation and/or Q waves in II, III, aVF, V1–V3
True posterior	Tall R waves in V1–V2 with ST depression in V1–V3. T waves remain upright in V1, V2. This can be confirmed with an esophageal lead if available (method similar to an NG tube). This usually occurs in conjunction with an inferior or lateral infarct
RV infarction	ST-segment elevation in the right precordial leads (V3R–V4R). Usually found in conjunction with inferior infarction. This may only be present in the early hours of infarction

Box 2.3 Conditions that may mimic ECG changes of a STEMI

- Left or right ventricular hypertrophy
- LBBB or left anterior fascicular block
- Wolff–Parkinson–White syndrome
- Pericarditis or myocarditis
- Cardiomyopathy (hypertrophic or dilated)
- Trauma to myocardium
- Cardiac tumors (primary and metastatic)
- Pulmonary embolus
- Pneumothorax
- Intracranial hemorrhage
- Hyperkalemia
- Cardiac sarcoid or amyloid
- Pancreatitis

- **PR-segment elevation/depression** and alterations in the contour of the P wave are generally indicative of atrial infarction. Most patients will also have abnormal atrial rhythms such as atrial fibrillation (AF) or flutter, wandering atrial pacemaker, and AV nodal rhythm.
- **T-wave inversion** may be immediate or delayed and generally persists after the ST elevation has resolved.
- **Nondiagnostic changes,** but ones that may be ischemic, include new LBBB or RBBB, tachyarrhythmias, transient tall-peaked T waves or T-wave inversion, axis shift (extreme left or right), or AV block.

Biochemical markers of cardiac injury

Serial measurements evaluating a temporal rise and fall should be obtained to allow a more accurate diagnosis. Creatine kinase (CK) and CK-MB from a skeletal muscle source tend to remain elevated for a greater time period in comparison to levels from a cardiac source.

CK (creatine kinase)

- Levels twice the upper limit of normal are considered abnormal.
- Serum levels rise within 4–8 hours post-STEMI and fall to normal within 3–4 days. The peak level occurs at about 24 hours but may be earlier (12 hours) and higher in patients who have had reperfusion (thrombolysis or percutaneous coronary intervention [PCI]).
- False-positive rates of ~15% occur in patients with alcohol intoxication, muscle disease or trauma, vigorous exercise, convulsions, IM injections, hypothyroidism, pulmonary embolism (PE), and thoracic outlet syndrome.

CK-MB isoenzyme is more specific for myocardial disease. Levels may be elevated despite a normal total CK. However, CK-MB is also present in small quantities in other tissues (skeletal muscle, tongue, diaphragm, uterus, and prostate) and trauma or surgery may lead to false-positive results. If there is doubt about myocardial injury with CK-MB levels obtained, a cardiac troponin must be measured.

Cardiac troponins (TnT, TnI)

- Both TnT and TnI are highly sensitive and specific markers of cardiac injury.
- Serum levels start to rise by 3 hours post-MI and elevation may persist up to 7–14 days. This is advantageous for diagnosis of late MI.
- In most STEMI cases, the diagnosis can be made using a combination of the clinical picture and serial CK/CK-MB levels. In the event of normal CK-MB levels and suspected noncardiac sources of CK, troponins can be used.
- Troponins can also be elevated in nonischemic myocyte damage, such as myocarditis, cardiomyopathy, and pericarditis.

Other markers

There are multiple other markers, but with increasing clinical availability of troponins, measurements of these markers are not recommended. These include aspartamine transferase (AST) (rise 18–36 hours post-MI) and lactate dehydrogenase (LDH) (rise 24–36 hours post-MI).

The time course of the various markers is seen in Figure 2.2.

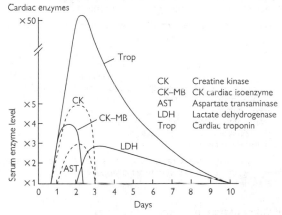

Figure 2.2 Graph of the appearance of cardiac markers in the blood vs. time of onset of symptoms.

Peak A: Early release of myoglobin or CK-MB isoforms after acute myocardial infarction (AMI).

Peak B: Cardiac troponin after AMI.

Peak C: CK-MB after AMI.

Peak D: Cardiac troponin after unstable angina.

Reprinted with permission from Wu AH, et al. (1999). *Clin Chem* 45(7):1104–1121.

STEMI: general measures

1. **Immediate stabilizing measures** are as outlined on p. 89 for all ACS.

2. **Control of cardiac pain**
- **Morphine** 2.5–10 mg IV is the drug of choice and may be repeated to ensure adequate pain relief, unless there is evidence of emerging toxicity (hypotension, respiratory depression). Nausea and vomiting should be treated with metoclopramide (10 mg IV) or a phenothiazine.
- **Oxygen** should be administered at 2–5 L/min for at least 2–3 hours. Hypoxemia is frequently seen post-MI due to ventilation–perfusion abnormalities secondary to LVF. In patients with refractory pulmonary edema, endotracheal intubation may be necessary. Beware of CO_2 retention in patients with COPD.
- **Nitrates** may lessen pain and can be given (sublingual or IV) provided that the patient is not hypotensive. These drugs should be used cautiously in inferior STEMI, especially with right ventricular infarction, as venodilation may decrease RV filling and precipitate hypotension. Nitrate therapy has no demonstrated effect on mortality (ISIS-4).

3. **Correction of electrolytes**
Both low potassium and low magnesium may be arrhythmogenic and must be supplemented, especially in the context of arrhythmias.

4. **Strategies to limit infarct size** (β-blockers, angiotensin-converting enzyme [ACE] inhibitors, and reperfusion).

β-Blockade
Early β-blockade has been shown to be beneficial by limiting infarct size, reducing mortality, and decreasing early malignant arrhythmias. All patients (including primary PCI and thrombolysis patients) should have early β-blockade. Patients with the following features may benefit most from β-blocker therapy:
- Hyperdynamic state (sinus tachycardia, hypertensive)
- Ongoing or recurrent pain or reinfarction
- Tachyarrhythmias such as AF

Absolute contraindications: heart rate (HR) <50, systolic blood pressure (SBP) <90 mmHg, moderate to severe heart failure, AV conduction defect, severe airways disease.

Relative contraindications: asthma, current use of calcium channel blocker and/or β-blocker, severe peripheral vascular disease with critical limb ischemia, large inferior MI involving the right ventricle.

Use a short-acting agent IV initially (metoprolol 5 mg at a time repeated at 5-minute intervals to a maximum dose of 15 mg) under continuous ECG and BP monitoring. Aim for a HR of 60 beats per minute (bpm) and SBP 100–110 mmHg. If hemodynamic stability continues 15–30 minutes after the last IV dose, start metoprolol 50 mg po bid. Esmolol is an ultra-short-acting IV β-blocker, which may be tried if there is concern whether the patient will tolerate β-blockers.

ACE inhibitors

After receiving aspirin, β-blockade (if appropriate), and reperfusion, all patients with STEMI/LBBB infarction should receive an ACE inhibitor within the first 24 hours of presentation.

- Patients with high risk or large infarcts, particularly with an anterior STEMI, a previous MI, heart failure, and impaired LV function on imaging, will benefit most.
- The effect of ACE inhibitors appears to be a class effect; therefore, one may use the drug that the physician is familiar with.

STEMI: reperfusion therapy (thrombolysis)

Rapid reperfusion is the cornerstone of current management of STEMI and is marked by normalization of ST segments on ECG. Primary percutaneous intervention (PCI, or angioplasty) and thrombolysis are the main reperfusion modalities. The best long-term outcome is achieved with primary PCI.

Time is of paramount importance and thrombolysis should be administered as soon as possible. Reperfusion occurs in 50%–70% of patients who receive thrombolysis within 4 hours of onset of pain. Thrombolysis reduces mortality, LV dysfunction, heart failure, cardiogenic shock, and arrhythmias.

However, the magnitude of the benefits obtained with thrombolysis is smaller than with PCI. Furthermore, often patients must undergo cardiac catheterization to delineate their coronary anatomy before further revascularization (whereas this is achieved at the same time with primary PCI).

Indications for thrombolysis

- Typical history of cardiac pain within previous 12 hours and ST elevation in two contiguous ECG leads (>1 mm in limb leads or >2 mm in V1–V6).
- Cardiac pain with newly presumed new LBBB on ECG.
- If ECG is equivocal on arrival, repeat at 15- to 30-minute intervals to monitor progression.
- Thrombolysis should not be given if the ECG is normal or if there is isolated ST depression (true posterior infarct must be excluded as described above).

Timing of thrombolysis

- Greatest benefit is achieved with early thrombolysis (especially if given within 1 1/2 hours of onset of first pain; see Box 2.4).
- Patients presenting between 12 and 24 hours from onset of pain should undergo thrombolysis only with persisting symptoms and ST-segment elevation.
- Elderly patients (>65 years) presenting within the 12- to 24-hour time period with symptoms are best managed by primary PCI, as thrombolysis has been demonstrated to result in increased incidence of cardiac rupture.

Choice of thrombolytic agent

- This is partly determined by each center's local thrombolysis strategy.
- Allergic reactions and episodes of hypotension are greater with streptokinase (SK).
- Bolus agents are easier and quicker to administer, with a decrease in drug errors in comparison to first-generation infusions.

- Recombinant tissue-type plasminogen activator (rtPA) has a greater reperfusion capacity and a marginally higher 30-day survival benefit than that of SK, but this agent has been associated with an increased risk of hemorrhage.
- More recent rtPA derivatives have demonstrated a higher 90-minute TIMI-III (coronary reperfusion scale) flow rate, but have shown similar 30-day mortality benefits to those with rtPA.
- An rtPA derivative (rather than SK) should be considered for any patient with any of the following:
  - Large anterior MI, especially if within 4 hours of onset
  - Previous SK therapy or recent streptococcal infection (as this has been shown to be a risk factor for allergic reactions to SK)
  - Hypotension (systolic BP <100 mmHg)
  - Low risk of stroke (age <55 years, systolic BP <144 mmHg)
  - Reinfarction during hospitalization where immediate PCI facilities are not available

The characteristics of the major thrombolytic agents are on p. 100.

Complications of thrombolysis

- Bleeding is seen in up to 10% of patients. Most incidents are minor and at sites of vascular puncture. Local pressure is generally sufficient to stop this bleeding but occasionally transfusion may be required. In extreme cases, SK may be reversed by tranexamic acid (10 mg/kg slow IV infusion).
- Hypotension during the infusion is common with SK. Treatment consists of placing the patient in a supine position and slowing/stopping infusion until the blood pressure rises. Treatment with cautious (100–500 mL) fluid challenges may be required, especially in inferior/RV infarction. Hypotension is not necessarily evidence of an allergic reaction and may not warrant treatment as such.
- Allergic reactions are common with SK and include a low-grade fever, rash, nausea, headaches, flushing, and, rarely (0.1%), anaphylaxis. Give hydrocortisone 100 mg IV with chlorpheniramine 10 mg IV.
- Intracranial hemorrhage is seen in ~0.3% of patients treated with SK and in ~0.6% with rtPA.
- Reperfusion arrhythmias (most commonly a short, self-limiting run of idioventricular rhythm) may occur.
- Systemic embolization may occur from lysis of thrombus within the left atrium, LV, or aortic aneurysm.

Box 2.4 Patients with greatest benefit from thrombolysis

- Anterior infarct
- Marked ST elevation
- Age >75 years
- Impaired LV function or LBBB
- Systolic BP <100 mmHg
- Patients presenting within 1 hour of onset of pain

Absolute contraindications to thrombolysis

- Active internal bleeding
- Suspected aortic dissection
- Recent head trauma and/or intracranial neoplasm
- Previous hemorrhagic stroke at any time
- Previous ischemic stroke within the past 1 year
- Previous allergic reaction to fibrinolytic agents
- Trauma and/or surgery within past 2 weeks at risk of bleeding

Relative contraindications to thrombolysis

- Trauma and/or surgery more than 2 weeks previously
- Severe uncontrolled hypertension (BP >180/110)
- Nonhemorrhagic stroke over 1 year ago
- Known bleeding diathesis or current use of anticoagulation within therapeutic range (INR ≥2)
- Prolonged (>10 minutes) cardiopulmonary resuscitation
- Prior exposure to SK (if planning to give SK, especially previous 6–9 months)
- Pregnancy or postpartum
- Lumbar puncture within previous 1 month
- Menstrual bleeding or lactation
- History of chronic severe hypertension
- Noncompressible vascular punctures (e.g., subclavian central venous lines)

Box 2.5 Doses and administration of thrombolytic agents

Streptokinase (SK)

- Give as 1.5 million units in 100 mL normal saline IV over 1 hour.
- There is no indication for routine heparinization after SK; there is no clear mortality benefit and there is a small increase in risk of hemorrhage.

Recombinant tissue-type plasminogen activator (rtPA, alteplase)

- The GUSTO trial suggested that the "front-loaded" or accelerated rtPA is the most effective dosage regimen.
- Give 15 mg bolus IV then 0.75 mg/kg over 30 minutes (not to exceed 50 mg), then 0.5 mg/kg over 60 minutes (not to exceed 35 mg).
- This should be followed by IV heparin.

Reteplase

- Give two IV bolus doses of 10 units 10 minutes apart.

Tenectaplase

- Give as injection over 10 seconds at 30–50 mg according to body weight (500–600 μg/kg).
- Maximum dose is 50 mg.

APSAC (anistreplase)

- Give as an IV bolus of 30 mg over 2–5 minutes.

STEMI: reperfusion by primary PCI

Time is of the essence for reperfusion, and each institution should have its recommended protocol. It is imperative that there are no delays in both the decision-making and implementation processes for reperfusion. In centers where primary PCI is chosen, a rapid response network should be in place such that one telephone call from the triage unit should ensure rapid assembly of the PCI team for treatment of the patient.

Primary PCI

Primary PCI is the current gold-standard reperfusion strategy for treatment of STEMI.

Primary PCI requires significant coordination among emergency services, community hospitals, and invasive centers. It must only be performed if 1) a primary PCI program is available and 2) the patient presents to an invasive center and can undergo catheterization without delay.

Indication for primary PCI

- All patients with chest pain and ST-segment elevation or new LBBB fulfill primary PCI criteria (compare with indications for thrombolysis).
- This includes a group of patients in whom ST-segment elevation may not fulfill all criteria for thrombolysis.
- In general, patients in whom thrombolysis is contraindicated should be managed by primary PCI. Patients in whom there is significant risk of bleeding must be managed individually.

Outcome in primary PCI

- Data from over 10 large randomized trials demonstrate a superior outcome in patients with STEMI who are treated with primary PCI in comparison to outcomes with thrombolysis.
- There is a significant short term, as well as long-term, reduction in mortality and major adverse cardiac events (MACE) (death, nonfatal reinfarction, and nonfatal stroke) in STEMI patients treated with primary PCI. Furthermore, primary PCI patients have overall better LV function, a higher vessel patency rate, and less recurrent myocardial ischemia.
- Multiple studies (including PRAGUE-2 and DANAMI-2) have also demonstrated that interhospital transportation for primary PCI (community hospital to invasive center) is safe, and primary PCI remains superior to thrombolysis despite the time delays involved.

Complications

- Bleeding from arterial puncture site, stroke, recurrent infarction, need for emergency coronary artery bypass grafting (CABG), and death are similar in frequency to that in nonemergent high-risk PCI cases (~1%).
- The best results are obtained from high-volume centers with significant experience in primary PCI.
- Each primary PCI center will have its own policy for management of cases, including the use of low-molecular-weight (LMW) or unfractionated (UF) heparin, antiplatelet agents (e.g., gpIIb/IIIa inhibitors), etc. It is generally accepted that in the acute phase only

the "culprit" lesion(s) and vessel(s) will be treated. The pattern of disease in the remainder of the vessels will determine whether further revascularization should be performed as an inpatient or an elective case in the future.

- STEMI patients treated with uncomplicated primary PCI can often be discharged safely within 72 hours of admission without the need for further risk stratification.
- Primary PCI is more cost-effective in the long term than thrombolysis with significant savings from fewer days in the hospital, less need for readmission, and less heart failure.
- Post-discharge care, secondary prevention, and rehabilitation remain identical to that for other MI cases.

Rescue PCI

Rescue PCI may be performed as an adjunct to thrombolysis but should be reserved for patients who remain symptomatic post-thrombolysis (failure to reperfuse) or develop cardiogenic shock. We recommend that all patients who continue to have post-thrombolysis symptoms and/or ongoing ST-elevation with or without symptoms be discussed with the local invasive cardiac center for urgent catheterization and revascularization.

Surgery for acute STEMI

Emergency surgical revascularization (CABG) cannot be widely applied to patients who suffer an MI outside the hospital. CABG in uncomplicated STEMI patients after 6 hours from presentation is contraindicated secondary to significant hemorrhage into areas of infarction. Unstable patients have a very high rate of perioperative mortality.

CABG in the context of an acute STEMI is of value in the following situations:

- High-risk coronary anatomy on catheterization (left main stenosis, left anterior descending [LAD] ostial disease).
- Complicated STEMI (acute mitral regurgitation, or ventricular rupture)
- STEMI patients (with or without successful thrombolysis) with additional coronary lesions whose anatomy is best served by CABG on prior or subsequent catheterization

STEMI: additional measures

Low-molecular-weight and unfractionated heparin
UFH
- There is no indication for "routine" IV heparin following SK.
- IV heparin (4000 U/max IV bolus followed by 1000 U/hr max adjusted for an aPTT ratio of 1.5–2.0 times control) should be used routinely following rtPA and its derivatives for 24–48 hours.

LMWH
- There is clinical trial data supporting the use of LMWH and thrombolysis (e.g., enoxaparin 30 mg IV bolus, then 1 mg/kg SC q12h).
- As an alternative to UFH, LMWH can be used at a prophylactic dose to prevent thromboembolic events in high-risk patients.

Clopidogrel
- This should be administered to all patients undergoing primary PCI (loading dose 300–600 mg po followed by 75 mg qd).
- The length of therapy is determined by the type of stent used. Drug-eluting stents require longer term use of clopidogrel than bare-metal stents (current guidelines for ACS is 1 year of Plavix).

Glycoprotein (gp) IIb/IIIa inhibitors
- There are multiple ongoing trials to evaluate the role of these agents in combination with thrombolysis and/or LMWH.
- These are recommended routinely in the context of STEMI patients treated with primary PCI. Lower doses of LMWH/UFH should be used (consult manufacturers information sheet for individual agents).
- They can also be used in the context of rescue PCI subsequent to failed thrombolysis, although there is a greater risk of bleeding. Current clinical use is determined on a case-by-case basis in most centers.

Calcium antagonists
- These are best avoided, especially in the presence of LV impairment.
- Diltiazem and verapamil started after day 4–5 in post-MI patients with normal LV function may have a small beneficial effect.
- Amlodipine is safe to use in patients with poor LV function post-MI.
- Nifedipine has been shown to increase mortality and should be avoided.

Right ventricular (RV) infarction

RV infarction results in elevated right-sided pressures (RA and RVEDP) and low left-sided pressures (resulting in low BP and cardiac output [CO]). It is common in inferior STEMI.

Diagnosis

- *Clinical:* signs of right heart failure (elevated jugular venous pulsations, Kussmaul's sign, and pulsus paradoxus) with absence of pulmonary edema in the context of a low output state (↓BP, cold extremities)
- *ECG:* in patients with inferior STEMI a 0.1 mV (>1 mm) ST-segment elevation in any one of leads V4R–V6R is highly sensitive and specific for RV infarction. See Figure 2.3 for different ECG patterns identified in right-sided precordial leads. Changes may be transient and present in the early stages only.
- *ECHO:* look for RV dilation and wall motion abnormalities.

Management

- Aim to maintain a high RV preload.
  - Initially give 1–2 L of IV fluids rapidly.
  - Avoid use of nitrates and diuretics as they reduce preload and can worsen hypotension.
  - In patients requiring pacing, AV synchrony must be maintained to ensure maximal CO (requires atrial and ventricular wires).
  - Cardiovert any arrhythmias (e.g., AF/flutter or ventricular rhythms).
- Reduce afterload.
  - This is particularly important if there is concomitant LV dysfunction.
  - Insert intra-aortic balloon pump (IABP)
  - Arterial vasodilators can be used with caution (Na nitroprusside, hydralazine) or ACE inhibitors.
- Inotropic support should ideally be avoided and used only if all other measures fail to restore hemodynamic status.
- Reperfusion of the right coronary artery (RCA) (PCI and thrombolysis) has been demonstrated to improve RV function and reduce mortality.
- In extreme cases, surgically implantable right ventricular assist devices (RVAD) may be used.

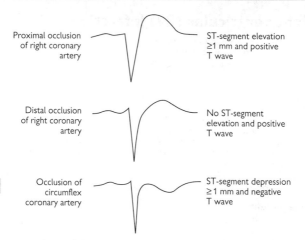

Proximal occlusion of right coronary artery — ST-segment elevation ≥1 mm and positive T wave

Distal occlusion of right coronary artery — No ST-segment elevation and positive T wave

Occlusion of circumflex coronary artery — ST-segment depression ≥1 mm and negative T wave

Figure 2.3 ST-elevation and T-wave configuration in lead V4R in inferoposterior acute MI. Proximal occlusion of the RCA produces ST elevation >1 mm and a positive T wave. Distal occlusion is characterized by a positive T wave but no ST elevation. Occlusion of the circumflex artery produces a negative T wave and ST depression of at least 1 mm. Reproduced with permission from Wellens HJ (1999). *N Engl J Med* 340(5):381–383. Copyright © 1999 Massachusetts Medical Society. All rights reserved.

STEMI: predischarge risk stratification

It is important to identify the subgroup of patients who have a high risk of reinfarction or sudden death. These patients may require further revascularization or placement of an automatic implantable cardioverter defibrillator (AICD) prior to discharge.

Primary PCI group

STEMI patients treated with primary PCI are at a much lower risk of developing post-MI complications than those without treatment or with thrombolytic therapy.

There is ongoing debate as to whether patients treated with primary PCI who are found to have additional high-grade coronary lesions at the time of angiography should have total revascularization as an inpatient or whether this can be achieved after functional testing on an outpatient basis.

Patients who should have electrophysiological assessment prior to discharge are listed below.

Thrombolysis group

Patients treated with thrombolysis should be risk stratified prior to discharge, and high-risk patients should have inpatient (or early outpatient) angiography (Fig. 2.4). High-risk patients are indicated by the following:
- Significant post-infarct angina or unstable angina
- Positive exercise test (modified Bruce protocol) with angina, >1 mm ST depression or fall in BP
- Cardiomegaly on CXR, poor LV function on ECHO (EF <40%)
- Documented episodes of ventricular ectopy or VT >24 hours post-infarction
- Frequent episodes of silent ischemia on Holter monitoring

Electrophysiological evaluation

All STEMI patients with 1) nonsustained VT and/or documented ejection fraction (EF) <40% or 2) sustained/pulseless VT/VF (regardless of EF) should be considered for implantation of an AICD for secondary preventions (AVID, CIDS trial). Patients post-MI with decreased LVEF (<35%) 4–6 weeks after index event should be considered for AICD implantation for primary prevention (MADIT and MUSTT trials).

Discharge and secondary prevention

- *Length of hospital stay in uncomplicated patients:* because the thrombolysis group needs to undergo risk stratification prior to discharge, they tend to have a mean hospital stay of 5–7 days. The primary PCI group generally has shorter hospital stay, between 3 and 4 days.
- Prior to discharge, an agreed-upon plan between the patient (patient's family) and physician is necessary to address modifiable risk factors, beneficial medication, and rehabilitation program.
- Modifiable risk factors include the following:
  - Management of lipids and use of statins
  - Detection and treatment of diabetes
  - Ensuring blood pressure is adequately controlled

- Counseling to discontinue smoking
- Advice on a healthy diet and weight loss
- It is vital that patients understand their prescribed medical regimen and, in particular, the importance of long-term treatment. Unless there are contraindications, all patients should be on a minimum of
  - Aspirin 325 mg qd (if true allergy, use clopidogrel 75 mg qd)
  - ACE inhibitor at the recommended dosage
  - Statin at the recommended dosage
  - The role of long-term formal anticoagulation is controversial.
- All patients should undergo a cardiac rehabilitation program.

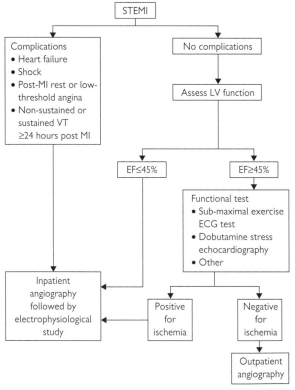

Figure 2.4 Suggested strategy post-STEMI in patients who have undergone thrombolysis to determine the need for inpatient angiography or electrophysiological study. This figure was published in Antman EM (2000). *Cardiovascular Therapeutics*, 2nd edition. Copyright Elsevier 2000.

STEMI: complications

Complications

- Continuing chest pain
- Fever
- A new systolic murmur may suggest ventricular septal defect (VSD), acute MR, or pericarditis.
- Dysrrhythmia (VT, AV block, ectopy, and bradycardia)
- Pump failure—hypotension, cardiac failure, and cardiogenic shock

Complications are encountered more commonly in patients post-STEMI, but can also be found in NSTEMI patients. In NSTEMI patients, complications are more common when multiple cardiac events have occurred.

Further chest pain

Chest pain post-MI is not necessarily angina. Careful history is needed to characterize the pain. If there is doubt about the etiology of pain in the absence of ECG changes, a stress test or thallium imaging may aid diagnosis.

A bruised sensation and musculoskeletal pains are common in the first 24–48 hours, especially in patients who have received CPR or repeated DC shock. Use topical agents for skin burns.

Recurrent infarction is an umbrella term including extension of infarction in the original territory or new infarct in a second territory.

- It is usually associated with recurrent ST elevation.
- If cardiac enzymes are not yet back to normal, a significant change is a twofold rise above the previous nadir.
- Patients should ideally undergo immediate PCI. Thrombolysis is an alternative but a less attractive approach. Standard thrombolysis criteria must be met. Bleeding is a risk (Note: SK should not be used in patients whose original STEMI was treated with SK).

Post-infarction angina (angina developing within 10 days of MI) should be treated with standard medical therapy. All patients with angina prior to discharge should undergo cardiac catheterization and revascularization as an inpatient.

Pericarditis presents as sharp, pleuritic, and positional chest pain, usually 1–3 days post-infarct. It is more common with STEMI. A pericardial friction rub may be audible. ECG changes are rarely seen.

Treat with high-dose aspirin (600 mg qid po) covering with a proton pump inhibitor (e.g., lansoprazole 30 mg qd po). Other nonsteroidal anti-inflammatory drugs (NSAIDs) have been associated with higher incidence of LV rupture and increased coronary vascular resistance and are probably best avoided.

Pericardial effusion is more common with anterior MI especially if complicated by cardiac failure. Detection is with a combination of clinical features and echocardiography. Most resolve gradually over a few months with no active intervention. Tamponade is rare and may be the result of ventricular rupture and/or hemorrhagic effusion.

Pulmonary thromboembolism can occur in patients with heart failure and prolonged bed rest. Routine use of prophylactic LMWH and UFH combined with early mobilization has reduced the incidence of PE. Sources include lower limb veins and/or RV.

Fever
- Often seen and peaks 3–4 days post-MI.
- Associated with elevated white blood cell count (WBC) and raised C-reactive protein (CRP).
- Other causes of fever should be considered (infection, thrombophlebitis, venous thrombosis, drug reaction, and pericarditis).

Ventricular septal defect post-MI

VSD is classically seen 24 hours (highest risk) to 10 days post-MI and affects 2%–4% of cases.

Clinical features

Features include rapid deterioration with a harsh pan-systolic murmur (maximal at the lower left sternal edge), poor perfusion, and pulmonary edema. The absence of a murmur in the context of a low-output state does not rule out a VSD.

Diagnosis

- Echocardiography—the defect may be visualized on 2-D ECHO, and color-flow Doppler shows the presence of left-to-right shunt. Anterior infarction is associated with apical VSD and inferior MI with basal VSD. Failure to demonstrate a shunt on ECHO does not exclude a VSD.
- Pulmonary artery (PA) catheter (especially in the absence of ECHO or inconclusive ECHO results)—a step-up in oxygen saturation from radial artery (RA) to right ventricle (RV) confirms the presence of a shunt, which may be calculated by

$$Qp:Qs = \frac{(Art\ sat - RA\ sat)}{(Art\ sat - PA\ sat)} \quad \text{where} \quad \begin{array}{l} Qp = \text{pulmonary blood flow} \\ Qs = \text{systemic blood flow} \end{array}$$

Management

Stabilization measures are all temporizing until definitive repair can take place. Hypotension and pulmonary edema should be managed as described elsewhere. Important principles are the following:

- Invasive monitoring (PA catheter and arterial line) to dictate hemodynamic management. RA and pulmonary capillary wedge pressure (PCWP) dictate fluid administration or diuretic use. Cardiac output, mean arterial pressure, and arterial resistance determine the need for vasodilator therapy.
- If SBP >100 mmHg, cautious use of vasodilator therapy, generally with nitroprusside, will lower the systemic vascular resistance and reduce the magnitude of the shunt (not be used with renal impairment.). Nitrates will cause venodilatation and increase the shunt and should be avoided.
- Give inotropes if severely hypotensive (initially dobutamine but epinephrine may be required depending on hemodynamic response). Increasing systemic pressure will worsen the shunt.
- In most cases, an intra-aortic balloon pump (IABP) should be inserted rapidly for counter-pulsation.
- Consult with surgeons early for possible repair. Operative mortality is high (20%–70%), especially in the context of perioperative shock, inferoposterior MI, and RV infarction. Current recommendations are for high-risk early surgical repair combined with CABG ± mitral valve (MV) repair or replacement.

- If the patient has been weaned off pharmacological and/or mechanical support, it may be possible to postpone surgery for 2–4 weeks to allow for some level of infarct healing.
- Patients should ideally undergo catheterization prior to surgical repair to ensure the culprit vessel(s) are grafted.
- Closure of the VSD with catheter placement of an umbrella-shaped device has been reported to stabilize critically ill patients until definitive repair is possible.

Acute mitral regurgitation post-MI

Mitral regurgitation (MR) due to ischemic papillary muscle dysfunction or partial rupture is seen 2–10 days post-MI. Complete rupture causes severe MR and is usually fatal. It is more commonly associated with inferior MI (which may affect the posteromedial papillary muscle) than anterior MI (anterolateral papillary muscle).

"Silent MR" is quite frequent and must be suspected in any post-MI patient with unexplained hemodynamic deterioration.

Diagnosis is by ECHO. In severe MR, PA catheterization will show a raised pressure with a large v wave.

Management (see p. 18)
- Treatment with vasodilators, generally nitroprusside, should be started as early as possible once hemodynamic monitoring is available.
- Mechanical ventilation may be necessary.
- Consult with surgeons early for possible repair.

Pseudoaneurysm and free wall rupture

- This is demonstrated in up to 6% of STEMI patients and leads to sudden death in two-third.
- A proportion is present subacutely with cardiogenic shock, allowing time for intervention.
- Diagnosis of subacute cases can be made on a combination of clinical features of pericardial effusion, tamponade, and echocardiography.
- Patients who have undergone early thrombolysis have a lower chance of wall rupture.
- Stabilization of the patient is similar to that for cardiogenic shock. The case must be discussed with surgeons immediately to facilitate early repair

Cocaine-induced MI

The incidence of cocaine-induced MI, LV dysfunction, and arrhythmias is on the increase. It is estimated that 14%–25% of young patients presenting to urban emergency departments with nontraumatic chest pain may have detectable levels of cocaine and its metabolites in their circulation (see Box 2.6). Of this group, 6% have enzymatic evidence of MI.

Diagnosis

- Diagnosis can be difficult and must be suspected in any young individual with chest discomfort and at low risk for ischemic heart disease.
- **Chest pain** occurs most commonly within 12 hours of cocaine use. Effects can return up to 24–36 hours later secondary to long-lasting active metabolites.
- **ECG** is abnormal with multiple nonspecific repolarization changes in up to 80% of cases, and approximately 40% may have diagnostic changes of STEMI qualifying for reperfusion therapy.
- **Biochemical markers of cardiac injury** can be misleading, as many patients will have elevated CK levels secondary to rhabdomyolysis. TnI is vital to confirm myocardial injury.

Management

General measures

- These are the same as for anyone presenting with an MI: oxygen: high flow 5–10 L unless there is a contraindication; analgesia; aspirin 325 mg qd.
- Nitroglycerin should be given at high doses as IV infusion (>10 mg/hr final levels) and dose titrated to symptoms and hemodynamic response.
- Benzodiazepines:to reduce anxiety.
- Calcium channel blockers.

Second-line agents

- **Verapamil** is given in high doses and has the dual function of reducing cardiac workload and hence restoring oxygen supply and demand, as well as reversing coronary vasoconstriction. It should be given cautiously as 1–2 mg IV bolus at a time (up to 10 mg total) with continuous hemodynamic monitoring. This should be followed by high-dose oral preparation to cover the 24-hour period for at least 72 hours after the last dose of cocaine (80–120 mg po tid).
- **Phentolamine** is an α-adrenergic antagonist and readily reverses cocaine-induced vasoconstriction (2–5 mg IV and repeated if necessary). It can be used in conjunction with verapamil
- **Labetalol** has both β- and α-adrenergic activity and can be used after verapamil and phentolamine if the patient remains hypertensive. It is effective in lowering cocaine-induced hypertension but has no effect on coronary vasoconstriction.
- **Reperfusion therapy:** evidence for use of thrombolysis is limited and generally associated with poor outcome secondary to hypertension-

induced hemorrhagic complications. If the patient fails to settle after implementing first-line measures, verapamil, and phentolamine, they should undergo immediate coronary angiography followed by PCI if appropriate (evidence of thrombus/vessel occlusion). In the event that angiography is not available, thrombolytic therapy can be considered.

- CAUTION: Other β-blockers must be avoided (e.g., propanolol). They may exacerbate coronary vasoconstriction by allowing unopposed action of the α-adrenergic receptors.

Box 2.6 Teaching points: cocaine-induced MI

Pathogenesis

- The cause of myocardial injury is multifactorial, including an increase in oxygen demand (increased HR, BP, and contractility) in the context of decreased supply caused by a combination of inappropriate vasoconstriction (in areas of minor atheroma), enhanced platelet aggregation, and thrombus formation.
- The effects can be delayed as the metabolites of cocaine are potent active vasoconstrictors and can remain in the circulation for up to 36 hours (or longer), resulting in recurrent waves of symptoms.

Other complications

- **Cocaine-induced myocardial dysfunction** is multifactorial and includes MI, chronic damage secondary to repetitive sympathetic stimulation (as in pheochromocytoma), myocarditis secondary to cocaine impurities/infection, and unfavorable changes in myocardial/ endothelial gene expression.
- **Cocaine-induced arrhythmias** include both atrial and ventricular tachyarrhythmias, as well as asystole and heart block (see post-MI arrhythmias
- **Aortic dissection**

Ventricular tachyarrhythmias post-MI

Accelerated idioventricular rhythm
- Common (up to 20%) in patients with early reperfusion in first 48 hours.
- Usually self-limiting and short lasting with no hemodynamic effects
- If symptomatic, accelerating sinus rate with atrial pacing or atropine may be of value.

Ventricular premature beats (VPB)
- Common and not related to incidence of sustained VT/VF
- Generally treated conservatively by correcting acid–base and electrolyte abnormalities (aim K^+ >4.0 mmol/L and Mg^{2+} >1.0 mmol/L)
- Peri-infarction β-blockade reduces VPB.

Nonsustained and monomorphic ventricular tachycardia (VT)
- Associated with worse clinical outcomes.
- Correct reversible features such as electrolyte abnormalities and acid–base balance.
- DC cardioversion for hemodynamic instability.
- Nonsustained VT and hemodynamically stable VT (slow HR <100 bpm) can be treated with amiodarone (300 mg bolus IV over 30 minutes, followed by 1.2 g infusion over 24 hours). Lidocaine is no longer recommended as first-line but may be used second- or third-line treatment. Procainamide is an effective alternative but may be pro-arrhythmic.
- For incessant VT on amiodarone, consider overdrive pacing.

Ventricular fibrillation (VF) and polymorphic VT
- Requires immediate defibrillation.
- In refractory VF consider vasopressin 40U IV bolus.
- Amiodarone 300 mg IV bolus to be continued as an infusion (see above) if output restored.

Atrial tachyarrhythmia post-MI

- Includes supraventricular tachycardia (SVT), AF, and atrial flutter
- If patient is hemodynamically unstable they must undergo immediate synchronized DC cardioversion.
- Hemodynamically stable patients can be treated with digoxin, β-blockers and/or calcium channel blockers.
- Amiodarone can be used to restore sinus rhythm. However, it is not very effective in controlling rate. Class I agents should generally be avoided as they increase mortality.
- In AF and flutter, patients should undergo anticoagulation to reduce embolic complications if there are no contraindications.

Bradyarrhythmias and indications for pacing

Isolated RBBB/LBBB does not need pacing (unless hemodynamically unstable or progression to higher levels of block). New bifasicular block (RBBB with either LAD or RAD) or BBB with first-degree AV block may require prophylactic pacing depending on the clinical picture. Indications for pacing should not delay reperfusion therapy. Venous access (femoral or internal jugular vein) should be obtained first and the pacing wire inserted later.

External temporary cardiac pacing, atropine (300 µg to 3 mg IV bolus), and isoproterenol can be used to temporarily stabilize patients.

Bradyarrhythmias post-MI

First-degree AV block

This is common and no treatment is required.

Second-degree AV block

This generally indicates a large infarction affecting the conduction system. Mortality is increased in this group of patients.

- Mobitz type I is self-limiting with no symptoms. Generally, it requires no specific treatment. If the patient is symptomatic or has progression to complete heart block they will need temporary pacing.
- Mobitz type II, 2:1, 3:1 should be treated with temporary pacing regardless of whether it progresses to complete heart block.

Third-degree AV block

- In the context of an inferior MI this can be transient and generally does not require temporary pacing unless there is hemodynamic instability or an escape rhythm of <40 bpm.
- Temporary pacing is required with anterior MI and unstable inferior MI.

Hypotension and shock post-MI

Important principles in managing hypotensive patients with MI are as follows:

- If the patient is well perfused peripherally, no pharmacological intervention is required.
- Try to correct any arrhythmia, hypoxia, or acidosis.
- Arrange for an urgent ECHO to exclude a mechanical cause for hypotension (e.g., mitral regurgitation, VSD, ventricular aneurysm, tamponade) that may require urgent surgery.

Patients may be divided into two subgroups

1. Hypotension with pulmonary edema

- Secure central venous access—internal jugular lines are preferable if the patient is treated with thrombolytic therapy.
- Begin inotropes.
- Use further invasive hemodynamic monitoring as available (PA pressures and wedge pressure monitoring, arterial line).
- Ensure optimal filling pressures, guided by physical signs and PA diastolic or wedge pressure. Significant mitral regurgitation will produce large v waves on the wedge trace and give high estimates of left ventricular end diastolic pressure (LVEDP).
- Ensure rapid coronary reperfusion (if not already done), either with thrombolytic therapy or primary PCI, where available.
- IABP counter-pulsation may allow stabilization until PCI can be performed.

2. Hypotension without pulmonary edema

- This may be due to either RV infarction or hypovolemia.
- Check the jugular venous pressure (JVP) and RA pressure. This will be low in hypovolemia and high in RV infarction.
- RV infarction on ECG is seen in the setting of inferior MI and ST elevation in right-sided chest leads (V3R–V4R).
- In either case, cardiac output will be improved by cautious plasma expansion. Give 100–200 mL of IV fluids over 10 minutes and reassess.
- Repeat once if there is some improvement in blood pressure and the patient has not developed pulmonary edema.
- Invasive hemodynamic monitoring with a PA catheter (Swan–Ganz) is necessary to ensure hypotension is not due to low left-sided filling pressures. Aim to keep PCWP 12–15 mmHg.
- Start inotropes if BP remains low despite adequate filling pressures.
- Use IV nitrates and diuretics with caution as venodilatation will compromise RV and LV filling and exacerbate hypotension.
- See p. 105 for management of RV infarction.

Cardiogenic shock

This affects between 5% and 20% of patients, and up to 15% of MI patients can present with cardiogenic shock.

Management involves a complex interaction between many medical, surgical, intensive care teams with multiple invasive and noninvasive measures. Despite significant advances, prognosis remains poor. Therefore, the absolute wishes of the patient with regard to such an invasive strategy should be respected from the outset.

Diagnosis

A combination of clinical and physiological measures:

- *Clinical:* marked, persistent (>30 minutes) hypotension with SBP <80–90 mmHg.
- *Physiological:* low cardiac index (<1.8 L/mm/m^2) with elevated LV filling pressure (PCWP >18 mmHg).

Management

- Management is complex and must be quick.
- Correct reversible factors:
  - Arrhythmias and aim to restore sinus rhythm
  - Acid–base, electrolyte abnormalities
  - Ventilation abnormalities—intubate if necessary
- Rapid hemodynamic, echocardiographic, and angiographic evaluation:
  - *Hemodynamic:* to ensure adequate monitoring and access including central venous lines, Swan–Ganz, arterial line insertion, urinary catheter
  - *Echocardiographic:* to assess ventricular systolic function and exclude mechanical lesions, which may need to be dealt with; for emergency cardiac surgery for mitral regurgitation, VSD, or ventricular aneurysm or pseudoaneurysm
  - *Angiographic:* with view to PCI or CABG, if appropriate
- Aim to improve hemodynamic status, achieving a SBP ≥90 mmHg, guided by physical signs and LV filling pressures. As a general guide:
  - **PCWP <15 mmHg**—cautious administration of IV fluids (colloids) in 100–200 mL aliquots.
  - **PCWP >15 mmHg**—inotropic support ± diuretics (if pulmonary edema).

Inotropes should be avoided if at all possible in acutely ischemic patients. The aim should be to rapidly restore or maximize coronary flow and off-load LV. Early revascularization is vital and has been shown to decrease mortality. IABP will help to achieve these goals.

If hemodynamic status does not improve after revascularization and IABP insertion, inotropes should be used. The choice of agent can be difficult and should be guided in part by local protocols and expertise. Generally accepted choices depend on the clinical picture:

- If the patient is hypotensive (± pulmonary edema) start with dopamine (up to 15 µg/kg/min), and if ineffective, one may substitute epinephrine and/or norepinephrine.

- If the patient has adequate blood pressure (± pulmonary edema) give dobutamine to increase cardiac output (starting at 2.5–5 µg/kg/min and increasing to 20 µg/kg/min), titrating to HR and hemodynamics. Phosphodiesterase inhibitors (PDIs) can be used as an alternative. If hypotension and tachycardia complicate dobutamine/PDI treatment, norepinephrine can be added as a second agent to achieve the desired hemodynamic effect.

Use of diuretics, thrombolysis, gp IIb/IIIa antagonists, and LMWH/UFH should follow normal principles and are based on the clinical picture.

Non-ST elevation myocardial infarction (NSTEMI)/unstable angina (UA)

UA and NSTEMI are closely related conditions with similar clinical presentation, treatment, and pathogenesis but of varying severity. If there is biochemical evidence of myocardial damage, the condition is termed NSTEMI; in the absence of damage it is termed UA.

Unlike patients with a STEMI, in whom diagnosis is generally made on presentation in the emergency department, diagnosis of NSTEMI/UA may not be definitive on presentation and evolves over the subsequent hours to days. Therefore, management of patients with NSTEMI/UA is a progression through a number of risk stratification processes dependent on history, clinical features, and investigative results. These in turn determine the choice and timing of a number of medical and/or invasive treatment strategies.

Figure 2.5 is a summary of a recommended **integrated care pathway** illustrating a management plan for diagnosis and risk-directed treatment of a patient with STEMI/UA.

Clinical presentation

There are three distinct presentations:
- **New-onset angina** (in a patient without prior angina)
- **Rest angina** (angina when patient is at rest; may occur in a patient with prior stable, exertional angina)
- **Increasing angina** (in a patient with previously diagnosed angina for whom angina has become more frequent or longer in duration or requires a lower threshold to elicit)

General examination must be undertaken to rule out pulmonary edema, assess hemodynamic stability, and look for cardiac valve abnormalities.

Integrated management plan

We recommend that all patients follow a local integrated care pathway on presentation. The various stages are broadly outlined below. See relevant pages for further information.

Initial stabilization
- Transfer patient to an area with continuous ECG monitoring.
- Strict bed rest is required.
- Give oxygen, aspirin 325 mg po, sublingual nitrates, and mild sedation if required.
- If pain persists, give morphine 2.5–5 mg IV prn with metoclopramide 10 mg IV for nausea.

General investigations are similar to those for STEMI patients, including blood for CBC, biochemical profile, markers of myocardial injury, and lipid. Arrange portable CXR (rule out LVF and mediastinal abnormalities).

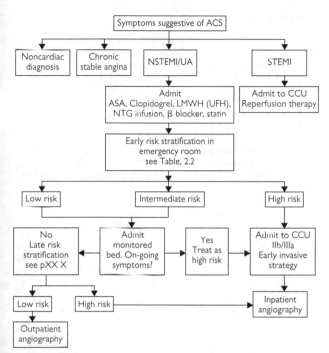

Figure 2.5 NSTEMI/VA—integrated care pathway. Reprinted with permission from ACC Practice Guidelines, *J Am Coll Cardiol*, 2000; 36:970–1062.

Confirm diagnosis

Risk stratification (see Fig. 2.5, above) to determine appropriate medical and invasive treatment strategies. High-risk patients should be admitted to a coronary care unit (CCU) and low- to intermediate-risk patients to monitored beds in a step-down unit.

Treatment is based on the patient's risk and includes the following:
• Medical treatment
  • Anti-ischemic
  • Antiplatelet
  • Antithrombic
• Invasive strategies (p. 131)

Secondary prevention and discharge

NSTEMI/UA: diagnosis

Diagnosis in NSTEMI/UA is an evolving process and may not be clear on presentation. **A combination of history, serial changes in ECG, and biochemical markers of myocardial injury** (usually over a 24- to 48-hour period) **determine the diagnosis**. Once a patient has been designated as having a diagnosis of ACS with probable or possible NSTEMI/UA they will require treatment outlined below.

1. Serial ECGs

Changes can be transient and/or fixed, especially if a diagnosis of NSTEMI is made.

- ST-segment depression of ≥0.05 mV is highly specific of myocardial ischemia (unless isolated in V1–V3, suggesting a posterior STEMI).
- T-wave inversion is sensitive but nonspecific for acute ischemia unless very deep (≥0.3 mV).
- Rarely, Q waves may evolve or there may be transient or new LBBB.

2. Serial biochemical markers of cardiac injury

These are used to differentiate between NSTEMI and UA, as well as to determine prognosis. We recommend levels at 0, 6, and 12 hours after the last episode of pain. A positive biochemical marker (CK, CK-MB, or troponin) in the context of one or more of the ECG changes listed above is diagnostic of NSTEMI. If serial markers over a 24-hour period from the last episode of chest pain remain negative, UA is diagnosed.

Cardiac troponin T and I

Both of these are highly cardiac specific and sensitive, can detect "micro-infarction" in the presence of normal CK-MB, are not affected by skeletal muscle injury, and convey prognostic information (worse prognosis if positive). Troponins can be raised in nonatherosclerotic myocardial damage (cardiomyopathy, myocarditis, pericarditis) and should thus be interpreted in the context of the clinical picture.

Both TnT and TnI rise within 3 hours of infarction. TnT may persist up to 10–14 days and TnI up to 7–10 days. Results must be interpreted with caution in patients with chronic renal failure (see Fig. 2.5).

- CK levels do not always reach the diagnostic twice upper-limit of normal and generally have little value in diagnosis of NSTEMI.
- CK-MB has low sensitivity and specificity. CK-MB isoforms improve sensitivity (CK-MB2>1 U/L or CK-MB2/CK-MB1 ratio >1.5), but isoform assays are not widely available clinically.
- Myoglobin is non–cardiac specific, but levels can be detected as early as 2 hours after onset of symptoms. A negative test is useful in ruling out myocardial necrosis.

3. Continuous ECG monitoring

can detect episodes of silent ischemia and arrhythmia, both of which have been shown to be more prolonged in NSTEMI than in UA.

NSTEMI/UA: risk stratification

NSTEMI/UA comprises a heterogeneous group of conditions with variable outcome. An assessment of risk for adverse outcome is vital to ensure formation of an adequate management plan.

Risk stratification should begin on initial evaluation and continue throughout the hospital stay. At each stage, patients with a high chance of a poor outcome should be identified and managed appropriately.

We recommend at least two formal risk stratification processes.

1. Early risk stratification (Table 2.2)

This should take place on presentation and forms part of the initial assessment used to make a diagnosis. It involves a combination of clinical features, ECG changes, and biochemical markers of cardiac injury. Patients are divided into high risk and intermediate/low risk.

• **High-risk patients** should be admitted to the CCU, follow an early invasive strategy, and be managed with a combination of
  • ASA, clopidogrel, LMWH (or UFH), and/or gpIIb/IIIa antagonists
  • Anti-ischemic therapy (first-line β-blocker, nitroglycerin)
  • Early invasive strategy (inpatient catheterization and PCI within 48 hours of admission)
• **Intermediate- to low-risk** patients should be admitted to a **monitored bed on a step-down unit and undergo a second inpatient risk stratification** once their symptoms have settled, to determine timing of invasive investigations. Initial management should include
  • ASA, clopidogrel, LMWH (or UFH)
  • Anti-ischemic therapy (first-line β-blocker, nitroglycerin)
  • Undergo a **late risk stratification in 48–72 hours** from admission

2. Late risk stratification

This involves a number of noninvasive tests to determine the optimal timing for invasive investigations in intermediate/low-risk patients. It is generally performed if there have been no further episodes of pain or ischemia at 24–48 hours after admission.

• Intermediate/low-risk patients who develop recurrent pain and/or ischemic ECG changes, heart failure, or hemodynamic instability (in the absence of a noncardiac cause) should be managed as a high-risk patient (see above).
• Table 2.2 is a summary of a recommended integrated care pathway combining diagnosis, risk stratification, and treatment.
• There are other risk stratification assessment scores, including Braunwald and TIMI. As recommended above, high-risk patients from these assessments should also follow an early invasive strategy and intermediate/low-risk patients, a more conservative strategy.

Table 2.2 Short-term risk of death nonfatal MI in patients with UA

Feature	High risk (at least 1 of the following features must be present)	Intermediate risk (no high-risk feature but must have 1 of the following)	Low risk (no high- or intermediate-risk feature) but may have any of the following features)
History	Accelerating tempo of ischemic symptoms in preceding 48 hours	Prior MI, peripheral or cerebrovascular disease or CABG, prior aspirin use	
Character of pain	Prolonged ongoing (>20 minutes) rest pain	Prolonged (>20 minutes) rest angina now resolved, with moderate or high likelihood of CAD	New-onset or progressive CCS Class III or IV angina the past 2 weeks without prolonged (>20 minutes) rest pain but with moderate or high likelihood of CAD
		Rest angina (<20 minutes) or relieved with rest or sublingual NTG	
Clinical findings	Pulmonary edema, most likely due to ischemia	Age >70 years	
	New or worsening MR murmur, S3, or new/ worsening rales Hypotension, bradycardia, tachycardia		
	Age >75 years		
ECG	Angina at rest with transient ST-segment changes >0.05 mV	T-wave inversions >0.2 mV	Normal or unchanged ECG during an episode of chest discomfort
	Bundle-branch block, new or presumed new sustained ventricular tachycardia	Pathological Q waves	
Cardiac markers	Elevated (e.g., TnT or TnI >0.1 ng/mL)	Slightly elevated (e.g., TnT >0.01 but <0.1 ng/mL)	Normal

Reprinted with permission from ACC Practice Guidelines, *J Am Coll Cardiol*, 2000; 36:970–1062.

NSTEMI/UA: late risk stratification

The highest risk of adverse outcome in patients who are designated inter-mediate/low risk on presentation is during the early phase of admission. Therefore, it is important that the second risk stratification process occurs within 24–48 hours of admission if the patient is stable.

Late risk stratification is based on one of the following noninvasive investigations.

A patient is regarded as being at high risk of adverse outcome if they fulfill one of the features listed below. These patients should have inpatient cardiac catheterization.

1. Exercise ECG test
- **Horizontal/down-sloping ST depression with**
  - Onset at HR <120 bpm or <6.5 METS
  - Magnitude of >2.0 mm
  - Post-exercise duration of changes >6 minutes
  - Depression in multiple leads reflecting multiple coronary distributions
- **Abnormal systolic BP response**
  - Sustained decrease of >10 mmHg or flat BP response with abnormal ECG
- **Other**
  - Exercise-induced ST-segment elevation
  - VT
  - Prolonged elevation of HR

2. Stress radionuclide myocardial perfusion imaging
- Abnormal tracer distribution in more than one territory
- Cardiac enlargement

3. LV imaging
- **Stress echocardiography**
  - Rest EF <40%
  - Wall motion score index of >1
- **Stress radionuclide ventriculography**
  - Rest EF <40%
  - Fall in EF >10%

NSTEMI/UA: medical management

Anti-ischemic therapy

All patients should be treated with adequate analgesia, IV nitrates, β-blockers, and statins (if no contraindications) to ensure adequate symptom control and a favorable hemodynamic status (SBP 100–110 mmHg, HR approximately 60 bpm). Other agents can also be added depending on the clinical picture.

1. Analgesia
- Morphine 2.5–5 mg IV. Acts as anxiolytic, reduces pain and systolic blood pressure through venodilatation and reduction in sympathetic arteriolar constriction. It can result in hypotension (responsive to volume therapy) and respiratory depression (reversal with naloxone 400 μg to 2 mg IV).

2. Nitrates
- Nitroglycerin infusion (50 mg in 50 mL normal saline at 1–10 mL/hr) titrated to pain and keeping SBP >100 mmHg. Tolerance to continuous infusion develops within 24 hours and the lowest efficacious dose should be used.

Common side effects are headache and hypotension both of which are reversible on withdrawal of medication. *Absolute contraindication* is use of sildenafil (Viagra) in the previous 24 hours. This can result in exaggerated and prolonged hypotension.

3. β-Blockers
- These should be started on presentation. Initially use a short-acting agent (e.g., metoprolol 12.5–100 mg po bid), which if tolerated, may be converted to a longer acting agent (e.g., atenolol 25–1000 mg qd). Rapid β-blockade may be achieved using short-acting IV agents such as metoprolol. Aim for HR of ~50–60 beats/min.

Mild LVF is not an absolute contraindication to β-blocker therapy. Pulmonary congestion may be secondary to ischemic LV systolic dysfunction and/or reduced compliance. If there is overt heart failure β-blockade is contraindicated.

By reducing heart rate and blood pressure, β-blockers reduce myocardial oxygen demand and thus angina. When used alone or in combination with nitrates and/or calcium antagonists, β-blockers are effective in reducing the frequency and duration of both symptomatic and silent ischemic episodes.

4. Calcium antagonists
- Diltiazem 60–360 mg po, verapamil 40–120 mg po tid. These aim to reduce HR and BP and are a useful adjunct to treatments 1–3 above. Amlodipine/felodipine 5–10 mg po qd can be used with pulmonary edema and in poor LV function.

Calcium antagonists alone do not appear to reduce mortality or risk of MI in patients with UA. However, when combined with nitrates and/or β-blockers they are effective in reducing symptomatic and silent ischemic episodes, nonfatal MI, and need for revascularization.

5. Statins (HMG-CoA reductase inhibitors)

High-dose statins (e.g., atorvastatin 80 mg qd) have been shown to reduce mortality and recurrent MI in the acute setting. The role of statins in primary and secondary prevention of cardiovascular events is well documented.

6. ACE inhibitors

Unlike patients with STEMI, in whom early introduction of an ACE inhibitor has significant prognostic benefits, specific trials in the NSTEMI/UA setting are lacking. However, there is good evidence that patients with low or high risk of cardiovascular disease will benefit from long-term ACE inhibition (HOPE and EUROPA Trials).

Antiplatelet therapy

All patients should be given aspirin and clopidogrel (unless contraindications)—gp IIb/IIIa antagonists to high-risk patients only.

1. Aspirin

- (325 mg po) should be administered immediately in the emergency department and continued indefinitely (unless there are contraindications).

In many trials, aspirin has been shown to consistently reduce mortality and recurrent ischemic events. In patients with aspirin hypersensitivity or major gastrointestinal intolerance, clopidogrel 75 mg qd should be used.

2. Thienopyridines

- Clopidogrel (75 mg qd) should be given on admission to all patients with proven NSTEMI/UA, regardless of risk, and continued for at least 1 month and ideally for 12 months.

Clopidogrel should be withheld in patients requiring CABG for 5–7 days to reduce hemorrhagic complications. Clopidogrel is preferred over ticlopidine because of its rapid onset of action and better safety profile.

3. Glycoprotein IIb/IIIa antagonists

There are multiple short- and long-acting commercially available molecules. These agents should be used in conjunction with aspirin, clopidogrel, and LMWH (or UFH).

- Eptifibatide and tirofiban should be used in high-risk patients with ongoing ischemia and elevated troponin in whom an early invasive management strategy is not planned or available (<24 hours).
- In patients with an early invasive strategy all gpIIb/IIIa antagonists can be used. Infusion is generally continued for 12 hours post-PCI.

Taken as a group, these agents protect NSTEMI/UA patients from death and nonfatal MI during the acute phase of their presentation and 24 hours post-intervention. See Box 2.7 for doses and administration regime.

Antithrombotic therapy

All patients should be given LMWH (UFH).

1. Low-molecular-weight heparins (LMWH)

These have been shown to be as good as, or superior to, UFH in short-term reduction of death, MI, and revascularization in patients with NSTEMI/UA. They should be used in conjunction with aspirin and clopidogrel in all patients on presentation and continued for 2–5 days after the last episode of pain and ischemic ECG changes.

Other advantages over UFH include subcutaneous administration, lack of monitoring, and reduced resistance and thrombocytopenia. Box 2.7 lists the doses of various agents in use for NSTEMI/UA.

2. Unfractionated heparin (UFH)

Multiple trials have demonstrated reduction of risk of death and MI in patients with UA/NSTEMI. UFH should be started on presentation as an alternative to LMWH in conjunction with aspirin and clopidogrel. Infusion should be continued for 2–5 days subsequent to the last episode of pain and/or ischemic ECG changes. Initial bolus of 60–70 U/kg (maximum 5000 U) should be followed by an infusion of 12–15 U/kg/h (1000 U/h). The infusion rate should be altered to achieve an aPTT value of 1.5–2.0 times control.

Coagulation should be checked initially every 6 hours followed by once every 24 hours after two consistent values have been obtained.

Thrombolysis

There is no evidence to suggest that combining thrombolytic agents with aspirin, LMWH, and conventional anti-ischemic therapy is of benefit in patients with NSTEMI. In the TIMI IIIB trial, the rtPA group had a worse outcome at 6 weeks, and risk of bleeding was also greater with the thrombolyis group.

Box 2.7 Doses of LMWH IIb/IIIa antagonists licensed for NSTEMI/UA

LMWH
- **Dalteparin**   120 U/kg bid (max 10,000 U twice daily)
- **Enoxaparin**   1 mg/kg bid (100 U/kg twice daily)

IIb/IIIa antagonists
- **Abciximab** (*Reopro®*) Bolus 250 µg/kg over 1 minute followed by IV infusion 125 ng/kg/min
- **Tirofiban** (*Aggrastat®*) 400 ng/kg/min for 30 minutes followed by IV infusion 100 ng/kg/min
- **Eptifibatide** (*Integrilin®*) Bolus 180 µg/kg followed by IV infusion 2 µg/kg/min

NSTEMI: invasive vs. noninvasive strategies

The current evidence supports early angiography and revascularization in patients who present with either high-risk features or intermediate/ low-risk features with ongoing symptoms. Furthermore, low- and intermediate-risk patients who settle on medical therapy should undergo symptom-limited noninvasive stress testing to identify a cohort of patients with an increased risk of adverse outcome. This second group will also benefit from an early invasive management.

Patients managed with an early conservative strategy tend to have an increased need for antianginal therapy and rehospitalization for angina, and many undergo coronary angiography within the year.

The following groups are recommended to benefit from an early invasive strategy (inpatient cardiac catheterization and PCI):

- **Patients with high-risk features of NSTEMI/UA**
  - Recurrent angina/ischemic ECG changes despite optimal medical therapy
  - Elevated troponin
  - New/presumed new ST-segment depression
  - Chest pain with clinical features of heart failure (pulmonary edema, new/worsening MR, S3 gallop)
  - Hemodynamic instability
  - Sustained ventricular tachycardia
- **Poor LV systolic function (EF <40%)**
- **Patients allocated to low/medium risk in whom, subsequent noninvasive testing demonstrates high-risk features**
- **PCI in previous 6 months**
- **Previous CABG**
- **Patients with other comorbidities** (e.g., malignancy, liver failure, renal disease) in whom risks of revascularization are not likely to outweigh benefits.

Discharge and secondary prevention

- **Length of hospital stay** will be determined by symptoms and the rate of progression through the NSTEMI/UA pathway. Generally patients are hospitalized for 3–7 days.
- **Secondary prevention** remains of paramount importance and is similar in principle to that for STEMI patients.

Chapter 3

Peripheral vascular disease

Introduction

In peripheral arterial disease (PAD), there is an obstruction to the blood supply of the upper or lower extremities. While this is most commonly caused by atherosclerosis, thrombosis, embolism, vasculitis, fibromuscular dysplasia, or entrapment can result in blood flow obstruction.

Peripheral vascular disease more broadly encompasses diseases that include renovascular and carotid disease, vasospasm, and venous disorders. PAD strongly correlates with risk of major adverse cardiovascular events. Unlike cardiovascular disease, PAD is frequently underdiagnosed and undertreated.

This chapter will focus on the diagnosis and management of peripheral vascular disease.

Epidemiology

The prevalence of PAD varies according to the study population. In large population-based studies conducted in the United States, Europe, and Middle East, the prevalence of PAD varied from 3.6% to 29%, based on abnormal ankle–brachial index (ABI).

PAD is more common in the elderly, present in 15%–20% of those older than 65 years. It is more prevalent in men than in women. PAD is more common in blacks than in non-Hispanic whites.

The incidence of critical limb ischemia is estimated at 400–450 per million population per year. The incidence of limb amputation is estimated at 112–250 per million population per year.

Classification of peripheral artery disease is commonly divided into the Fontaine stages, introduced by Dr. Rene Fontaine in 1954, and Rutherford categories (see Table 3.1).

Table 3.1 Classification of peripheral artery disease (PAD)

Fontaine	Rutherford		
Stage/clinical	Grade	Category	Clinical
I: Asymptomatic	0	0	Asymptomatic
IIa: Mild pain on walking	I	1	Mild claudication
IIb: Moderate to severe pain on walking relatively short distances (intermittent claudication)	I	2	Moderate claudication
	I	3	Severe claudication
III: Ischemic rest pain	II	4	Ischemic rest pain
IV: Ulceration or gangrene	III	5	Minor tissue loss
	III	6	Major tissue loss

Reprinted from Dormandy JA, Rutherford RB (2000). Management of peripheral arterial disease (PAD). TASC Working Group. TransAtlantic Inter-Society Concensus (TASC). *J Vasc Surg* 31:S1.

Risk factors

Traditional risk factors for cardiovascular disease contribute to atherosclerosis of the peripheral circulation. The risk of PAD is increased by cigarette smoking, diabetes mellitus, dyslipidemia, and hypertension (see Table 3.2).

Table 3.2 Risk of peripheral artery disease by risk factor

Risk factor	Odds ratio
Cigarette smoking	2.0–2.7
Diabetes mellitus	1.9–4.0
Hypertension	1.3–2.2
Hypercholesterolemia	1.05–1.1
Fibrinogen	2.2–2.5
C reactive protein	2.1–2.8
Hyperhomocysteinemia	1.7–6.8

Natural history

The 2005 American College of Cardiology/American Heart Association (ACC/AHA) guidelines on PAD estimated the following rates of limb and cardiovascular outcomes at 5 years in patients with noncritical claudication:

- For limb morbidity: stable claudication in 70%–80%, worsening claudication in 10%–20%, and critical limb ischemia in 1%–2% (Fig. 3.1).
- For cardiovascular morbidity and mortality: nonfatal myocardial infarction (MI) or stroke in 20%, and death in 15%–30% (three-quarters due to cardiovascular causes). An association between cardiovascular disease and PAD has been noted in multiple studies and this association cannot be overemphasized.

Among the 1%–2% of patients with critical limb ischemia, the guidelines estimated the following outcomes at 1 year:
- Alive with two limbs: 50%
- Amputation: 25%
- Cardiovascular mortality: 25%

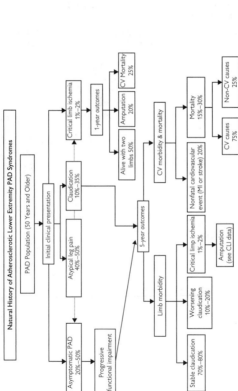

Figure 3.1 The natural history of atherosclerotic lower extremity peripheral arterial disease (PAD). Individuals with atherosclerotic lower extremity PAD may a) be asymptomatic (without identified ischemic leg symptoms, albeit with a functional impairment); b) present with leg symptoms (classic claudication or atypical leg symptoms); or c) present with critical limb ischemia. All individuals with PAD face a risk of progressive limb ischemic symptoms, as well as a high short-term cardiovascular ischemic event rate and increased mortality. These event rates are most clearly defined for individuals with claudication or critical limb ischemia (CLI), and less well defined for individuals with asymptomatic PAD. CV, cardiovascular; MI, myocardial infarction. Adapted from 1) ACC/AHA Practice Guidelines. Hirsch et al. (2006). *Circulation* 113:e463– e465 and 2) Weitz JI, Byrne J, Clagett GP, et al. (1996). *Circulation* 94(11):3026–3049.

Pathophysiology

The balance of circulatory supply of nutrients to skeletal muscle and the oxygen and nutrient demand of skeletal muscle are key features in the pathophysiology of PAD. The symptoms of claudication develop when the oxygen and nutrient supply is less than the demand in skeletal muscle as during exercise. Local sensory receptors are activated by the accumulation of lactate and other metabolites.

Typically, resting blood flow is preserved until critical limb ischemia develops and the resting blood supply diminishes to the point that the nutritional needs of the limb can no longer be met. Ultimately, there is impaired vasodilation, accentuated vasoconstriction, and abnormal rheology, all of which contribute to critical limb ischemia.

While most commonly this is due to atherosclerosis and frequently multiple obstructive lesions exist, there are other causes of claudication, listed in Table 3.3.

Table 3.3 Causes of claudication

Major cause
Atherosclerosis (arteriosclerosis obliterans)
Other causes
Acute arterial disease (dissection, embolism, thrombosis, trauma)
Adventitial cystic disease
Aortic coarctation
Arterial fibrodysplasia
Arterial tumor
Ergot toxicity
Iliac endofibrosis of athletes
Occluded limb aneurysms
Popliteal-artery entrapment
Pseudoxanthoma elasticum
Radiation fibrosis
Retroperitoneal fibrosis
Takayasu's arteritis
Temporal arteritis
Thoracic outlet obstruction
Thromboangiitis obliterans (Buerger's disease)
Vasospasm

Clinical presentation

Symptoms
- Intermittent claudication and rest pain with critical limb ischemia
- Discomfort often with walking or exertion and resolves at rest

The site of pain correlates with the location of stenosis:
- Buttock and hip: aortoiliac disease
- Thigh: common femoral artery or aortoiliac
- Upper two-thirds of the calf: superficial femoral artery
- Lower one-third of the calf: popliteal artery
- Foot claudication: tibial or peroneal artery
- Parasthesias
- Skin sensitivity

On examination
Features may include the following:
- Normal findings
- Diminished or absent pulses
- Poor wound healing
- Bruit
- Shiny skin
- Prolonged venous filling
- Hair loss, skin atrophy, nail changes
- Unilateral cool extremity
- Foot pallor with elevation of the leg and with leg in the dependent position, a dusky red flush spreading proximally from the toes (Buerger test)
- Muscle atrophy
- Ulceration (arterial typically have a pale base and involve the toes, heel of the foot, or pressure sites) (Table 3.4)
- Gangrene

Table 3.4 Differential diagnosis of common foot and leg ulcers

Origin	Cause	Location	Pain	Appearance
Main arteries	Atherosclerotic lower extremity PAD, Buerger's disease, acute arterial occlusion	Toes, foot	Severe	Irregular, pink base
Venous	Venous disease	Malleolar	Mild	Irregular, pink base
Skin infarct	Systemic disease, embolism, hypertension	Lower third of leg	Severe	Small after infarction, often multiple
Neurotrophic	Neuropathy	Foot sole	None	Often deep, infected

Adapted from 1) the ACC/AHA Practice Guidelines. Hirsch et al. (2006). *Circulation* 113:e463–e465, and 2) Differential Diagnosis of Critical Limb Ischemia. *J Vasc Surg* 2000; 31(1) Supplement 1:S184–S188.

Testing for peripheral artery disease

Ankle–brachial index (ABI)

The ABI provides a measure of PAD and is simple and inexpensive to perform (see Fig. 3.2). Calculation is by measuring the systolic blood pressure (by Doppler probe) in the brachial, posterior tibial, and dorsalis pedis arteries. The higher ankle measurement is divided by the higher brachial measurement.

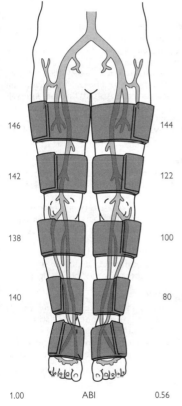

146	144
142	122
138	100
140	80
1.00	ABI 0.56

Figure 3.2 Ankle–brachial indices (ABI).

- ABI 1.0–1.3 is the normal value. Values >1.3 suggest a noncompressible calcified vessel.
- ABI below 0.9 is associated with a >50% stenosis in one or more major vessels and has a 95% sensitivity for detecting angiogram-positive PAD.
- ABI 0.4–0.9 suggests arterial obstruction often associated with claudication.
- ABI <0.4 represents advanced ischemia.

ABIs typically correlate with the clinical measures of lower extremity function such as walking distances, balance, and overall physical activity. Lower ABIs correlate with a higher risk of coronary artery disease (CAD), stroke, progressive renal insufficiency, and all-cause mortality.

Treadmill exercise testing

Exercise decreases vascular resistance and enhances blood flow to exercising extremities. According to Poiseuille's law, the pressure gradient across the stenosis increases in direct proportion to flow.

Exercise in lesions with <70% stenosis may induce a systolic pressure gradient across the stenosis or increase the systolic pressure gradient. This change can be detected by serial post-exercise ABIs at 1-minute intervals for 5 minutes after exercise. This is particularly useful in patients who have normal resting ABIs and typical symptoms of claudication.

In addition, treadmill testing allows for an objective measure of the patient's walking capacity.

Duplex ultrasound imaging

Ultrasound examination of the lower extremity includes localization of stenosis with color Doppler, B-mode imaging, pulse-wave Doppler, and continuous-wave Doppler.

Examinations begin with the common femoral artery and proceed distally to the popliteal artery. A twofold or greater increase in peak systolic velocity at the site of an atherosclerotic plaque indicates a 50% or greater stenosis. Similarly, a threefold increase in velocity indicates a 75% or greater stenosis. In an occluded artery there is no Doppler signal.

When using contrast angiography as a gold standard, duplex ultrasound imaging has a sensitivity of 80%–90% and specificity of 95%. See Figure 3.3.

Magnetic resonance angiography

Magnetic resonance angiography (MRA) can be used to noninvasively image the aorta and vascular territories. The resolution of MRA with gadolinium approaches that of contrast digital subtraction angiography.

In patients at risk for complications from conventional angiography, MRA provides an accurate noninvasive tool prior to planning endovascular or surgical intervention.

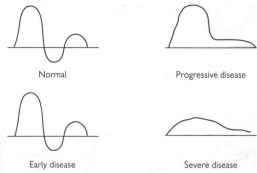

Normal	Progressive disease
Early disease	Severe disease

Figure 3.3 Ultrasonography in peripheral arterial disease. Schematic representation of peripheral arterial waveforms in duplex Doppler ultrasonography in peripheral vascular disease. The normal peripheral arterial velocity waveform is triphasic and consists of a forward flow systolic peak, reversal of flow in early diastole, and forward flow in late diastole (top left). With progressive peripheral vascular disease, there is elimination of the reverse flow (top right), a decrease in systolic peak and an increase in flow in diastole (bottom right). Reproduced with permission from Mohler III, ER (2009). Noninvasive diagnosis of peripheral arterial disease. In Basow DS (Ed.), *UpToDate*, Waltham, MA. Copyright © 2009 UpToDate, Inc. For more information visit www.uptodate.com.

Computed tomographic angiography (CTA)

Multidetector CT scanners allow for rapid acquisition of high-resolution images. The addition of IV contrast allows visualization of the aorta and peripheral arteries.

Multidetector technology has improved the spatial resolution of images over a relatively short period of time. In addition, evolving software applications enable three-dimensional display and post-processing techniques that can aid in visualization of stenoses.

Contrast angiography

This remains the gold standard in evaluation of peripheral vascular disease. Digital subtraction techniques following contrast administration are typically used to enhance resolution.

While the femoral approach is most common, brachial, axillary, or translumbar approaches can be used to attain aortic access.

Summaries of diagnosis of PAD, asymptomatic PAD and leg pain, and claudication are given in Figures 3.4, 3.5, and 3.6.

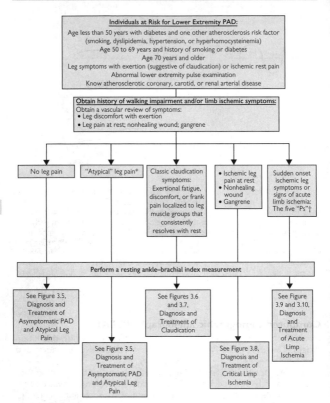

Figure 3.4 Steps toward the diagnosis of peripheral arterial disease (PAD).
*"Atypical" leg pain is defined by lower extremity discomfort that is exertional but that does not consistently resolve with rest, consistently limit exercise at a reproducible distance, or meet all "Rose questionnaire" criteria.
†The five "Ps" are defined by the clinical symptoms and signs that suggest potential limb jeopardy: pain, pulselessness, pallor, parasthesias, and paralysis (with polar being a sixth "P").
Reprinted with permission from the ACC/AHA Practice Guidelines. Hirsch et al. (2006). *Circulation* 113:e463–e465.

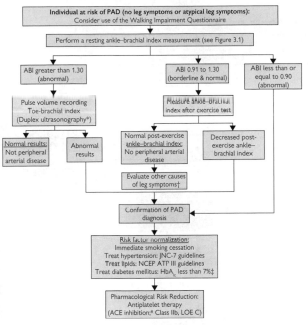

Figure 3.5 Diagnosis and treatment of asymptomatic peripheral arterial disease (PAD) and atypical leg pain.

*Duplex ultrasonography should generally be reserved for use in symptomatic patients in whom anatomic diagnostic data are required for care.

† Other causes of leg pain may include lumbar disk disease, sciatica, radiculopathy, muscle strain, neuropathy, and compartment syndrome.

‡ It is not yet proven that treatment of diabetes mellitus will significantly reduce PAD-specific (limb ischemic) end points. Primary treatment of diabetes mellitus should be continued according to established guidelines.

The benefit of angiotensin-converting enzyme (ACE) inhibition in individuals without claudication has not been specifically documented in prospective clinical trials but has been extrapolated from other at-risk populations.

ABI, ankle–brachial index; HbA1C, hemoglobin A1C; JNC-7, Seventh Report of the Joint National Committee on Prevention, Detection, Evaluation, and Treatment of High Blood Pressure; LOE, level of evidence; NCEP ATP III, National Cholesterol Education Program Adult Treatment Panel III.

Adapted from 1) Hiatt WR (2001). *N Engl J Med* 344:1608–1621 and 2) ACC/AHA Practice Guidelines. Hirsch et al. (2006). *Circulation* 113:e463–e465.

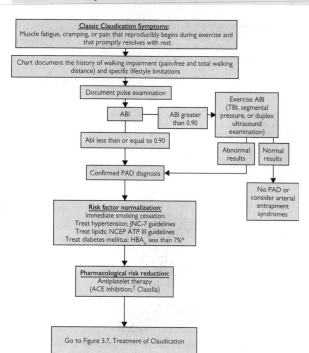

Figure 3.6 Diagnosis of claudication and systemic risk treatment.
* It is not yet proven that treatment of diabetes mellitus will significantly reduce peripheral arterial disease (PAD)-specific (limb ischemic) end points. Primary treatment of diabetes mellitus should be continued according to established guidelines.
† The benefit of angiotensin-converting enzyme (ACE) inhibition in individuals without claudication has not been specifically documented in prospective clinical trials but has been extrapolated from other "at-risk" populations.
ABI, ankle–brachial index; HbA1C, hemoglobin A1C; JNC-7, Seventh Report of the Joint National Committee on the Prevention, Detection, Evaluation, and Treatment of High Blood Pressure; LOE, level of evidence; NCEP ATP III, National Cholesterol Education Program Adult Treatment Panel III.
Reprinted with permission from the ACC/AHA Practice Guidelines. Hirsch et al. (2006). *Circulation* 113:e463–e465.

Prognosis in peripheral artery disease

Many studies have shown an increased cardiovascular risk in patients with PAD, in addition to a risk of limb loss and decreased quality of life. Patients with abnormal ABIs are two to three times more likely to have had a history of MI, angina, heart failure, and/or cerebrovascular accident (CVA).

From 60% to 80% of patients with PAD have angiographically significant CAD. Nearly 25% of patients with critical limb disease die within a year. In patients who have undergone amputation, the mortality may be as high as 45% at 1 year, and 25% of patients complaining of claudication develop worsening symptoms.

Mobility loss occurs more frequently in patients with PAD. Critical limb ischemia develops in nearly 8% of patients with claudication in the first year after diagnosis and at a rate of 2.2% annually thereafter. Both smoking and diabetes independently predict disease progression.

Treatment

The treatment goals for PAD include reduction in cardiovascular morbidity and mortality with aggressive risk factor modification, pharmacological and revascularization therapies, and improvement in quality of life by decreasing the symptoms of claudication (Figs. 3.7 and 3.8).

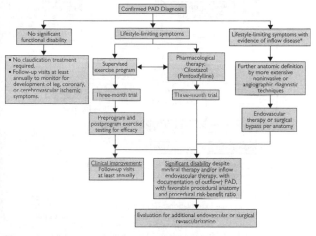

Figure 3.7 Treatment of claudication.
*Inflow disease should be suspected in individuals with gluteal or thigh claudication and femoral pulse diminution or bruit and should be confirmed by noninvasive vascular laboratory diagnostic evidence of aortoiliac stenoses.
†Outflow disease represents femoropopliteal and infrapopliteal stenoses (the presence of occlusive lesions in the lower extremity arterial tree below the inguinal ligament from the common femoral artery to the pedal vessels).
Reprinted with permission from the ACC/AHA Practice Guidelines. Hirsch et al. (2006). *Circulation* 113:e463–e465.

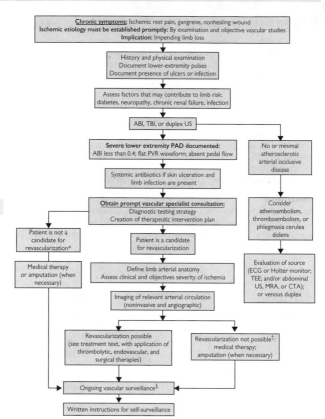

Figure 3.8 Diagnosis and treatment of critical limb ischemia.

*Based on patient comorbidities.

† Based on anatomy or lack of conduit.

‡ *Risk factor normalization*: immediate smoking cessation, treat hypertension per the Seventh Report of the Joint National Committee on Prevention, Detection, Evaluation, and Treatment of High Blood Pressure guidelines; treat lipids per National Cholesterol Education Program Adult Treatment Panel III guidelines; treat diabetes mellitus (HbA1C [hemoglobin A1C] less than 7%; Class IIa). It is not yet proven that treatment of diabetes mellitus will significantly reduce PAD-specific (limb ischemic) end points. Primary treatment of diabetes mellitus should be continued according to established guidelines.

ABI, ankle–brachial index; CTA, computed tomographic angiography; ECG, electro-cardiogram; MRA, magnetic resonance angiography; PVR, pulse volume recording; TBI, toe–brachial index; TEE, transesophageal echocardiography; US, ultrasound. Reprinted with permission from the ACC/AHA Practice Guidelines. Hirsch et al. (2006). *Circulation* 113:e463–e465.

Risk factor modification

Similar to CAD, studies have shown the importance of risk factor modification to the reduction of cardiovascular mortality and morbidity associated with PAD. In particular, robust statin data suggest a reduction in cardiovascular event rates with therapy included in patients with PAD.

Similarly, smoking cessation is imperative. Not only do survival rates increase in patients with PAD who do not smoke, but smoking cessation reduces the rate of critical limb ischemia.

While aggressive diabetes control reduces the risk of microvascular events, there are limited data to support benefit in regard to macrovascular complications.

Antihypertensive therapy reduces the risk of cardiovascular events. Blood pressure should treated according to the current guidelines, which suggest a target of <140/90 for patients with PAD and <130/80 in patients with diabetes.

Antiplatelet therapy

Antiplatelet therapy has been shown in a large meta-analysis to yield a 22% odds reduction for vascular death, MI, or stroke. In the CHARISMA trial, dual antiplatelet therapy with aspirin and clopidogrel was compared to aspirin alone in patients with known CAD, CVA, or PAD as well as patients with CAD risk factors. Dual antiplatelet therapy provided no significant benefit over aspirin alone on the primary composite end point of MI, stroke, or cardiovascular death.

Current guidelines recommend patients with PAD be treated with either acetylsalicylic acid (ASA) or Plavix. Anticoagulation with warfarin is not recommended as it is not more effective than antiplatelet therapy and has more bleeding complications.

Pharmacotherapy

Vasodilator therapy has not demonstrated efficacy in the treatment of PAD. Physiologically this may be explained by a relative steal phenomenon that can develop with dilation of proximal vascular beds with vasodilator use, which reduces resistance, blood flow, and perfusion pressure. Distal to the stenosis there would be minimal effect, as these vascular beds would be endogenously dilated. In addition, in skeletal muscle vasodilators do not reduce oxygen demand.

Pentoxyphilline and cilostazol are drugs approved by the U.S. Food and Drug Administration (FDA) for use in patients with claudication. Pentoxyphilline, a xanthine derivative, is thought to decrease blood viscosity and improve erythrocyte flexibility. It may also have anti-inflammatory and antiproliferative effects. In two meta-analyses, pentoxyphilline was shown to increase absolute claudication distance by 45–50 meters compared with placebo.

Cilostazol is a quinilone derivative and acts as a phosphodiesterase III inhibitor. It therefore decreases cyclic adenosine monophosphate degradation, which increases its concentration in platelets and blood vessels. Several trials have reported an increase in absolute claudication distance by 40%–50% compared with placebo. A comparison study of placebo, pentoxyphilline, and cilostazol showed that cilostazol had the most improvement in absolute walking distances while the former two were equivalent.

Other drugs have been studied in the treatment of claudication and include statins, angiotensin-converting enzyme (ACE) inhibitors, serotonin antagonists, calcium channel blockers, L-arginine, vasodilator prostaglandins, and angiogenic growth factors, to name a few. A recent study showed ramipril improved maximal claudication time. Preliminary trials of serotonin antagonists and L-arginine have not been effective in improving walking distances. Similarly, preliminary trials of vasodilator prostaglandins and angiogenic growth factors have been disappointing.

Exercise rehabilitation

A supervised exercise rehabilitation program improves symptoms in patients with PAD. Meta-analyses have shown significant improvement, with up to 150% increase in walking distance with regular 30-minute sessions at least several times a week for 6 months.

It is thought that formation of collateral vessels, improved endothelium-dependent vasodilation, hemorheology, and muscle metabolism are possible mechanisms for this improvement.

Percutaneous transluminal angioplasty and stents

In patients with lifestyle-limiting claudication, peripheral catheter-based interventions are indicated if a trial of exercise rehabilitation and pharmacotherapy has failed. Percutaneous intervention should also be considered when patients have inflow disease with symptoms of thigh or buttock claudication or diminished femoral artery pulses.

Procedural patency rates and durability of the procedure are related to lesion morphology and patient characteristics. Shorter vs. longer, larger arteries vs. smaller, and single vs. multiple occlusions have better patency rates.

Peripheral arterial surgery

Aortobifemoral bypass is the most frequent operation for patients with aortoiliac disease. A knitted or woven prothesis made of Dacron or polytetrafluoroethylene (PTFE) is anastamosed proximally from the distal aorta to each common femoral artery distally.

The surgical operation planned must take into account both inflow and outflow in order to maintain graft patency. Similar to percutaneous procedures, the location of obstruction along with patient clinical factors contribute to surgical success.

In some high-risk patients with critical limb ischemia, extra-anatomic reconstructive procedures are performed in which the aortoiliac circulation is circumvented and instead, axillobifemoral bypass, iliobifemoral bypass, and femoral femoral bypass are performed. Long-term patency rates are lower for these grafts. Five-year patency rates range from 50 to 70% for the axillobifemoral bypass. The operative mortality for extra-anatomic surgical procedures is 3%–5%.

Femoral popliteal, femoral tibial, and femoral peroneal artery bypass are potential reconstructive surgeries for infrainguinal arterial disease. Grafts made of PFTE or in situ or reversed saphenous vein are used for the infrainguinal reconstructive surgery. Patency rates are better for autologous saphenous vein grafts than for synthetic grafts and better for above-than for below-knee popliteal anastamosis.

In patients with claudication, 5-year patency for femoral popliteal reconstruction is 75%–80%, while in patients with critical limb ischemia the patency is 45%–60% for synthetic vs. autologous vein grafts, respectively. The 5-year patency for synthetic grafts in the infrapopliteal location is 65% in patients with claudication and 33% in patients with critical limb ischemia.

Graft stenoses can result from technical errors made during surgery, such as retained valve cuffs, intimal flap, or valvotome injury. Fibrous intimal hyperplasia can result usually within 6 months from surgery. Finally, atherosclerosis can develop. This usually results 1–2 years from surgery.

Graft surveillance programs in which color duplex ultrasonography is performed at regular intervals have enabled the early evaluation of graft stenosis. This allows for early graft revision and avoids graft failure. Antiplatelet and Coumarin datives also increase graft patency rates.

Acute limb ischemia

Acute limb ischemia develops when there is sudden reduction in arterial blood flow that jeopardizes limb viability. On physical exam, the symptoms and signs can be remembered by the five Ps: pain, pulselessness, pallor, parethesias, and paralysis.

The 5-year survival rate after acute limb ischemia caused by thrombosis is close to 45% and less than 20% after embolism. The risk of limb loss depends on the time elapsed before revascularization and the severity of ischemia.

The causes of limb ischemia include arterial embolism, thrombosis in situ, dissection, and trauma. The history and physical exam typically establish the diagnosis (see Fig. 3.9).

Treatment includes analgesic medications for pain, lowering the foot of the bed to increase blood flow by gravitational effects, sheep skin to reduce pressure on the heels, and warm room temperature to reduce cutaneous vasoconstriction (see Fig. 3.10). IV heparin should be administered as soon as the diagnosis is made.

If symptoms persist or viability of the limb is threatened, revascularization is indicated. Intra-arterial thrombolytic therapy, percutaneous mechanical thrombectomy, and surgical revascularization are options for restoring blood flow.

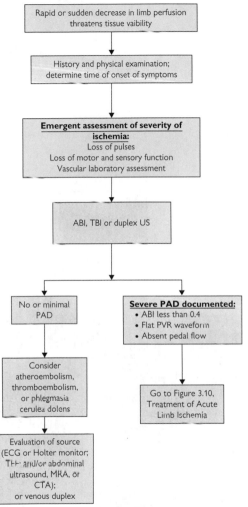

Figure 3.9 Diagnosis of acute limb ischemia. ABI, ankle–brachial index; CTA, computed tomographic angiography; ECG, electrocardiogram; MRA, magnetic resonance angiography; PVR, pulse volume recording; TBI, toe–brachial index; TEE, transesophageal echocardiography; US, ultrasound. Adapted from 1) the ACC/AHA Practice Guidelines. Hirsch et al. (2006). *Circulation* 113:e463–e465 and 2) Rutherford RB, Baker JD, Ernst C, et al. (1997). *J Vasc Surg* 26(3):517–538.

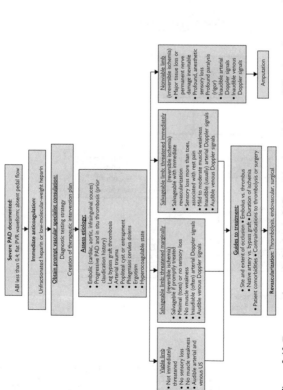

Figure 3.10 Treatment of acute limb ischemia. PAD, peripheral arterial disease; PVR, pulse volume recording; US, ultrasonography. Adapted from 1) the ACC/AHA Practice Guidelines. Hirsch et al. (2006). *Circulation* 113:e463–e465 and 2) Rutherford RB, Baker JD, Ernst C, et al. (1997). *J Vasc Surg* 26(3):517–538.

Severe PAD documented:
ABI less than 0.4; flat PVR waveform; absent pedal flow

Immediate anticoagulation:
Unfractionated heparin or low-molecular-weight heparin

Obtain prompt vascular specialist consultation:
Diagnostic testing strategy
Creation of therapeutic intervention plan

Assess etiology:
• Embolic (cardiac, aortic, infrainguinal souces)
• Progressive PAD and in situ thrombosis (prior claudication history)
• Leg bypass graft thrombosis
• Arterial trauma
• Popliteal cyst or entrapment
• Phlegmasia cerulea dolens
• Ergotism
• Hypercoagulable state

Viable limb
• Not immediately threatened
• No sensory loss
• No muscle weakness
• Audible arterial and venous US

Salvageable limb: threatened marginally
(reversible ischemia)
• Salvageable if promptly treated
• Minimal (toes) or no sensory loss
• No muscle weakness
• Inaudible (often) arterial Doppler signals
• Audible venous Doppler signals

Salvageable limb: threatened immediately
(reversible ischemia)
• Salvageable with immediate revascularization
• Sensory loss more than toes, associated with rest pain
• Mild to moderate muscle weakness
• Inaudible (usually) arterial Doppler signals
• Audible venous Doppler signals

Nonviable limb
(irreversible ischemia)
• Major tissue loss or permanent nerve damage inevitable
• Profound, anesthetic sensory loss
• Profound paralysis (rigor)
• Inaudible arterial Doppler signals
• Inaudible venous Doppler signals

Guides to treatment:
• Site and extent of occlusion • Embolus vs. thrombus
• Native artery vs. bypass graft • Duration of ischemia
• Patient comorbidities • Contraindications to thrombolysis or surgery

Revascularization: Thrombolysis, endovascular, surgical

Amputation

Cerebrovascular disease

Stroke is the leading cause of disability in the United States. Carotid artery disease is common in patients with coronary artery disease. Each year there are approximately 750,000 strokes and 150,000 deaths related to cerebrovascular disease.

An asymptomatic carotid bruit is present in 13% of the population and incidence increases with age. Transient ischemic attacks are defined as a focal loss of function related to cerebral ischemia lasting less than 24 hours and localized to a limited area of the brain, whereas stroke is a permanent neurological deficit. Causes of stroke are listed in Table 3.5.

Duplex sonography is an important tool in diagnosing carotid artery stenosis and is able to provide both hemodynamic and anatomic information. MRA can also be used to accurately diagnose extra- and intracranial arterial disease. It is indicated for patients with symptomatic carotid artery disease to further characterize cerebral anatomy. Standard angiography can also be performed and is associated with a 1% risk of stroke.

Carotid endarterectomy has been shown to be superior to medical therapy in patients with symptomatic carotid disease and a high-grade stenosis. In patients with mild carotid artery disease, medical therapy is preferred; treatment for those with moderate disease remains controversial.

The Asymptomatic Carotid Atherosclerosis Study (ACAS) demonstrated that carotid endarterectomy is superior to medical therapy in people with asymptomatic carotid stenosis >60%, with a combined perioperative mortality <3%. In patients with symptomatic carotid stenosis <60%, the current medical management includes anticoagulation for 3 months, followed by antiplatelet therapy (ASA or Plavix) indefinitely.

Carotid artery stenting has gained acceptance in patients whose operative mortality is elevated. In high-risk patients, surgical mortality may be as high as 18%. Using a standard percutaneous approach, the carotid artery can be stented.

The SAPPHIRE trial is the only published randomized trial that has compared carotid endarterectomy with carotid artery stenting. Patients had at least one high-risk surgical feature and were included with symptomatic carotid stenosis of >50% or asymptomatic carotid stenosis of >80%. While the primary end point was complex, the carotid-stent arm of the trial had significantly less composite stroke, MI, and death within 30 days.

An ongoing trial of carotid revascularization endarterectomy vs. stent trial (CREST) is reviewing both treatment strategies in 1400 patients with a goal of 4-year follow-up.

Table 3.5 Causes of stroke

Intracardiac thrombus
Intracardiac mass lesions
Valvular heart disease
Infectious endocarditis
Paradoxic emboli
Large vessel occlusive disease
Small-vessel disease (hypertension, DM, arteritis)
Carotid atherosclerosis
Polycythemia vera
Thrombocytosis
Antiphospholipid antibody syndrome
Cryoglobulinemia
Air and fat emboli
Cortical vein thrombosis

Renovascular disease

Obstructive renovascular disease can be caused by atherosclerosis or fibromuscular dysplasia (FMD). Renal FMD tends to occur in younger patients. There is a female preponderance.

FMD typically involves the secondary or distal branches. Renal artery revascularization with surgery or percutaneous angioplasty techniques can be curative of hypertension.

While the true prevalence of atherosclerotic renal artery disease is not known, in patients identified as having atherosclerosis in other vascular beds the prevalence is between 10% and 30%. The true natural history of renal atherosclerotic disease, outcomes after revascularization, and appropriate populations for intervention still require clarification.

Clinical signs include known atherosclerosis in alternate vascular beds, onset of hypertension (HTN) prior to age 30 (FMD) or after age 55, worsening of previously controlled HTN, malignant or resistant hypertension, abdominal or flank bruit, discrepancy in renal size, unexplained azotemia or renal function worsened by ACE inhibitors or angiotensin II receptor blockers (ARBs), and recurrent heart failure or flash pulmonary edema in a hypertensive patient with preserved LV function.

Diagnostic testing

MRA, CTA, and duplex Doppler ultrasonography can be used in the diagnosis of renal artery stenosis (RAS) (see Fig. 3.11). Captopril renal scintigraphy, selective renal vein renin measurements, and plasma renin activity are not useful screening tests for RAS.

Both MRA and CTA have lower diagnostic accuracy, with sensitivity in 20%–30% range, for lesions caused by FMD. This is likely secondary to their anatomic location.

Magnetic resonance angiography

Multiple series have shown the high diagnostic accuracy of MRA and increasingly this is becoming the first-line diagnostic test. Because of links to administration of gadolinium in patients with moderate to severe renal disease to nephrogenic systemic fibrosis, MRA is not recommended in patients with a glomerular filtration rate (GFR) <30.

CT angiography

Spiral CT with administration of contrast allows for highly accurate non-invasive imaging of renal arteries. Sensitivity and specificity are roughly in the high 70% and mid 90% range, respectively.

Duplex Doppler ultrasonography

This allows for both functional and anatomic assessment of RAS. Direct visualization is combined with Doppler measurements for hemodynamic assessment. The sensitivity and specificity are 85% and 92%, respectively.

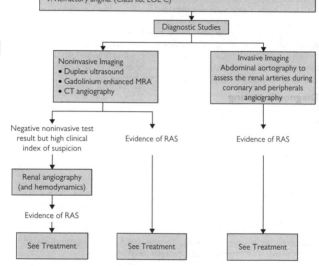

Figure 3.11 Clinical clues to the diagnosis of renal artery stenosis (RAS).
* For definition of hypertension, please see Chobanian AV, Bakris GL, Black HR, et al. (2003). The Seventh Report of the Joint National Committee on Prevention, Detection, Evaluation, and Treatment of High Blood Pressure: the JNC-7 report. *JAMA* 289:2560–2572.
† For example, atrophic kidney due to chronic pyelonephritis is not an indication for RAS evaluation.
ACE, angiotensin-converting enzyme; ARB, angiotensin receptor blocking agent; CT, computed tomography; LOE, level of evidence; MRA, magnetic resonance angiography.
Reprinted with permission from the ACC/AHA Practice Guidelines. Hirsch et al. (2006). *Circulation* 113:e463–e465.

Revascularization

Angiographic lesions >75% in one or both renal arteries suggest reno-vascular disease. It is important to remember that such findings may be present in patients with or without hypertension who have other vascular disease.

The clinical history is particularly important in helping to select patients who are appropriate for percutaneous revascularization (Fig. 3.12). By repeat duplex sonography, while RAS lesion severity may increase over time in most patients, the progression to renal failure is uncommon.

The decision to revascularize an RAS is based on the assumption that clinical benefit will be derived from the intervention. The evaluation of resistive index (1-end diastolic velocity divided by peak systolic velocity) prior to angioplasty may predict which patients will have a successful revascularization procedure. A higher resistive index, >8, may indicate irreversible intrarenal vascular arteriosclerosis.

The procedure is performed from a femoral approach and technical success varies based on the location of the lesion.

In general, results are much better with FMD, with <15% procedural failure and infrequent restenosis rate. In atherosclerotic disease, the failure rate approximates 20%–30% and the restenosis rate is between 8% and 30%. The efficacy of angioplasty improves by insertion of a stent.

While clinical trials are limited, anecdotal experience suggests that drug-eluting stents may significantly reduce restenosis rates. The current ACC/AHA guidelines recommend stenting for ostial atherosclerotic lesions in patients who meet clinical criteria. However, for FMD the guidelines rec-ommend balloon angioplasty with bailout stent placement, if necessary.

The procedural complication rate is between 5% and 15%. Complications include puncture site hematoma, renal artery dissection, renal artery thrombosis or perforation, and acute renal failure from atheroembolism or contrast-induced nephropathy. Distal embolic protection devices have been advocated to help to reduce the complications of atheroembolism.

Surgical revascularization is recommended by ACC/AHA guidelines for patients who have indications for revasculrization, have small renal arteries, or require aortic reconstruction near the renal arteries for other indications. While surgery is generally more effective in treating athero-sclerotic renovascular disease, the mortality rate may be as high as 5%–8% in older patients.

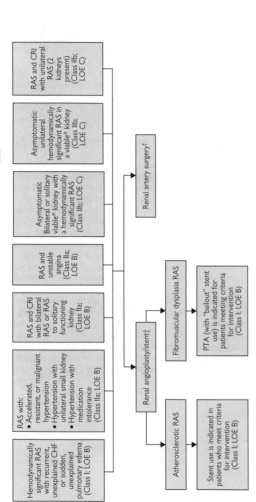

Figure 3.12 Indications for renal revascularization.

* "Viable" means kidney linear length >7 cm.

† It is recognized that renal artery surgery has proven efficacy in alleviating renal artery stenosis (RAS) due to atherosclerosis and fibromuscular dysplasia. Currently, however, its role is often reserved for individuals in whom less invasive percutaneous RAS interventions are not feasible. CHF, congestive heart failure; CRI, chronic renal insufficiency; LOE, level of evidence; PTA, percutaneous transluminal angioplasty. Reprinted with permission from the ACC/AHA Practice Guidelines. Hirsch et al. (2006). *Circulation* 113:e463–e465.

Aortic disease

Aortic atheroembolism

This represents an important cause of micro- and macroemboli in both the cerebral and systemic circulation. Cerebral embolism suggests the source of embolism is intracardiac or within the ascending/transverse aorta, whereas peripheral embolism is most commonly caused by abdominal aortic aneurysm or diffuse atherosclerotic disease.

Clinical features include livedo reticularis, blue toes, palpable pulses, hypertension, renal insufficiency, elevated erythrocyte sedimentation rate, and eosinophilia.

Thoracic aortic atherosclerotic plaque is most accurately assessed by TEE. Plaque thickness >4 mm or mobile plaque of any size is associated with an increased risk of embolization.

Treatment includes the use of antiplatelet medications and statin therapy, as well as identification and, if possible, surgical resection of the source of embolism.

Thoracic aortic aneurysm (TAA)

TAAs are most commonly caused by atherosclerosis. They can also occur with systemic hypertension, Marfan syndrome, bicuspid aortic valve, giant cell arteritis, Takayasu disease, infections (syphilis), and trauma.

Most TAAs are asymptomatic and discovered incidentally and can be diagnosed noninvasively with CT, MRI, and TEE.

Surgical resection should be considered if symptoms attributable to the aneursym are present, if the aneursym is rapidly enlarging, if pseudoaneurysm is present, if there is a post-traumatic aneurysm, and if the aneursym size is >6 cm in low-risk patients and 4.5 cm or greater in Marfan patients.

Abdominal aortic aneursym (AAA)

In high-risk patients, screening tests are recommended because the physical exam lacks sensitivity. A single screening abdominal ultrasound over the age of 65 can diagnose the majority of AAAs. The United States Prevention Services Task force recommends a one-time screening ultrasound in men ages 65–75 who have ever smoked.

In siblings and first-degree relatives of patients with AAA, screening typically begins at age 50.

- Elective surgical repair is indicated when the aneurysm diameter is between 5.5 and 6.0 cm in good-risk patients (Fig. 3.13).
- Surgery is also recommended for AAAs that are symptomatic, traumatic, or infectious in origin or are expanding >0.5 cm/year.
- In high-risk patients, surgical therapy is individualized. In those patients, endovascular approach with a stent-anchored Dacron prosthetic graft provides an alternate therapeutic option (Fig. 3.14).

All patients with endovascular repair will need continued lifelong tomographic imaging.

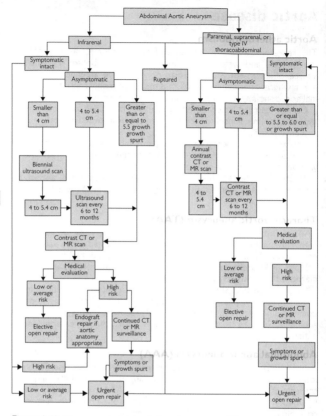

Figure 3.13 Management of abdominal aortic aneuryms. CT, computed tomography; MR, magnetic resonance imaging. Reprinted with permission from the ACC/AHA Practice Guidelines. Hirsch et al. (2006). *Circulation* 113:e463–e465.

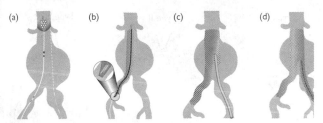

Figure 3.14 Diagram of deployment of an aortic stent graft. a) The catheter placement and proximal stabilization are achieved via right femoral access. b) The body and right limb of the stent graft are positioned and deployed. c) The cannula for deployment of the left limb of the graft is placed via left femoral access. d) The left limb of the graft is deployed, completing the endovascular repair of the aortic aneurysm with left iliac involvement. This figure was published in Libby et al., *Braunwald's Heart Disease*, 8th ed., p. 1462, Copyright Elsevier 2007.

Aortic dissection

The most common predisposing factors for dissection include advanced age, male gender, hypertension, Marfan syndrome, and bicuspid/unicuspid aortic valve. Iatrogenic aortic dissection can occur with surgical and invasive angiographic procedures (Fig. 3.15).

Clinical features include severe pain in the anterior chest, back, or abdomen; hypertension; aortic diastolic murmur; pulse deficits or blood pressure differential; and neurological changes.

Syncope can occur when there is extension of the dissection into the pericardial sac with resulting cardiac tamponade. Congestive heart failure occurs from severe aortic regurgitation. CXR may reveal widened mediastinum, discrepancy in the sizes of ascending vs. descending aorta, and deviation of the trachea to the right.

Definitive diagnosis can be made with prompt imaging, including echocardiography, CT, MRI, and aortography. In a patient with acute suspected aortic dissection, test selection should depend on the most readily available test at your institution.

Type I and II dissections should have emergent surgery. Medical therapy includes IV antihypertensive medications to decrease mean arterial pressure.

Penetrating aortic ulcer

This occurs when atherosclerotic plaque undergoes ulceration and penetrates the internal elastic lamina. It can result in several consequences: formation of an intramural hematoma, formation of saccular aneursym, formation of pseudoaneurysm, or transmural rupture.

The clinical features are similar to those of aortic dissection; however, pulse deficits, neurological signs, and acute cardiac disease are not seen with penetrating aortic ulcer.

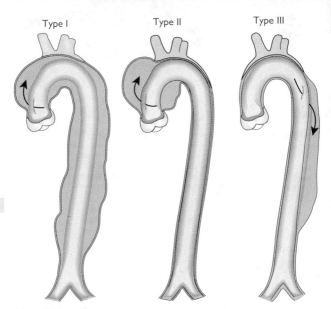

Figure 3.15 Commonly used classification systems for aortic dissection. This figure was published in Libby et al., *Braunwald's Heart Disease*, 8th ed., p. 1470. Copyright Elsevier 2007.

The diagnosis can be made with CT, MRI, TEE, or aortography. The treatment is nonoperative only if a intramural hematoma is present, whereas surgical treatment is recommended for patients with ascending aorta involvement, saccular aneursym, or pseudoaneursym, or for patients with intramural hematoma with persisting symptoms, increasing aortic diameter, or poorly controlled hypertension.

Incomplete aortic rupture

This results from deceleration injuries and typically involves the thoracic aorta at the isthmus.

While this is seen most frequently in patients who have been in a motor vehicle accident, it should be considered in any patient where there is evidence of chest wall trauma, decreased or absent leg pulses, left-sided hemothorax, or widening of the superior mediastinum on CXR.

The diagnosis can be confirmed by TEE, CT, MRI, or angiography. Treatment is emergent surgical repair.

Type A Endovascular treatment of choice

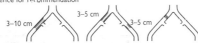

Type B Currently, endovascular treatment is more often used but insufficient evidence for recommendation

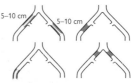

Type C Currently surgical treatment is more often used but insufficient evidence for recommendation

Type D Surgical treatment of choice

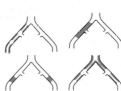

Figure 3.16 Summary of preferred options in interventional management of iliac lesions.
Reprinted with permission from Dormandy JA, Rutherford RB. TASC Working Group (2000). Endovascular procedures for intermittent claudication. *J Vasc Surg* 31(1) Supplement 1:S97–S113.

Noninvasive and invasive vascular diagnostic tools

Noninvasive and invasive vascular diagnostic tools: benefits and limitations

Diagnostic tool*	Benefits	Limitations
Ankle–brachial indices (ABIs)	A quick and cost-effective way to establish or refute the lower extremity PAD diagnosis (see text)	May not be accurate when systolic blood pressure cannot be abolished by inflation of an air-filled blood pressure cuff (non-compressible pedal arteries), as occurs in a small fraction of diabetic or very elderly individuals
Toe–brachial indices	A quick and cost-effective way to establish or refute the lower extremity PAD diagnosis (see text)	Requires small cuffs and careful technique to preserve accuracy
	Can measure digital perfusion when small-vessel arterial occlusive disease is present	
	Useful in individuals with noncompressible posterior tibial or dorsalis pedis arteries	
Segmental pressure examination	Useful to establish or refute the PAD diagnosis (see text)	May not be accurate when systolic blood pressure cannot be measured by inflation of an air-filled blood pressure cuff owing to noncompressible pedal arteries, as occurs in a small fraction of diabetic or very elderly individuals
	Useful to provide anatomic localization of lower extremity PAD when data are required to create a therapeutic plan	
	Can provide data to predict limb survival, wound healing, and patient survival	
	Useful to monitor the efficacy of therapeutic interventions	
Pulse volume recording	Useful to establish diagnosis of PAD in vascular laboratories or office practice	Usefulness maintained in patients with noncompressible vessels (ABI value >1.3)
	Helpful in predicting outcome in CLI and risk of amputation	Qualitative, not quantitative, measure of perfusion
	Can be used to monitor limb perfusion after revascularization procedures	May not be accurate in more distal segments
		Less accurate than other non-invasive tests in providing arterial anatomic localization of PAD
		May be abnormal in patients with low cardiac stroke volume

Diagnostic tool*	Benefits	Limitations
Continuous-wave Doppler ultrasound	Useful to assess lower extremity PAD anatomy, severity, and progression Can provide localizing information in patients with poorly compressible arteries Can provide quantitative data after successful lower extremity revascularization	"Pulse normalization" downstream from stenoses can diminish test sensitivity Test specificity greater for patent superficial femoral arteries than for aortoiliac occlusive disease Does not provide visualization of arterial anatomy Limited accuracy in tortuous, overlapping, or densely calcified arterial segments, and insensitive for iliac arteries (in context of obesity, bowel gas, and vessel tortuosity)
Duplex ultrasound	Can establish the lower extremity PAD diagnosis, establish anatomic localization, and define severity of focal lower extremity arterial stenoses Can be useful to select candidates for endovascular or surgical revascularization	Useful tool to provide graft surveillance after femoral-popliteal or femoral tibial or pedal surgical bypass with venous (but not prosthetic) conduit Accuracy is diminished in proximal aortoiliac arterial segments in some individuals (e.g., due to obesity or presence of bowel gas) Dense arterial calcification can limit diagnostic accuracy Sensitivity is diminished for detection of stenoses downstream from a proximal stenosis
Toe-tip exercise testing, with pre-exercise and post-exercise ABIs	Useful to diagnose lower extremity PAD when resting ABI values are normal Can be performed without a treadmill, with increased convenience and low cost	Diminished predictive value in surveillance of prosthetic bypass grafts Provides qualitative (rather than quantitative) exercise diagnostic results Lower workload may not elicit symptoms in all individuals with claudication
Treadmill exercise testing, with and without pre-exercise and postexercise ABIs	Helps differentiate claudication from pseudoclaudication in individuals with exertional leg symptoms Useful to diagnose lower extremity PAD when resting ABI values are normal	Requires use of a motorized treadmill, with or without continuous ECG monitoring, as well as staff familiar with exercise testing protocols

Diagnostic tool*	Benefits	Limitations
	Objectively documents magnitude of symptom limitation in patients with claudication, especially when used with a standardized treadmill protocol	
	Demonstrates safety of exercise and provides data to individualize exercise prescriptions in individuals with claudication before initiation of a formal program of therapeutic exercise training	
	Useful to measure objective functional response to claudication therapeutic interventions	
Magnetic resonance angiography (MRA)	Useful to assess PAD anatomy and presence of significant stenoses	Tends to overestimate degree of stenosis·
	Useful to select patients who are candidates for endovascular or surgical revascularization	May be inaccurate in arteries treated with metal stents
		Cannot be used in patients with contraindications to the magnetic resonance technique (e.g., pacemakers, defibrillators, intracranial metallic stents, clips, coils, and other devices)
Computed tomographic angiography (CTA)	Useful to assess PAD anatomy and presence of significant stenoses	Single-detector computed tomography lacks accuracy for detection of stenosis
	Useful to select patients who are candidates for endovascular or surgical revascularization	Spatial resolution lower than that of digital subtraction angiography
	Helpful to provide associated soft tissue diagnostic information that may be associated with PAD presentation (e.g., aneurysms, popliteal entrapment, and cystic adventitial disease)	Venous opacification can obscure arterial filling
		Asymmetrical opacification of the legs may obscure arterial phase in some vessels
	Patients with contraindications to MRA (e.g., pacemakers or defibrillators) may be safely imaged	Accuracy and effectiveness are not as well determined as with MRA
		Treatment plans based on CTA have not been compared with those of catheter angiography
		Requires iodinated contrast and ionizing radiation (although radiation exposure is less than with catheter angiography)

Diagnostic tool*	Benefits	Limitations
	Metal clips, stents, and metallic prostheses do not cause significant CTA artifacts	Because CTA requires administration of iodinated contrast, use is limited in individuals with established renal dysfunction
	Scan times are significantly faster than for MRA	
Contrast angiography	Definitive method for anatomic evaluation of PAD when revascularization is planned	Invasive evaluation is associated with risk of bleeding, infection, vascular access complications (e.g., dissection or hematoma), athero-embolization, contrast allergy, and contrast nephropathy
		May provide limited visualization of tibial-pedal vessels in patients with CLI and poor inflow to the leg
		Below-knee vessels may be difficult to identify by digital subtraction angiography
		Multiple projections may be necessary to visualize eccentric lesions

*Tools are listed in order from least invasive to most invasive and from least to most costly.

CLI, critical limb ischemia; PAD, peripheral arterial disease.

Reprinted with permission from the ACC/AHA Practice Guidelines. Hirsch et al. (2006). *Circulation* 113:e463–e465.

Further reading

Aboyans V, Criqui MH, Denenberg JO, et al. (2006). Risk factors for progression of peripheral arterial disease in large and small vessels. *Circulation* 113:2623–2629.

Ailawadi, G, Eliason JL, Upchurch GR Jr (2003). Current concepts in the pathogenesis of abdominal aortic aneurysm. *J Vasc Surg* 38:584.

Barani J, Nilsson JA, Mattiasson I, et al (2005). Inflammatory mediators are associated with 1-year mortality in critical limb ischemia. *J Vasc Surg* 42:75–80.

Braunwald E, et al. (2004). *Braunwald's Heart Disease: A Textbook of Cardiovascular Medicine.* St. Louis: WB Saunders.

Creager MA, Dzau VJ, Loscalzo J, ed. (2006). *Vascular Medicine: A Companion to Braunwald's Heart Disease,* Philadelphia: Elsevier; pp. 934–960.

Criqui, MH (2001). Peripheral arterial disease—epidemiological aspects. *Vasc Med;* 6:3–7.

Criqui MH, Langer, RD, Franek, A, et al. (1992). Mortality over a period of 10 years in patients with peripheral arterial disease. *N Engl J Med* 326:381.

Criqui MH, Ninomiya J: The epidemiology of peripheral arterial disease. In: MA Creager, Dzau VJ, Loscalzo J, ed. *Vascular Medicine: A Companion to Braunwald's Heart Disease,* Philadelphia: Elsevier; 2006:223–238.

Criqui MH, Vargas V, Denenberg JO, et al. (2005) Ethnicity and peripheral arterial disease: The San Diego Population Study. *Circulation* 112:2703–2707.

Diehm C, Schuster A, Allenberg JR, et al. (2004). High prevalence of peripheral arterial disease and co-morbidity in 6880 primary care patients: Cross-sectional study. *Atherosclerosis* 172:95–105.

Hiatt WR, Brass EP (2006). Pathophysiology of intermittent claudication. In Creager MA, Dzau VJ, Loscalzo J (Eds.), *Vascular Medicine: A Companion to Braunwald's Heart Disease.* Philadelphia: Elsevier; pp. 239–247.

Hirsch AT, Criqui MH, Treat-Jacobson D, et al. (2001). Peripheral arterial disease detection, awareness, and treatment in primary care. *JAMA* 286:1317.

Hirsch AT, Haskal ZJ, Hertzer NR, et al. (2006). ACC/AHA 2005 guidelines for the management of patients with peripheral arterial disease (lower extremity, renal, mesenteric, and abdominal aortic): Executive summary a collaborative report from the American Association for Vascular Surgery/Society for Vascular Surgery, Society for Cardiovascular Angiography and Interventions, Society for Vascular Medicine and Biology, Society of Interventional Radiology, and the ACC/ AHA Task Force on Practice Guidelines (Writing Committee to Develop Guidelines for the Management of Patients With Peripheral Arterial Disease) endorsed by the American Association of Cardiovascular and Pulmonary Rehabilitation; National Heart, Lung, and Blood Institute; Society for Vascular Nursing; TransAtlantic Inter-Society Consensus; and Vascular Disease Foundation. *J Am Coll Cardiol* 47:1239–1312.

Jude EB, Oyiba SO, Chalmers N, Boulton AJ (2001). Peripheral arterial disease in diabetic and nondiabetic patients: a comparison of severity and outcome. *Diabetes Care* 24:1433.

Libby P, et al. (2008). *Braunwald's Heart Disease: A Textbook of Cardiovascular Medicine.* Philadelphia: Elsevier.

Lu JT, Creager MA (2004). The relationship of cigarette smoking to peripheral arterial disease. *Rev Cardiovasc Med* 5:189–193.

Marso SP, Hiatt WR (2006). Peripheral arterial disease in patients with diabetes. *J Am Coll Cardiol* 47:921–929.

McDermott MM, Greenland P, Liu K, et al. (2001). Leg symptoms in peripheral arterial disease: associated clinical characteristics and functional impairment. *JAMA* 286:1599.

McDermott MM, Kerwin DR, Liu K, et al. (2001). Prevalence and significance of unrecognized lower extremity peripheral arterial disease in general medicine practice. *J Gen Intern Med* 16:384.

McDermott MM, Liu K, Greenland P, et al. (2004). Functional decline in peripheral arterial disease: associations with the ankle brachial index and leg symptoms. *JAMA* 292:453.

Murabito JM, D'Agostino RB, Silbershatz H, Wilson WF (1997). Intermittent claudication. A risk profile from The Framingham Heart Study. *Circulation* 96:44–49.

Norgren L, Hiatt WR, Dormandy JA, et al. (2007). Inter-Society Consensus for the Management of Peripheral Arterial Disease (TASC II). *J Vasc Surg* 45:S5–S67.

O'Hare, AM, Katz, R, Shilpak, MG, et al. (2006). Mortality and cardiovascular risk across the ankle-arm index spectrum: results from the Cardiovascular Health Study. *Circulation* 113:388.

Olin JW (2005). Hypertension and peripheral arterial disease. *Vasc Med* 10:241–246.

Ouriel, K (2001). Peripheral arterial disease. *Lancet* 358:1257.

Pasternak RC, Criqui MH, Benjamin EJ, et al. (2004). Atherosclerotic vascular disease conference: Writing Group I: epidemiology. *Circulation* 109:2605.

Rimmer, JM, Gennari, FJ (1993). Atherosclerotic renovascular disease and progressive renal failure. *Ann Intern Med* 118:712.

Selvin E, Erlinger TP (2004). Prevalence of and risk factors for peripheral arterial disease in the United States: Results from the National Health and Nutrition Examination Survey, 1999–2000. *Circulation* 110:738–743.

Smith SC Jr, Milani RV, Arnett DK, et al. (2004). Atherosclerotic vascular disease conference: Writing Group II: risk factors. *Circulation* 109:2613.

Wattanakit K, Folsom AR, Selvin E, et al. (2005). Risk factors for peripheral arterial disease incidence in persons with diabetes: The Atherosclerosis Risk in Communities (ARIC) Study. *Atherosclerosis* 180:389–397.

Wildman RP, Muntner P, Chen J, et al. (2005). Relation of inflammation to peripheral arterial disease in the national health and nutrition examination survey, 1999–2002. *Am J Cardiol* 96:1579–1583.

Chapter 4

Valvular heart disease

General considerations

Development

Cardiac valves develop from the mesodermal germ layer between the fourth and seventh weeks of gestation. Factors affecting embryogenesis during this time can influence valve development, such as infection (rubella) or drugs.

Anatomy

The human heart contains four valves: two on the left side of the heart (mitral and aortic) and two on the right (tricuspid and pulmonic, or pulmonary) (Fig. 4.1).

The mitral and tricuspid valves, also referred to as atrioventricular (AV) valves, are supported by a fibrous skeleton and separate the atrial and ventricular chambers, ensuring unidirectional flow of blood during diastole. The mitral valve is composed of two leaflets (anterior and posterior) while the tricuspid valve (as the name implies) contains three leaflets (anterior, posterior, and septal).

Both the mitral and tricuspid valve leaflets are attached by chordae tendinae to papillary muscles in their respective ventricles, the contraction of which ensures valve competency.

The aortic and pulmonic valves, also referred to as semilunar valves, separate the left and right ventricles from the aorta and pulmonary artery, respectively, ensuring unidirectional forward blood flow during systole. The aortic and pulmonic valves each contain three cusps.

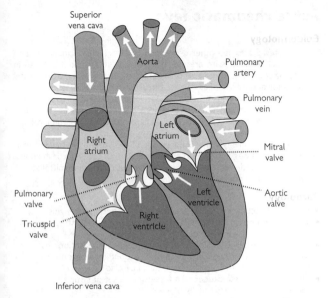

Figure 4.1 Heart valves as viewed from above with the atria removed (top) and in a coronal section (bottom).

Acute rheumatic fever

Epidemiology

In the United States and other developed countries, the incidence is 2 to 14 cases per 100,000, with around 10 cases per 1000 school children in developing countries. Although it is now rare in the developed world, it still accounts for almost half of all cardiac disease in the developing world.

Declining incidence in the developed world is likely due to improved economic standards and housing conditions, decreased crowding in houses and schools, improved access to medical care, and effective antimicrobials, especially penicillin.

Those affected are typically children aged 5–15 years from lower socio-economic class living in crowded conditions; 20% of cases occur in adults.

There is no gender difference in incidence, but chorea and mitral stenosis (MS) are more common in females.

Pathology

- It typically occurs several weeks after streptococcal pharyngitis.
- The most common pathogen is group A beta-hemolytic streptococci (*Streptococcus pyogenes* serotype M).
- Antigenic mimicry is implicated in the pathogenesis as antibodies to carbohydrates in the cell wall (anti-M antibodies) of group A *Streptococcus* cross-react with proteins in cardiac valves.
- Time from acute streptococcal infection to onset of symptomatic rheumatic fever (RF) is usually 3–4 weeks.
- RF is thought to complicate up to 3% of untreated streptococcal sore throats.
- Previous episodes of RF predispose to recurrences.
- Other areas of cross-reactivity may explain noncardiac findings (e.g., involvement of connective tissue in joints causing arthritis, caudate nucleus in brain leading to Sydenham's chorea).
- RF commonly causes a *pancarditis*.
- *Pericarditis* rarely causes hemodynamic instability/tamponade or constriction.
- *Myocarditis* may cause acute heart failure and arrhythmias.
- *Endocarditis* affects the mitral valve (65%–70%), aortic valve (25%), and tricuspid valve (10%, never in isolation), causing acute regurgitation and heart failure but chronic stenosis.
- Pericardium, perivascular regions of myocardium, and endocardium develop foci of eosinophilic collagen surrounded by lymphocytes, plasma cells, and macrophages called *Aschoff bodies*.

Clinical features

- *Sore throat* occurs 1–5 weeks prior in two-thirds of cases.
- Fever, abdominal pain, and epistaxis.
- Migratory large-joint *polyarthritis* starting in the lower limbs in 75% of cases. Duration is <4 weeks at each site. There is severe pain and tenderness in contrast to a mild degree of joint swelling.

- *Pancarditis* occurs in 50% of cases with features of acute heart failure, mitral and aortic regurgitation, and pericarditis.
- *Chorea* occurs in 10%–30%, usually occurs 1–6 months after pharyngitis. Patients exhibit difficulties in writing and speaking, generalized weakness, choreiform movements, and emotional lability. Joints are hyperextended with hypotonia, diminished tendon reflexes, tongue fasciculation, and a relapsing grip (alternate increases and decreases in tension). Full recovery is usually in 2–3 months.
- *Erythema marginatum* is an evanescent rash with serpiginous outlines and central clearings on the trunk and proximal limbs. It is seen in 5%–13% of cases. It begins as erythematous, nonpruritic papules or macules that spread outward. It fades and reappears in hours and persists throughout the disease course. See Fig. 4.2.
- *Subcutaneous nodules* are seen in 0–8% of cases usually several weeks after the onset of pancarditis. They occur mainly over bony surfaces or joint prominences and tendons and usually last 1–2 weeks.
- There is a risk of overdiagnosing RF in children admitted with fever, soft murmurs, and arthralgia, all of which are common in childhood. Evidence for an antecedent streptococcal infection is required for the definitive diagnosis—see Box 4.1.

Treatment

- Oral penicillin V for 10 days or intramuscular penicillin G (single dose of 1.2 million units) to treat the acute infection. If patient is penicillin allergic, use oral erythromycin, azithromycin, or cephalexin for 10 days.
- Oral aspirin 4–8 g daily until ESR and CRP are normal
- Systemic corticosteroids for 2–4 weeks for moderate–severe carditis
- Standard medical therapy (i.e., diuretics, ACE inhibitors, and digoxin) for heart failure

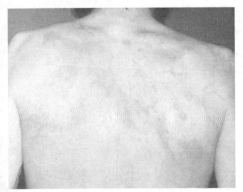

Figure 4.2 Erythema marginatum in rheumatic fever.

Box 4.1 Diagnostic criteria for rheumatic fever (Jones criteria)

- Evidence of group A streptococcal pharyngitis
- Either a positive throat culture or rapid streptococcal antigen test, or an elevated or rising streptococcal antibody titer (samples taken 2 weeks apart).
- Plus two major or one major and two minor Jones criteria:

Major criteria
- Polyarthritis
- Carditis
- Chorea
- Erythema marginatum
- Subcutaneous nodules

Minor criteria
- Fever
- Arthralgia
- Prolonged PR interval
- Elevated ESR and CRP

Prognosis
- Determined by severity of cardiac involvement.
- Acute-phase duration is about 3 months in 80% of cases.
- Mortality is 1%–10% in developing countries.
- Recurrence rates are high and are most common in the first 2 years following acute infection. Chronic valve disease occurs in one-third without and two-thirds with recurrent infections.
- Murmurs resolve in 50% of cases up to 5 years after index infection.
- *Antibiotic prophylaxis* against group A streptococcal infection is used to prevent recurrence of RF. It is usually continued for at least 10 years or until young adulthood. Daily oral penicillin or intramuscularly penicillin injection every 3–4 weeks are standard regimens. Erythromycin can be used in penicillin-allergic patients.

World Health Organization 2001 guidelines for prophylaxis
- Patients without proven carditis: at least 5 years of antibiotic prophylaxis following diagnosis of acute RF or until age 18.
- Patients with mild mitral regurgitation: at least 10 years of prophylaxis or until age 25.
- Patients with severe valve disease and/or after valve surgery: lifelong prophylaxis.

Mitral stenosis

The most common etiology is rheumatic heart disease. Other causes are rare and include the following:

- Congenital (isolated lesion or in association with an atrial septal defect [ASD]—Lutembacher's syndrome, or other left-sided obstructive lesions (Shone complex)
- Carcinoid syndrome (stenosis usually not severe and associated with regurgitation)
- Fen-phen valvulopathy (stenosis usually not severe and associated with regurgitation)
- Mucopolysaccharidoses (e.g., Hurler's syndrome)
- Endocardial fibroelastosis
- Radiation
- Mitral annular calcification (doesn't usually cause severe stenosis)
- Iatrogenic following mitral valve repair for mitral regurgitation (MR)
- Prosthetic mitral valve obstruction

Stenosis occurs at three levels: chordae (fuse, thicken, and shorten), cusps (thicken and calcify), and commissures (fuse with the valve cusps still mobile). Left atrial myxoma and cor triatrium can cause similar pathophysiology by obstructing left ventricular (LV) inflow.

Pathophysiology

Elevated left atrium (LA) pressure is required to drive blood through the narrowed mitral valve orifice during diastole, leading to pulmonary venous hypertension and exertional dyspnea. Secondary pulmonary arterial hypertension leads to right ventricular (RV) hypertrophy and failure.

LV systolic function is preserved but as filling is impaired, adequate cardiac output (CO) cannot always be maintained, especially with exercise and tachycardia. Onset of atrial fibrillation (AF) is associated with abrupt clinical deterioration due to both the loss of atrial systole and the fast heart rate, which shortens the diastolic filling period.

Clinical features

- Dyspnea on exertion, orthopnea, paroxysmal nocturnal dyspnea.
- Acute pulmonary edema may be precipitated by uncontrolled AF, exercise, pulmonary infection, anesthesia, and pregnancy.
- AF increases the risk of thromboembolism. Systemic embolism occurs in 20%–30% and usually originates in the dilated LA and LA appendage.
- Fatigue is due to reduced cardiac output reserve.
- Hemoptysis can occur for a variety of reasons: alveolar capillary rupture (pink frothy pulmonary edema); bronchial vein rupture (larger hemorrhage); blood-stained sputum of chronic bronchitis; pulmonary infarction (low CO, immobile patient).
- Chest pain similar to angina may occur in patients with pulmonary hypertension and RV hypertrophy, even with normal coronaries.
- The enlarging LA may compress surrounding structures, producing hoarse voice (left recurrent laryngeal nerve compression—Ortner's syndrome), dysphagia (esophageal compression), and left lung collapse (left main bronchus compression).

Physical exam findings (see Fig. 4.3)
- Mitral facies or malar flush
- Prominent a-waves in jugular venous pressure (JVP) if in sinus rhythm
- Small-volume arterial pulse
- Irregularly irregular pulse in AF
- "Tapping" apex beat—palpable S1
- Diastolic thrill at apex
- Left parasternal heave (due to RVH), palpable pulmonic closure

Auscultation

S1 is loud if in sinus rhythm and the valve is pliable (Fig. 4.4). P2 is accentuated. Opening snap (OS) of the MV is heard best at or medial to the apex in expiration. The A2–OS interval varies inversely with severity of stenosis.

Low-pitched, rumbling, mid-diastolic murmur with presystolic accentuation (if in sinus rhythm) is heard best at the apex with patient in left lateral position. Early diastolic murmur due to pulmonary regurgitation from pulmonary hypertension (Graham–Steell murmur) may be heard.

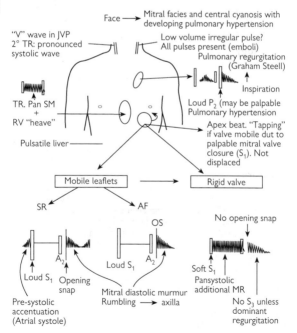

Figure 4.3 Physical signs in mitral stenosis. Reproduced with permission from Swanton RH. *Cardiology Pocket Consultant*, 5th ed. Copyright Wiley-Blackwell 2003.

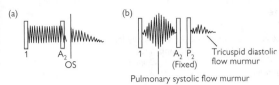

(a) (b)

1 A₂ OS

1 A₂ P₂ (Fixed) Tricuspid diastolic flow murmur

Pulmonary systolic flow murmur

Figure 4.4 Similarity on auscultation between (a) mixed mitral valve disease and (b) ASD. Reproduced with permission from Swanton RH. *Cardiology Pocket Consultant*, 5th ed. Copyright Wiley-Blackwell 2003.

Table 4.1 Radiographic features of mitral stenosis

PA film	Lateral film
• Straight or convex L heart border	• LA or RV enlargement
• Double shadow of LA behind RA	• Valvular calcification
• Splaying of carina (>90)	• McCallum's patch (LA calcification)
• Dilated upper lobe veins	• Esophageal indentation on barium swallow
• Prominent pulmonary conus	
• Pulmonary hemosiderosis	

Testing

- **ECG** shows LA abnormality (P mitrale) if in sinus rhythm. AF is common. Right axis deviation and RV hypertrophy. RA abnormality (P pulmonale) occurs with severe pulmonary hypertension/cor pulmonale.
- **CXR** shows straightening of the left heart border, prominent upper lobe veins, pulmonary artery enlargement, Kerley B lines—interstitial edema. Large left atrium is visible as a double shadow (Table 4.1).
- **TTE** is the diagnostic modality of choice. Parasternal long-axis (PLAX) view shows enlarged left atrium and doming of the valve leaflets due to commissural fusion. In parasternal short-axis (PSAX) view, mitral valve orifice can be measured by planimetry. Valvular and subvalvular thickening and calcification can be seen. M-mode shows restricted valve leaflet separation due to commissural fusion. Continuous wave (CW) Doppler can be used to measure transvalvular pressure gradient and valve area, as well as estimate pulmonary artery pressure from TR jet. It is important to evaluate for coexistent MR or other valvular disease.
- **Stress ECHO** to assess for exertional pulmonary hypertension
- **TEE** provides better anatomic detail and can visualize thrombi in the LA and LA appendage, which is especially important prior to percutaneous mitral balloon valvotomy (PMBV).
- **Cardiac catheterization:** increased PCWP to LV end diastolic pressure gradient. If the mean mitral gradient is low at rest, repeat measurements following exercise in cath lab (e.g., straight-leg raising or lifting bags of saline). Assess for coexisting coronary and valvular lesions.

Treatment

Medical

- Asymptomatic patients—observe clinically for development of AF, pulmonary hypertension, or symptoms.
- Mild symptoms—salt intake restriction and oral diuretics as needed
- Atrial fibrillation—β-blocker, nondihydropyridine calcium channel blocker, or digoxin for rate control. Restoration of sinus rhythm may be attempted if appropriate.
- Anticoagulants—at least 1 year for those with thromboembolism and lifelong if in AF. Patients with low-output states and R heart failure should also be anticoagulated. There is no proven benefit if the patient is in sinus rhythm.
- Antibiotic prophylaxis for mitral stenosis is no longer indicated.

Percutaneous mitral balloon valvotomy (PMBV)

Moderate to severe symptoms or development of pulmonary hypertension (>50 mmHg at rest or >60 mmHg with exercise) warrants mechanical relief of mitral valve obstruction, and PMBV is the preferred approach to achieve this. In PMBV, a guide wire is placed in LA after trans-septal puncture and a balloon (Inoue balloon) is directed across the valve and inflated at the orifice.

This procedure is suitable for patients with pliable valves with minimal MR, no subvalvular distortion, and without heavy calcification. An ECHO-derived Wilkins score <8 predicts procedural success and should be determined in each case.

Surgical (see Box 4.2)

- *Closed valvotomy.* Fused cusps separated by a dilator introduced through LV apex. Results are inferior to PMBV so it is now rarely performed.
- *Open valvotomy* with cardiopulmonary bypass is preferred to closed valvotomy. Cusps are separated under direct vision. Any fusion of subvalvular apparatus is loosened.
- *Mitral valve replacement* is used if there is significant MR or the valve is severely diseased or heavily calcified.

Box 4.2 ACC/AHA 2006 guidelines* for surgery in mitral stenosis

- *Class I:* Symptomatic (NYHA Class III/IV) patients with moderate to severe MS when PMBV is not available or is contraindicated (i.e., LA thrombus, significant mitral regurgitation)
- *Class IIA:* Patients with NYHA Class I–II symptoms and severe pulmonary hypertension not candidates for PMBV
- *Class IIB:* Recurrent systemic emboli despite anticoagulation
- *Class III:* Patients with mild MS. Closed comissurotomy should not be performed in patients undergoing surgery for MS.

*Bonow, RO, et al. (2006). ACC/AHA 2006 guidelines for the management of patients with valvular heart disease. J Am Coll Cardiol 48:598–675.

Mitral regurgitation

Causes

Acute
- Infective endocarditis
- Acute myocardial infarction (MI) (usually inferior wall) from papillary muscle dysfunction or acute rupture
- Trauma

Chronic
- Mitral valve prolapse
- Rheumatic heart disease
- Ischemic heart disease
- Left ventricular dilatation of any cause
- Hypertrophic cardiomyopathy
- Carcinoid syndrome
- Fen-phen valvulopathy
- Congenital lesions (i.e., cleft mitral valve).

Pathophysiology

The LV unloads into the LA during systole. In acute MR, the LA size is usually normal initially because of normal compliance, and this results in raised LA pressure and acute pulmonary edema. In longstanding severe MR, the LA enlarges, which accommodates the volume overload with minimal rise in LA pressure. In this case, symptoms usually occur with exertion or tachycardia, which causes further increases in LA pressure.

Symptoms

- In acute severe MR, pulmonary edema is common.
- In chronic MR, fatigue (due to impaired forward CO), exertional dyspnea, orthopnea, and systemic embolization (less common than in MS) occur. Palpitations are due to premature atrial beats or AF. Symptoms of pulmonary hypertension/RV failure occur in later stages.

Physical examination

- Rapid upstroke in arterial pulse
- Prominent a-waves in JVP in patients in sinus rhythm
- Large v-waves if associated tricuspid regurgitation (TR)
- Forceful apex displaced laterally
- Pansystolic murmur loudest at the apex and radiating into the axilla
- Systolic thrill at apex
- Soft first heart sound
- Wide splitting of S2 due to premature aortic valve closure
- Prominent low-pitched S3
- A mid-diastolic flow murmur may follow S3.
- Mid-systolic click in mitral valve prolapse (MVP)

Testing

- *ECG* shows features of LA enlargement, left ventricular hypertrophy (LVH), and RA enlargement in pulmonary hypertension. AF is common in chronic MR.
- *CXR* shows cardiomegaly. There is LA and LV enlargement. Pulmonary venous congestion, and calcified mitral annulus may be seen.
- *TTE* is the diagnostic test of choice. Dilated LA, hyperdynamic LV (until late when LV failure occurs) can be found, as can features of MVP, ischemic MR (i.e., leaflet tethering). Color Doppler is used to detect and quantify the MR, including jet direction. Assess LV size and function (EF, end systolic diameter, end diastolic diameter). CW Doppler is used to assess velocity of the regurgitant jet and estimate PA pressure from the TR jet. Assess for presence of vegetations in infective endocarditis as well as associated valve disease (i.e., TR).
- *TEE* shows the anatomy in greater detail and allows accurate assessment of the feasibility of valve repair. It has higher sensitivity for detecting vegetations in infective endocarditis. It should be performed prior to surgery.
- **Cardiac catheterization** confirms the severity of the lesion. Elevated v-waves are on PCWP tracing. Contrast left ventriculography can quantify MR as 1+ (mild) to 4+ (severe) based on the degree of LA opacification. Coronary angiography is used to assess for obstructive CAD prior to MV surgery.

Prognosis

Outcome is poor in severe symptomatic mitral regurgitation, with a 33% survival at 8 years without surgical intervention. Death is usually due to heart failure or is arrhythmia related (i.e., sudden cardiac death, stroke).

Management

Medical management

Infective endocarditis prophylaxis is no longer required according to the 2007 ACC/AHA guidelines. Asymptomatic patients with severe MR can be managed conservatively with serial echocardiograms (every 6–12 months) to assess for LV dysfunction (dilation, drop in EF) and pulmonary hypertension, as well as adequate clinical follow-up to evaluate for the onset of symptoms or AF.

There is no beneficial role for vasodilator therapy in asymptomatic patients with chronic MR. Vasodilators may be used acutely in *symptomatic* patients to increase forward CO and reduce regurgitant volume.

Patients with congestive heart failure (CHF) should also receive diuretics for symptom relief, though outcome without surgery is poor. Chronic medical therapy with vasodilators and diuretics is only recommended in patients who are not surgical candidates.

In atrial fibrillation, β-blockers and/or calcium channel blockers or digoxin should be given for rate control, and these patients should receive anticoagulation, unless contraindicated. Rhythm control in AF should be attempted in those patients who remain symptomatic despite adequate attempts at rate control.

Surgical treatment

Surgery is indicated in patients with severe MR who are symptomatic (Box 4.3). Asymptomatic patients with severe MR may need surgery if there is LV enlargement or LV systolic dysfunction. Pulmonary hypertension and new-onset AF are other indications for surgery.

Timing of the surgery is very important. Reduction of the left ventricular ejection fraction (LVEF) <60% or end systolic dimension (ESD) >45 mm indicates LV systolic dysfunction and the need for surgery.

- Mitral valve repair is preferred to valve replacement if technically feasible. Long-term anticoagulation and risk of hemorrhage and thromboembolism can be avoided.
- Mitral valve replacement with a prosthesis, either mechanical or bioprosthetic, is needed if valve leaflets are severely damaged or heavily calcified.

Box 4.3 2006 ACC/AHA guidelines* for surgery in MR

Class I

- Symptomatic severe acute MR
- Severe symptomatic chronic MR in the absence of severe LV dysfunction (LVEF <30% or ESD >55 mm)
- Asymptomatic severe chronic MR with LVEF of 30%–60% and/or ESD ≥40 mm
- Mitral valve repair is preferred to replacement in most patients.

Class IIa

- Mitral valve repair in asymptomatic severe chronic MR with preserved LV function (LVEF >60% and ESD <40 mm) if likelihood of successful repair ≥90%
- Asymptomatic severe chronic MR and preserved LVEF with new-onset AF or pulmonary hypertension (PASP >50 mmHg at rest or >60 mmHg with exercise)
- If mitral valve repair is highly likely, severe symptomatic chronic MR due to a primary abnormality in the mitral valve apparatus and severe left ventricular dysfunction (LVEF <30% or ESD >55 mm)

Class IIb

- Mitral valve repair for severe MR due to severe LV dysfunction (LVEF <30%) in patients with persistent symptoms despite optimal medical therapy for heart failure

Class III

- Isolated valve surgery for mild to moderate MR
- Asymptomatic patients with preserved LV function if MV repair not feasible

* Bonow RO, et al. (2006) ACC/AHA 2006 guidelines for the management of patients with valvular heart disease. *J Am Coll Cardiol* 48:598–675.

Mitral valve prolapse

(Barlow's syndrome, floppy mitral valve syndrome)

Causes

Primary or classic mitral valve prolapse (MVP) is an idiopathic valvular abnormality characterized by myxomatous degeneration of the mitral valve leaflets and subvalvular apparatus in the absence of any recognizable systemic connective tissue disorder. It can be inherited as an autosomal dominant phenotype with incomplete penetrance.

Secondary MVP occurs in the setting of known connective tissue disorders, including Marfan's syndrome, Ehlers–Danlos syndrome, pseudoxanthoma elasticum, and osteogenesis imperfecta. MVP is also frequently associated with atrial septal defects and Ebstein's anomaly. One can also see acquired leaflet prolapse (i.e., functional MVP) in ischemic heart disease and dilated cardiomyopathy. Overall prevalence is approximately 2% and is similar in men and women.

Pathophysiology

Myxomatous degeneration and excess mucopolysaccharide accumulation lead to large, "floppy" valve leaflets. Prolapse can be caused by papillary muscle dysfunction, elongated or ruptured chordae tendinae, a dilated mitral annulus, and/or redundant leaflets. MV leaflet (usually posterior) prolapses into the LA during ventricular systole.

Mitral regurgitation results from leaflet malcoaptation; this is the most common cause of MR in adults.

Symptoms

Most patients are asymptomatic, though some have a constellation of nonspecific symptoms such as atypical chest pain, palpitations, and panic attacks. These symptoms are probably related to autonomic dysfunction rather than the mitral valve abnormality.

Patients may also develop symptoms of MR if it becomes significant, which occurs in roughly 7% patients with classic MVP.

Examination

Mid-systolic click is due to tensing of the chordae tendinae and the prolapsed leaflet. The click may occur closer to S1 with maneuvers that decrease LV volume, such as standing from a squatting position.

A *mid-late systolic murmur* may be heard if there is associated MR.

Testing

TTE is the most useful noninvasive test to establish the diagnosis and assess for the presence and severity of MR.

Classic MVP is defined as systolic displacement of one or both MV leaflets by ≥2 mm into the LA beyond the high points of mitral annulus in the PLAX view and leaflet thickness ≥5 mm.

Leaflet thickness <5 mm is referred to as *nonclassic MVP*.

Treatment

Infective endocarditis prophylaxis is no longer recommended. β-Blockers can provide symptomatic relief from atypical chest pain and palpitations.

Rate or rhythm control and anticoagulation are needed in patients with AF.

MV repair (rarely replacement) is indicated for severe MR if symptomatic or for LV dysfunction.

Prognosis

This condition is benign in most patients and determined largely by the severity of MR; moderate to severe MR is the most important predictor of adverse outcomes. Complications of MVP occur in 1% patients per year and include significant MR, infective endocarditis, cerebrovascular events, and arrhythmias.

Although a variety of arrhythmias may occur in patients with MVP, the incidence of sudden cardiac death is quite low (1.9 per 10,000 per year) in the absence of hemodynamically significant MR.

Aortic stenosis

Incidence

Aortic stenosis (AS) is the most common acquired valvular lesion in adults. Incidence is increasing as the population ages and with improvements in diagnostic modalities, primarily Doppler echocardiography.

Symptoms and prognosis are related to the degree of left ventricular outflow tract (LVOT) obstruction.

Differential diagnosis of LVOT obstruction

- *Valvular stenosis*: calcific AS is the most common etiology.
- *Supravalvular stenosis*: tubular narrowing of proximal ascending aorta is commonly associated with William's syndrome.
- *Subvalvular stenosis*: discrete membrane or a tubular muscular narrowing. Dynamic obstruction can occur in hypertrophic obstructive cardiomyopathy (HOCM).

Causes of valvular AS

Acquired

Calcific AS

Calcific AS (senile degenerative) is most common, affecting 2% of people >65 years old, with an increasing incidence with age. End-stage renal disease and Paget's disease of bone are also associated with valvular calcification.

Risk factors for atherosclerosis, such as diabetes, hypertension, hyperlipidemia, and smoking, play a role in the underlying inflammatory process. This leads to heavy leaflet calcification, thickening, and immobility with reduced systolic opening.

Aortic sclerosis without LVOT obstruction is common and occurs in 25% patients >65 years of age and may precede stenosis, with 9% of patients developing stenosis in 5 years.

Rheumatic AS

This usually occurs in conjunction with mitral valve disease. Commissural fusion and retraction of valve leaflets leads to systolic doming and impaired leaflet coaptation. One often sees associated aortic regurgitation.

Congenital

Bicuspid aortic valve

This is seen in 2% of the population. There is often familial clustering and autosomal dominant inheritance with incomplete penetrance.

This condition results in chronic turbulent flow, which leads to accelerated leaflet calcification and fibrosis. It usually presents clinically with significant stenosis at ages 45–65 years. It is often associated with aortic pathology (aneurysm, dissection, or coarctation), so all patients should be screened for aortic involvement at time of diagnosis.

Unicuspid aortic valve

This presents in infancy.

Pathophysiology

Progressive valvular narrowing and obstruction to left ventricular outflow lead to pressure overload and compensatory concentric hypertrophy to lessen the increased wall stress. Diastolic dysfunction and decreased ventricular compliance lead to elevated LV diastolic pressure, which reduces the coronary perfusion gradient, resulting in ischemia. Ischemia can also result from increased myocardial O_2 consumption due to increased LV mass and prolonged systolic ejection time.

When valve obstruction becomes critical, LV systolic failure can occur.

Symptoms and presentation

- There is a long latent asymptomatic period.
- *Angina* is due to myocardial ischemia from O_2 supply–demand mismatch. Only half of the affected patients have significant epicardial coronary stenosis.
- *Syncope* is due to arrhythmias, abnormal vasodepressor reflexes, and LVOT obstruction/hypotension.
- *Exertional dyspnea/CHF* is usually due to diastolic heart failure.
- Sudden cardiac death occurs rarely as the initial presentation of symptomatic AS (incidence is 0.4%/year in asymptomatic patients with severe AS).
- Exercise treadmill testing may be helpful if presence of symptoms or functional status is equivocal from the patient's history.

Physical exam

- Small-volume, slow rising pulse *(pulsus parvus et tardus)* is best felt at the carotid. BP—narrow pulse pressure; in advanced AS systolic BP is decreased. Prominent a-wave on JVP. Sustained apical impulse. Systolic thrill is felt in the aortic area (second intercostal space on right) during full expiration.
- Auscultation—S1 normal or soft. S2 normal in mild AS. As severity of AS worsens, A2 is delayed by prolonged systolic ejection time and S2 may be paradoxically split (P2 before A2), although it is usually soft or absent in severe AS. An S4 (atria contracting into stiff ventricle) and systolic ejection click (if valve pliable, especially bicuspid valves) may also be heard. Systolic ejection murmur is heard throughout precordium but is best heard in the aortic area in full expiration and usually radiates to carotids. The murmur intensity peaks later in systole as AS worsens.

The following exam findings are most specific for severe AS:
- Late-peaking systolic murmur
- Delayed carotid upstroke
- Soft or absent S2

Aortic stenosis: management

Diagnostic testing

- *ECG* shows LVH with strain; branch bundle block (BBB) (either R or L). One may see AF.
- *CXR* shows calcification involving valve or aortic root, poststenotic dilatation in the ascending aorta.
- *TTE* is the diagnostic test of choice. It will show a calcified valve with restricted opening (2D and M-mode); also evaluate for congenital abnormalities and aortic pathology. Assess for LVH and LV systolic and diastolic function.
- *Color Doppler* is used to look for concomitant AR and/or MR.
- *CW Doppler* is used to measure transvalvular pressure gradient and calculate valve area using the continuity principle.
- *Dobutamine stress ECHO* can distinguish low-gradient true severe aortic stenosis from pseudoaortic stenosis due to low cardiac output.
- *Cardiac catheterization* is used to assess for concomitant coronary artery disease prior to aortic valve surgery. There is no need to assess valve gradient (significant risk of embolic events with this; CW Doppler accurately assesses gradient and LV function) unless there is a discrepancy between echocardiogram and clinical findings.
- *TEE* is used for calculation of the valve area by planimetry if TTE is nondiagnostic and to assess for aortic pathology (especially in patients with bicuspid valves).

Severity

Severity is classified according to pressure gradient and valve area (Table 4.2). Echocardiography with Doppler is the preferred modality to acquire these measurements.

Prognosis

AS is a progressive condition that gradually worsens over time. Symptoms are usually not present until stenosis is severe. Once symptoms occur, prognosis without surgery is poor: of patients who present with symptoms of angina, 50% will die within 5 years; if patients present with syncope, 50% will die in 3 years; if patients present with congestive heart failure, 50% will die within 2 years.

Treatment

Surgery

Aortic valve replacement (AVR) is the mainstay of therapy for symptomatic patients and can be performed with a very low (1%) operative mortality (see Box 4.4).

Medical therapy

Medical therapy offers very little to symptomatic patients in terms of improved outcomes. These patients should be referred promptly for surgery. Medical therapy (i.e., diuretics) may provide temporary and palliative symptomatic relief to patients who are not surgical candidates, but must be administered with caution to avoid hypovolemia and hypotension.

Table 4.2 ACC/AHA classification* of AS severity

Severity	Gradient (mmHg)	Velocity (m/sec)	Valve area (cm^2)
Mild	<25	<3.0	>1.5
Moderate	25–40	3.0–4.0	1.0–1.5
Severe	>40	>4.0	<1.0

* Bonow, RO, et al. (2006) ACC/AHA 2006 guidelines for the management of patients with valvular heart disease. *J Am Coll Cardiol* 48:598–675.

Box 4.4 2006 ACC/AHA guidelines* for AVR in AS

Class I

- Symptomatic patients with severe AS
- Patients with severe AS undergoing CABG or aortic or other valvular surgery
- Patients with severe AS and LVEF <50%

Class IIa

- Patients with moderate AS undergoing CABG or aortic or other valvular surgery

Class IIb

- Severe AS in asymptomatic patients who have an abnormal response to exercise such as the development of symptoms or hypotension
- Severe AS in asymptomatic patients with a high likelihood of rapid progression
- Severe AS in asymptomatic patients in whom surgery might be delayed at the time of symptom onset
- Mild AS in patients undergoing CABG surgery in whom there is evidence, such as moderate to severe valve calcification, that progression may be rapid
- Extremely severe AS (aortic valve area <0.6 cm^2, mean gradient >60 mmHg, and aortic jet velocity >5.0 m/sec) in asymptomatic patients in whom the expected operative mortality is ≤1%

Class III

- For the prevention of sudden cardiac death in asymptomatic patients who have none of the class IIa or IIb findings

* Bonow, RO, et al. (2006). ACC/AHA 2006 guidelines for the management of patients with valvular heart disease. *J Am Coll Cardiol* 48:598–675.

Use of medications (particularly HMG-CoA reductase inhibitors) to delay AS progression in asymptomatic patients has been studied and the results thus far are inconclusive.

Transcatheter techniques

Balloon aortic valvuloplasty was introduced as a nonsurgical alternative treatment for AS and is integral to the management of congenital AS in the pediatric population. Results in the adult population are not as good as anticipated because of procedural complications and high restenosis rates.

Aortic valvuloplasty is currently not an acceptable alternative to surgical AVR and its use should be restricted to palliative therapy in patients deemed nonoperable and as a bridge to AVR in hemodynamically unstable patients.

Percutaneous aortic valve replacement is currently being performed at experienced centers and may be a valuable treatment approach in the future. Current use is restricted to patients who are not surgical candidates.

Aortic regurgitation

Causes

Valvular

- *Rheumatic fever* leads to fibrosis, fusion, and retraction of cusps such that they cannot appose properly.
- *Infective endocarditis* causes destruction of valve leaflets.

Aortic root disease

Dilatation, aneurysm, and dissection cause failure of coaptation of cusps. One may see diastolic cusp prolapse in dissection.

Causes

- Hypertension
- Marfan's syndrome
- Osteogenesis imperfecta
- Syphilis
- Spondyloarthritides (ankylosing spondylitis, Reiter's, etc.)
- Trauma
- Bicuspid aortic valve

Incidence

Aortic regurgitation (AR) is less common than AS. Valvular causes are becoming less frequent and aortic root causes now account for >50% of cases.

Pathophysiology

As the aortic valve becomes incompetent, more stroke volume regurgitates into LV during diastole, causing LV *volume overload*. Cardiac output is maintained by increasing stroke volume at the expense of increased LV end-diastolic volume. Eventually, with further LV dilatation, myocyte function deteriorates and LV failure occurs.

Symptoms

Symptoms include dyspnea/CHF, angina, and symptoms of an underlying cause (i.e., chest pain in aortic dissection, fever in infective endocarditis).

Physical examination

There is very wide pulse pressure with associated signs: collapsing (water-hammer) pulse, *Corrigan's sign* (visible carotid pulsation), *De Musset's sign* (head nodding with each pulse), *Müller's sign* (visible pulsation of uvula), *Traube sign* (also called "pistol shot femorals"—loud noises heard with the stethoscope over the femoral artery), *Quincke sign* (visible capillary pulsation in the nailbed), and *Durozicz sign* (heard over the femoral artery when the artery is digitally compressed).

Apex beat is displaced inferolaterally and is diffuse/hyperdynamic.

Auscultation

A2 may be normal (or louder) if AR is due to aortic root pathology; it may be soft or absent if AR is due to aortic valve pathology. S3 may be heard with dilated LV. A systolic ejection murmur similar to AS may be audible (due to either mixed AR/AS or turbulent flow from increased stroke volume).

Murmur of AR is a high-pitched early diastolic murmur immediately following A2, heard best along the left sterna border with the patient sitting up and leaning forward in expiration. Duration of the murmur in diastole correlates with severity of AR.

Austin Flint murmur is a mid-diastolic murmur heard at the apex due to antegrade flow across a mitral valve orifice that has been narrowed by a combination of rising LV pressure and jet of AR directed at the anterior MV leaflet.

Diagnostic testing

- *ECG* shows LVH with strain; left axis deviation.
- *CXR:* In chronic AR, an enlarged cardiac shadow is evident. There may also be dilated ascending aorta with aortic root pathology.
- *TTE:* Color Doppler and CW Doppler confirm the diagnosis and are used to assess the severity of regurgitation. 2D/M-mode measures aortic root and LV dimensions.
- *Cardiac catheterization* is used to assess for concomitant coronary artery disease prior to aortic valve/root surgery. An aortogram in left anterior oblique (LAO) projection shows aortic root size and severity of AR.

Prognosis

Chronic AR can be well tolerated for many years and is associated with a good prognosis: 5-year survival is ~75%, 10-year survival is ~50%. Prognosis worsens as symptoms develop (see Table 4.3).

Acute severe AR, however, is associated with a high mortality from LV failure, and early surgical intervention is indicated.

Table 4.3 Natural history of aortic regurgitation

Asymptomatic patients with normal LV function	
Progression to symptoms/signs of CHF	<6%/year
Progression to asymptomatic LV dysfunction	<3.5%/year
Sudden death	<0.2%/year
Asymptomatic patients with LV systolic dysfunction	
Progression to cardiac symptoms	>25%/year
Symptomatic patients	
Mortality rate	>10%/year

Reprinted with permission from Bonow RO, et al. (1998). ACC/AHA guidelines for the management of patients with valvular heart disease. *J Am Coll Cardiol* 32:1486–1582. ©1998, American Heart Association, Inc.

Treatment
Medical
- Asymptomatic mild to moderate AR with normal LV: routine follow-up (every 1–2 years) with ECHO
- Asymptomatic severe AR with normal LV: frequent (6-month) follow-up, or sooner if symptoms intervene.

Symptoms of CHF may respond to medical therapy (i.e., loop diuretics) while arrangements are made for surgery. Vasodilators (ACE inhibitor, calcium channel blockers) offer symptomatic relief and may improve hemodynamics. Anginal chest pain can be treated with nitrates but use β-blockers with caution.

Concomitant hypertension can worsen AR and should be treated with standard therapies. Antibiotic prophylaxis is not indicated in AR.

Surgical
Because of the relatively benign nature of asymptomatic chronic AR with normal LV function, these patients should be managed conservatively with close follow-up. Once symptoms have developed or evidence of significant LV dysfunction appears, referral for AVR/root replacement should be considered (see Box 4.5). In borderline cases frequent (2- to 4-month) follow-up is indicated.

Box 4.5 2006 ACC/AHA guidelines* for AVR in AR

Class I

- Symptomatic patients with severe chronic AR
- Asymptomatic patients with severe chronic AR and an LVEF ≤50% at rest
- Patients with severe chronic AR who undergo CABG or surgery on the aorta or other heart valves

Class IIa

- Asymptomatic patients with severe chronic AR and an LVEF >50% who have severe left ventricular dilatation (EDD >75 mm or ESD >55 mm)

Class IIb

- Patients with moderate chronic AR who undergo CABG or surgery on the ascending aorta
- Asymptomatic patients with severe chronic AR, an LVEF >50%, and an EDD >70 mm or ESD >50 mm, and there is evidence of progressive left ventricular dilatation, declining exercise tolerance, or an abnormal hemodynamic response to exercise

Class III

- Asymptomatic patients with mild, moderate, or severe chronic AR and an LVEF >50% at rest and an EDD <70 mm or ESD <50 mm.

*Bonow, RO, et al. ACC/AHA 2006 guidelines for the management of patients with valvular heart disease. J Am Coll Cardiol 2006; 48: 598–675.

Right heart valve lesions

Tricuspid stenosis (TS)

Causes include rheumatic fever (almost always associated with MS), congenital, carcinoid, and pacemaker lead.

Symptoms are fatigue, anorexia, and peripheral edema.

Examination

Look for wasting, edema, hepatomegaly, and elevated JVP with prominent a-waves. Rumbling mid-diastolic murmur is heard best at lower left sternal border (LLSB) in inspiration.

Investigation

- *ECG:* sinus rhythm, RA enlargement (tall peaked p-waves in II, V1 often coincides with signs of LA enlargement because of MS) but no RVH.
- *CXR:* enlarged RA but normal PA size.
- *TTE:* 2D image can show thickened restricted leaflets. CW Doppler is diagnostic of increased transvalvular gradient. If diagnosis of TS is made, always look for coexistent MS.

Treatment

Salt restriction and diuretics may markedly improve symptoms. If coexistent MS is being operated on, then surgical valvuloplasty may help.

Tricuspid valve (TV) replacement is occasionally performed. Bioprosthetic valves give better results than mechanical valves.

TV balloon valvuloplasty is an alternative to surgery.

Tricuspid regurgitation (TR)

Causes

These include any cause of RV dilatation (MV disease, congenital heart disease, RV infarction, pulmonary embolism, pulmonary hypertension), infective endocarditis (particularly IV drug abuse), Marfan's syndrome, Ebstein anomaly, rheumatic fever, and carcinoid causes.

Symptoms

Symptoms are usually mild. As right heart failure develops, patients complain of edema, ascites, nausea, anorexia, and abdominal pain (tender, congested liver).

Examination

Look for cachexia/wasting, jaundice, and edema. AF is common, along with elevated JVP with systolic V waves and tender pulsatile hepatomegaly. On auscultation RV S3 is often heard, and systolic murmur is audible at LSB (increases with inspiration). Murmur is loudest in TR secondary to pulmonary hypertension

Investigation
- *ECG*: nonspecific may show evidence of underlying condition, RA enlargement.
- *CXR*: cardiomegaly in patients with functional TR, RA/RV enlargement, occasional distended azygos vein, pleural effusion.
- *TTE*: color Doppler confirms diagnosis. CW Doppler of TR jet can assess RV systolic pressure. Flow reversal in hepatic vein suggests severe TR. 2D images may reveal etiology of TR (RV infarction, ASD/VSD, Ebstein's, etc.).

Treatment
In the absence of pulmonary hypertension, TR is well tolerated and may not require specific treatment (in infective endocarditis of TV, valve excision is sometimes performed with good recovery). Symptoms of RV failure respond to diuretics and fluid/salt restriction.

If coexistent MV disease is being operated on and TR is mild (with minimally elevated PA pressure), TR usually improves following surgery as PA pressure falls. In patients with severe TR due to annular dilatation, TV annuloplasty may be indicated.

TR secondary to valve pathology (Ebstein's, carcinoid) may require valve replacement, preferably with a large bioprosthesis to minimize risk of thrombosis.

Pulmonic stenosis
Causes include congenital, carcinoid, and rheumatic causes and extrinsic compression. Stenosis may be valvular or supravalvular.

Symptoms
Usually there are none. With severe stenosis there is exertional dyspnea and light-headedness. Eventually symptoms of RV failure may develop.

Examination
Look for prominent a-wave in JVP, RV heave, and occasional thrill in second left intercostal space. On auscultation there is a widely split S2 (as pulmonary valve [PV] closure becomes delayed), P2 becomes softer (unless stenosis is supravalvular), and systolic ejection murmur at left upper sternal border (LUSB), heard best in inspiration.

Investigation
- *ECG*: RVH and RA abnormality.
- *CXR*: dilated pulmonary arteries, occasionally with calcification of valve; if severe then oligemic lung fields.
- *TTE* confirms the diagnosis and level of obstruction (valvular, supravalvular, or RV outflow tract) and measures pressure gradient. It can also demonstrate associated conditions (ASD, PDA, TOF, etc.).
- *Cardiac catheterization* is used to assess the severity of obstruction and hemodynamic effects.

Treatment

In general, invasive intervention is recommended when the gradient across the valve is >50 mmHg at rest or when symptoms occur.

- *Medical therapy* includes supportive/symptomatic treatment of RV failure (diuretics, salt and fluid restriction).
- *Balloon valvuloplasty* is the treatment of choice for stenosis at the valvular level. It is highly effective and safe with good long-term results.
- *Surgical valvotomy* is very effective with minimal recurrence, though significant pulmonary regurgitation may occur.
- *Pulmonary valve replacement* is indicated if the patient is not suitable for above treatments or develops severe PR following intervention.

Pulmonary regurgitation

Causes

These include pulmonary hypertension (causes dilatation of valve ring), infective endocarditis (rarely involves pulmonic valve), connective tissue disease (e.g. Marfan's), and iatrogenic (following valvotomy, valvuloplasty or PA catheter placement) carcinoid causes.

Symptoms

Patients are often asymptomatic. Symptoms develop when pulmonary hypertension or RV failure occurs and include dyspnea on exertion, lethargy, peripheral edema, and abdominal pain.

Examination

Look for RV heave, occasionally a thrill in pulmonary area. On auscultation P2 may be delayed (large stroke volume), loud (if pulmonary hypertension), or soft (if PV stenosis). Murmur of pulmonary regurgitation (PR) is heard best in the third to fourth intercostal space along the LSB and increases with inspiration.

Investigation

- *ECG*: RVH (if pulmonary hypertension), RBBB/rsR pattern in V1
- *CXR*: enlarged PA and RV
- *TTE*: 2D images may show RV dilatation/hypertrophy. There is abnormal septal motion with RV volume overload. PR is seen on color Doppler and quantified with pulsed Doppler.

Treatment

Usually, supportive treatment suffices. Treat RV failure in the usual way (diuretics, etc.). If PR is due to PV ring dilatation secondary to pulmonary hypertension, treating the cause of pulmonary hypertension can relieve this and decrease the severity of PR (e.g., mitral valve surgery).

If there is severe right heart failure then PV replacement can be considered.

Prosthetic heart valves

Types
- *Mechanical:* ball and cage (Starr–Edwards) or tilting disc (single leaflet—Medtronic Hall, Bjork–Shiley; bileaflet—St. Jude Medical, Carbomedics) (see Fig. 4.5)
- *Bioprosthetic:* porcine or bovine (Carpentier–Edwards)
- *Homograft:* preserved human cadaveric valve

Mechanical valves
These valves are very durable (often last >20 years). They are thrombogenic, therefore require lifelong warfarin therapy (± aspirin if high risk).

Ball and cage valves are earlier models that are very durable but also highly thrombogenic and require more intensive anticoagulation. More recent tilting disc valves are less thrombogenic (bileaflet valves are less thrombogenic than single-leaflet valves).

The most commonly used prosthesis in practice today is the bileaflet valve.

Tissue valves
Tissue valves (bioprosthetic or homograft) have the advantage of not requiring long-term anticoagulation but are not as durable as mechanical valves (15-year failure rate of 10%–20% for homografts and 20%–30% for bioprostheses, and higher rates for patients <40 years of age).

Consequently, mechanical valves tend to be placed in younger patients (<65 years) or those with another reason for warfarin (AF, hypercoagulable state). Bioprostheses are generally implanted in older patients or those who refuse warfarin (see Table 4.4).

Valve hemodynamics
Different prosthetic valves have unique profiles and valve areas. For any given valve dimension, bioprosthetic valves and ball and cage valves have the smallest effective valve orifice area, and homografts have the largest valve area (comparable to native valve area).

Assessment of prosthetic valve function
Clinically
Each prosthetic valve produces a distinctive sound. Dysfunction may be indicated by new sounds, a change in sound or volume of sound, or a new (or changing) murmur.

Imaging modality
Fluoroscopy can be used to assess mechanical valve leaflet movement. Diminished leaflet motion is seen in valve thrombosis whereas excessive movement of the base ring may indicate prosthetic valve dehiscence.

TTE is of limited use because of shadowing caused by metallic leaflets in mechanical valves. It can be used to look at valve ring motion (in mechanical valves), leaflet motion (in tissue valves), and regurgitation (with Doppler).

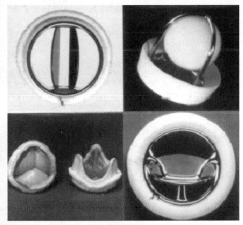

Figure 4.5 Common types of heart valve prostheses (from top left clockwise): St. Jude's Medical bileaflet, Starr–Edwards ball and cage, Bjork–Shiley tilting disk, stented porcine prosthesis. Reproduced with permission from Bloomfield P (2002). *Heart* 87(6):583–589.

Table 4.4 Class I and II AHA/ACC recommendations for choice of prosthetic valve*

Recommendations for valve replacement with a mechanical prosthesis	
Patients with expected long lifespan	I
Patients with a mechanical valve already in place in a different position than the valve being replaced	I
Patients with renal failure on hemodialysis or with hypercalcemia	II
Patients requiring anticoagulation due to risk factors for thromboembolism[†]	IIa
Patients <65 years for AVR and <0 years for MVR	IIa
Recommendations for valve replacement with a bioprosthesis	
Patients who cannot or will not take warfarin treatment	I
Patients >65 years needing AVR with no risk factors for thromboembolism[†]	I
Patients considered to have possible compliance problems with warfarin	IIa
Patients > 70 years needing MVR with no risk factors for thromboembolism[†]	IIa
Valve replacement for thrombosed mechanical valve	IIb

* Reproduced with permission from Bloomfield P (2002). *Heart* 87(6):583–589.

[†] Risk factors: atrial fibrillation, severe LV dysfunction, previous thromboembolism, hypercoagulable condition. AVR (aortic valve replacement); MVR (mitral valve replacement).

TEE is better at assessing prosthetic mitral valve function than it is for prosthetic aortic valves.

MRI is safe for modern mechanical valves, but is expensive and time consuming, therefore reserved for cases when TTE/TEE is inconclusive.

Cardiac catheterization

This modality can be used to assess valve gradient (and thus valve area). It can quantify the degree of regurgitation.

Because there is a risk of passing the catheter across mechanical valves, it is used prior to reoperation or when noninvasive tests are inconclusive.

Prosthetic heart valves: complications

Valve thrombosis

- *Incidence:* 0.1%–5.7% per patient-year.
- *Risks:* inadequate anticoagulation and mitral prostheses. There are similar rates for bioprosthetic valves and mechanical valves receiving adequate anticoagulation. There is no difference in rates between different types of mechanical valves receiving adequate anticoagulation.
- *Clinical presentation:* pulmonary edema, systemic embolism, sudden death
- *Investigation:* decreased intensity of valve sounds, decreased leaflet motion on TTE or fluoroscopy, and increased valve gradient on TTE
- *Treatment:* anticoagulation with heparin. If thrombus is <5 mm on TTE then anticoagulation may suffice. If >5 mm, then will need further treatment (thrombolysis, thrombectomy or valve replacement).
- *Prognosis:* valve replacement for valve thrombus has a mortality rate of <15%, thrombolysis has a mortality rate of <10% (with embolization in <20%). Thrombolysis is more effective for aortic valve thrombosis and in recent (<2 week) onset.

Systemic embolization

The most common manifestation is TIA or stroke.

- *Incidence:* 4% per patient-year with no anticoagulation, 2% per patient-year on aspirin, and 1% per patient-year on warfarin.
- *Risks:* AF, age >70 years, depressed LV function, mitral prostheses, ball and cage valves, >1 valve, suboptimal anticoagulation, infective endocarditis.

Hemolysis

A low level of background hemolysis is common in patients with mechanical prostheses (even when functioning normally). Severe hemolysis is uncommon and is usually secondary to valve dysfunction (paravalvular leak, dehiscence, infection). Hemolysis is uncommon in tissue prostheses.

- *Investigation:* anemia, elevated LDH, low serum haptoglobin level, reticulocytosis, schistocytes on peripheral smear.
- *Treatment:* treat underlying problem (including further valve surgery if needed); give blood transfusion, folic acid, and iron supplementation.

Endocarditis

Prevalence

Endocarditis occurs at some point in 3%–6% of patients with prosthetic valves. Risk is greatest <3 months after implantation.

Early endocarditis occurs within 60 days of valve surgery and late endocarditis occurs >60 days since surgery.

Early prosthetic valve endocarditis (PVE) usually arises from skin or wound infections or indwelling IV catheters and is commonly due to S. aureus, S. epidermidis, gram-negative bacteria, and fungi. Late PVE has similar microbiology to that of native valve endocarditis. The risk is similar for tissue and mechanical valves.

All patients with prosthetic valves should receive antibiotic prophylaxis during dental procedures.

Infective endocarditis

Epidemiology
There are approximately 15,000 new cases diagnosed in the United States annually with a male predominance (M:F 2.5:1). Mitral valve prolapse with MR and degenerative aortic valve disease are the leading predisposing conditions.

The incidence of nosocomial and iatrogenic infections is rising due to the increased use of dialysis catheters, permanent pacemakers, and other indwelling central venous catheters (see Table 4.5). The mitral valve is most commonly involved, followed by the aortic valve.

Right-sided endocarditis, usually tricuspid valve, generally occurs in IV drug users. The majority of patients (75%) with infective endocarditis (IE) have underlying structural heart disease.

Pathogenesis
Valvular endothelium is damaged from local trauma, turbulence or metabolic changes leading to platelet and fibrin deposition, which results in nonbacterial thrombotic lesions. These areas are subsequently colonized during an episode of bacteremia resulting from trauma to mucous membranes or other colonized tissue.

Once colonization of the valve occurs, bacterial division and further platelet/fibrin deposition results in a mature vegetation that can lead to valve ring abscess, valve regurgitation, and valve perforation.

Staphylococci and streptococci account for most cases (Table 4.6). Vegetations are usually localized downstream from regurgitant flow along lines of valve closure. Both humoral and cellular immunity are stimulated.

Symptoms
Noncardiac symptoms are constitutional and include malaise, anorexia, weight loss, fever, rigors, and night sweats.

Cardiovascular symptoms depend on the valve involved and the severity of valve destruction and include CHF, syncope, and chest pain from pericarditis or myocardial ischemia.

Patients may also have pulmonary symptoms in right-sided endocarditis. Embolic phenomena are common (up to 1/3 patients) and may be asymptomatic.

Physical exam
In addition to nonspecific findings associated with systemic infection (i.e., fever, tachycardia), the following findings are unique (see also Table 4.7):
- *Osler node*: small, painful nodular lesions on the pads of fingers and toes. They are often multiple and are due to immune complex deposition.
- *Janeway lesions:* hemorrhagic macular painless plaques seen on the palms and soles. They are due to peripheral embolization.
- *Splinter hemorrhage*: narrow, reddish-brown lines of blood beneath the nails due to vasculitis or microemboli.
- *Roth spots*: oval, pale retinal lesions surrounded by hemorrhage. They are located near the optic disk.

Table 4.5 Risk factors for infective endocarditis

High risk	Prosthetic valves
	Previous bacterial endocarditis
	Aortic valve disease
	Mitral regurgitation or mixed mitral disease
	Cyanotic congenital heart disease
	Patent ductus arteriosis
	Uncorrected L-to-R shunt
	Intracardiac and systemic-pulmonary shunts
Moderate risk	MVP with regurgitation or valve thickening
	Isolated mitral stenosis
	Tricuspid valve disease
	Pulmonic stenosis
	Hypertrophic cardiomyopathy
	Bicuspid aortic valve disease
	Degenerative valve disease in elderly
	Mural thrombus (e.g., post-infarction)
Low risk	MVP without regurgitation
	Tricuspid incompetence without structural abnormality
	Isolated ASD
	Surgically corrected L-to-R shunt with no residual shunt
	Calcification of MV annulus
	Ischemic heart disease and/or previous CABG
	Permanent pacemaker
	Atrial myxoma

Other predisposing factors

- Arterial prostheses or arteriovenous fistulas
- Recurrent bacteremia (e.g., IV-drug users, severe periodontal disease, colon carcinoma)
- Conditions predisposing to infections (e.g., diabetes, renal failure, alcoholism, immunosuppression)
- Recent central line

In many cases no obvious risk factor is identified.

Table 4.6 Microbiology of infective endocarditis

40%	Streptococci (especially *Strep. viridans* group)
	Enterococci
10%	Staphylococci
30%–40%	*S. aureus* – coagulase positive
	S. epidermidis = coagulase negative
5–10%	Culture negative
<1%	Gram-negative bacilli
<1%	Multiple organisms
<1%	Diptheroids
<1%	Fungi

Table 4.7 Extracardiac manifestations in infective endocarditis

Central nervous system
- Cerebral emboli/infarction, arteritis, abscess, mycotic aneurysm, intracerebral hemorrhage, cerebritis/meningitis

Kidney
- Glomerulonephritis, infarcts, abscess

Spleen
- Abscess, infarct

Lung
- Pulmonary emboli, pleural effusion

Skin
- Osler nodes, Janeway lesions, splinter hemorrhages, palatal petechiae

Eye
- Roth spots, conjunctival petechiae

Musculoskeletal
- Mono- or oligoarthritis

Patients with significant cardiac complications may have rales, S3 (if CHF), pericardial rub (if abscess, pericarditis), hypotension, tachycardia, altered mental status, decreased urine output (if cardiogenic shock), and wide pulse pressure (in severe acute AR). Unique exam findings may be seen following systemic embolization (i.e., focal neurological deficits).

Cardiac complications

These occur in up to 50% of patients and include the following:
- *CHF:* due to acute valvular insufficiency, aortic > mitral. This is the leading cause of death in patients with IE.
- *Perivalvular abscess: S. aureus* is most common. Abscess is associated with increased mortality. Aortic valve involvement and IV drug use are risk factors. It may extend into the septum and cause conduction abnormalities, including AV block.
- *Myocardial infarction:* rare complication of IE due to coronary emboli
- *Pericarditis:* associated with myocardial abscess.
- *Hemopericardium/fistulas:* due to rupture of mycotic aneurysm on sinus of Valsalva. These have a high mortality of >40%.

Systemic embolization

This is a common complication, occurring in one-third of patients. Left-sided endocarditis, especially mitral valve, is the most common predisposing lesion. Other factors associated with increased risk include vegetation size >10 mm; highly mobile vegetations; *S. bovis, S. aureus,* and *Candida* infection; and antiphospholipid antibodies.

Anticoagulation is not indicated and may increase the risk of hemorrhagic stroke and death.

Diagnosis

Diagnosis is based on clinical history and physical exam as well as blood culture and echocardiographic findings. The modified Duke criteria system (Box 4.6) is the most widely used classification scheme and is highly specific (99%) and sensitive (92%).

Echocardiography

TTE has a low sensitivity of <50% but a high specificity of 98% for the diagnosis of infective endocarditis. TEE has a sensitivity of 75%–95% and a specificity of 85%–98% and is the recommended diagnostic imaging test in patients with prosthetic valves, cases rated at least possible IE by clinical criteria, and patients with complications. TEE is also recommended when the clinical suspicion for IE is high despite a negative TTE.

Box 4.6 Duke criteria

Definite endocarditis	Direct evidence of endocarditis from histological or microbiological findings from surgical or autopsy specimens. Clinical diagnosis requires 2 major criteria, 1 major and 3 minor criteria, or 5 minor criteria.
Possible endocarditis	Findings that fall short of definite endocarditis but are not rejected. Requires 1 major and 1 or 2 minor clinical criteria or 3 minor criteria
Rejected diagnosis	Firm alternative diagnosis, or sustained resolution of clinical features with <4 days of antibiotic therapy

Major criteria

- Positive blood culture
  - Typical microorganism for IE from two separate blood cultures
  - Persistently positive blood culture
  - Single positive blood culture or titer for Q fever
- Evidence of endocardial involvement
  - Positive echocardiogram.
    —Oscillating intracardiac mass (vegetation)
    —Abscess
    —New partial dehiscence of prosthetic valve
  - New valve regurgitation

Minor criteria

- Predisposing condition or IV drug use
- Fever >38°C
- Vascular phenomena: arterial emboli, septic pulmonary infarcts, mycotic aneurysm, intracranial and conjunctival hemorrhage, Janeway lesions
- Immunological phenomena: glomerulonephritis, Osler's nodes, Roth spots, rheumatoid factor
- Positive blood cultures not meeting major criteria

Medical therapy

Intravenous bactericidal antibiotics are the cornerstone of therapy and should be guided by the suspected organism and local resistance patterns (see Table 4.8). Blood culture data, including antibiotic susceptibility and minimum inhibitory concentration, should be used to tailor therapy to the causative organisms.

Antibiotics are typically continued for 4–6 weeks. Surveillance blood cultures should be obtained to document clearance of the bacteremia.

Indications for surgery

- Hemodynamic instability (CHF, AV block)
- Severe valvular insufficiency
- Abscess, fistulas
- Fungal endocarditis
- Other organisms (*Pseudomonas aeruginosa, Brucella* species, *Coxiella burnetii*)
- Recurrent emboli
- Persistent bacteremia despite antibiotics
- Large, mobile vegetations >10 mm in size
- Prosthetic valve endocarditis if dehiscence, valve obstruction or worsening regurgitation

Prognosis

Overall mortality can be as high as 20%–25% and depends on co-morbidities, the presence of cardiac complications, and the causative organism. *S. aureus*, fungi, and gram-negative organisms are associated with higher mortality than that with streptococcal species.

Antibiotic prophylaxis during dental procedures

Current recommendations (2007 AHA guidelines) for antimicrobial prophylaxis for dental and other procedures are limited to cardiac conditions associated with the highest risk for adverse outcomes from endocarditis:
- Prosthetic cardiac valve or prosthetic material used for valve repair
- Previous infective endocarditis
- Congenital heart disease
  - Unrepaired cyanotic lesions
  - Repaired defects using prosthetic material or devices for 6 months
  - Residual defects following repair
- Cardiac transplant recipients with valvulopathy
- Dental procedures involving gingival manipulation and respiratory tract procedures involving incision or biopsy require prophylaxis.

Routine prophylaxis is no longer recommended for gastrointestinal or genitourinary procedures. The primary antibiotic regimen for most patients is amoxicillin, 2 g po 30–60 minutes before the procedure.

Cephalexin, azithromycin, or clindamycin can be used in penicillin-allergic patients.

Table 4.8 Antibiotic regimens

Penicillin-susceptible streptococci (MIC ≤0.12 µg/mL)	Penicillin G or ceftriaxone or vancomycin for 4 weeks
Penicillin-intermediate susceptible streptococci (MIC >0.12 µg/mL but <0.5 µg/mL)	Either penicillin G or ceftriaxone for 4 weeks plus gentamicin for 2 weeks, or monotherapy with vancomycin 4 weeks
Penicillin-susceptible enterococci	Gentamicin for 4–6 weeks plus either penicillin G, ampicillin, or vancomycin for 4–6 weeks
Penicillin-resistant enterococci Vancomycin/penicillin/ aminoglycoside resistant enterococci	Gentamicin for 6 weeks plus either ampicillin-sulbactam (if β-lactamase producing) or vancomycin for 6 weeks
E. faecium	Linezolid ≥8 weeks or quinupristin-dalfopristin ≥8 weeks
E. faecalis	Imipenem/cilastatin plus ampicillin ≥8 weeks or ceftriaxone plus ampicillin ≥8 weeks
Oxacillin-susceptible staphylococci	Nafcillin, oxacillin, or cefazolin for 6 weeks plus gentamicin for 3–5 days
Oxacillin resistant staphylococci	Vancomycin for 6 weeks
HACEK organisms	Ceftriaxone, ampicillin-sulbactam, or ciprofloxacin for 4 weeks
Culture-negative endocarditis	Ampicillin-sulbactam plus gentamicin for 4–6 weeks or vancomycin plus gentamicin plus ciprofloxacin 4–6 weeks

Adapted from AHA Scientific Statement on Infective Endocarditis, *Circulation* 2005; 111(23):3167–3184.

Heart failure

Introduction

Definition

Heart failure (HF) is a progressive condition with several stages as outlined by the ACC/AHA Task Force (stages A–D, see Fig. 5.1). *Heart failure* can be defined as a clinical syndrome that results from any structural or functional abnormality of the heart that impairs the ability of the left ventricle to fill with or to eject blood. It is characterized by dyspnea and/or fatigue on exertion (and occasionally at rest) and evidence of fluid retention that may lead to peripheral edema or pulmonary congestion.

A clinical response to treatment directed at heart failure *alone* (e.g., diuretic use) is not sufficient for diagnosis.

Epidemiology and prognosis

The development of new therapeutic innovations for coronary artery disease coupled with an aging population has led to an increase in the prevalence of heart failure. There are currently over 5 million cases in the United States and an estimated 23 million people with heart failure worldwide. Nearly one million new cases are diagnosed annually worldwide.

The lifetime risk of developing heart failure for all comers over the age of 40 is 20%. The prevalence increases with age, with the mean age of the heart failure population being in their mid-70s.

Despite improvement in prognosis in coronary artery disease, the prognosis in heart failure remains poor with over 50% of all patients hospitalized for the first time with heart failure dying within 5 years.

Patients with heart failure can die suddenly (as the result of ventricular tachyarrhythmias) or with worsening heart failure symptoms and fluid overload.

Pathophysiology

The origin of symptoms in heart failure is poorly understood. An initial event (infarction, inflammation, pressure/volume overload) causes myocardial damage resulting in an increase in myocardial wall stress. This is followed by the activation of multiple neuroendocrine systems including the renin–angiotensin–aldosterone system, the sympathetic nervous system, and the release of cytokines such as tumor necrosis factor (TNF).

Neuroendocrine activation is also accompanied by structural and metabolic changes in the peripheral skeletal muscle and by abnormalities in cardiopulmonary reflex function, such as the baroreflex and chemoreflex. These produce further wall stress perpetuating this vicious cycle (see Fig. 5.2).

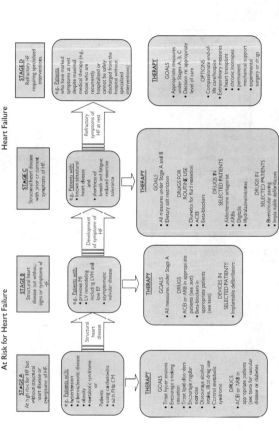

Figure 5.1 Stages of heart failure. ACE-, angiotensin-converting enzyme inhibitor; ARB, angiotensin receptor blocker; HF, heart failure. Reprinted with permission from the ACC/AHA Guidelines 2005. *Circulation* 2005; 112:e154–e235. ©2005, American Heart Association, Inc.

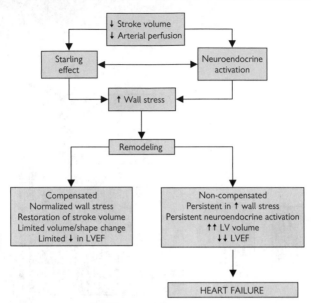

Figure 5.2 Pathophysiology of heart failure.

Forms of heart failure

Acute vs. chronic heart failure
The clinical manifestations depend on the speed with which the syndrome develops. Acute heart failure is often used to describe the patient with acute-onset dyspnea and pulmonary edema, but it can also apply to cardiogenic shock where the patient is hypotensive and oliguric. Compensatory mechanisms have not yet become operative.

Acute deterioration may be a consequence of myocardial infarction (MI), arrhythmia, or acute valve dysfunction (e.g., endocarditis).

Systolic vs. diastolic heart failure
Most patients with heart failure have impaired LV systolic function: there is a failure of the LV to eject blood.

However, there is a group of patients with signs and symptoms of heart failure but apparently preserved LV systolic function. These patients are said to have diastolic heart failure: there is an abnormality in the ability of the LV to fill in diastole. This may be transient (e.g., acute ischemia) or persistent (restrictive or infiltrative cardiomyopathy, or LVH).

Right vs. left heart failure
Right and *left heart failure* refers to whether the patient has either predominantly systemic venous congestion (swollen ankles, hepatomegaly) or pulmonary venous congestion (pulmonary edema), respectively. These terms do not necessarily indicate which ventricle is most seriously affected.

Fluid retention in heart failure is due to a combination of factors: reduced GFR (glomerular filtration rate) and activation of the renin–angiotensin–aldosterone system and sympathetic system. However, there are causes for swollen ankles other than heart failure (gravitational disorder, e.g., immobility; venous thrombosis or obstruction; varicose veins; hypoproteinemia, e.g., nephrotic syndrome or liver disease; or lymphatic obstruction; see also Box 5.1).

High-output vs. low-output heart failure
A variety of high-output states may lead to heart failure, e.g., thyrotoxicosis, Paget's disease, beriberi, and anemia. High-output failure is characterized by warm extremities and normal or widened pulse pressure.

In contrast, low-output states are characterized by cool, pale extremities, cyanosis due to systemic vasoconstriction, and low pulse volume.

The mixed venous oxygen saturation (a marker of the ability of the heart to deliver oxygen to the metabolizing tissues) is typically abnormally low in low-output states but normal or even high in high-output states.

Box 5.1 Conditions mimicking heart failure

- Obesity
- Chest disease, including lung, diaphragm, or chest wall
- Venous insufficiency in lower limbs
- Drug-induced ankle swelling (e.g., dihydropyridine calcium blockers)
- Drug-induced fluid retention (e.g., NSAIDs)
- Hypoalbuminemia
- Intrinsic renal disease
- Intrinsic hepatic disease
- Pulmonary embolic disease
- Depression and/or anxiety disorders
- Severe anemia
- Thyroid disease
- Bilateral renal artery stenosis

Causes and precipitants

In all patients with heart failure it is important to carefully consider the underlying etiology, as there may be specific exacerbating factors or other diseases that influence the patients' management. A nonexhaustive list is given in Box 5.2.

Patients with compensated heart failure have a high rate of readmission to hospital with acute exacerbations. A number of studies have demonstrated that a precipitating cause for emergency admission to the hospital with heart failure can be identified in up to two-thirds of patients.

- *Inappropriate reduction in therapy:* self-discontinuation or iatrogenic withdrawal of diuretics, ACE-I, digoxin, and dietary excess of salt are recognized precipitants. Education of the patient and family is important.
- *Cardiac arrhythmias:* most commonly AF, but any tachyarrhythmia will further reduce LV filling and stroke volume, and may exacerbate ischemia. Marked bradycardia reduces cardiac output especially if stroke volume cannot increase any further.
- *Myocardial ischemia or infarction* exacerbates LV dysfunction and may worsen mitral regurgitation due to ischemia of papillary muscles.
- *Infection:* respiratory infections are a common precipitant, but any systemic infection can precipitate heart failure through a combination of factors, including direct myocardial depression from inflammatory cytokines, sinus tachycardia, and fever.
- *Anemia:* this causes a high-output state that may precipitate acute heart failure and may exacerbate underlying ischemia.
- *Concomitant drug therapy:* drugs that directly depress myocardial function (e.g., calcium antagonists—verapamil, diltiazem; many antiarrhythmics, anesthetics, overenthusiastic initiation of β-blockers, etc.) as well as drugs causing salt and water retention (e.g., NSAIDs, estrogens, steroids, COX-2 antagonists) may precipitate heart failure.
- *Alcohol:* this is directly toxic and in excess can depress myocardial function and predispose to arrhythmias.
- *Pulmonary embolism:* the risk increases in the immobile patient with low-output state and atrial fibrillation.

It is very important to look for precipitating causes in all patients with heart failure (see Table 5.1). Once the precipitant has been identified and treated, appropriate measures (patient and family education, adjustment of therapy) should be put into place to prevent recurrence.

Box 5.2 Etiology of heart failure

- Ischemic heart disease (most common cause in developed world)
- Dilated cardiomyopathy
- Post viral
- Alcohol
- Hypothyroidism
- Hypertension
- Hemachromatosis
- Familial
- Infiltration (amyloid/sarcoid)
- Valve disease
- Postpartum
- Chemotherapy
- Radiotherapy
- Infections (Chagas disease)
- Nutritional (beriberi)

Table 5.1 Population-attributable risk of heart failure related to various risk factors*

Risk factor	Attributable risk (%)
Coronary disease	61.6
Cigarette smoking	17.1
Hypertension	10.1
Physical inactivity	9.2
Male sex	8.9
Less than high school education	8.9
Overweight	8.0
Diabetes	3.1
Valvular heart disease	2.2

* Reproduced with permission from He J, Ogden LG, Bazzano LA, et al. (2001). *Arch Intern Med* 161:996. Copyright © 2001 American Medical Association. All rights reserved.

Diagnosis and initial workup

Signs and symptoms

The diagnosis of heart failure is a clinical diagnosis, using the history, physical exam, chest X-ray (CXR) and other diagnostic tests (i.e., transthoracic echocardiogram [TTE]) to make the diagnosis. Box 5.3 provides a list of some of the most common signs and symptoms of heart failure.

Symptoms alone can be used to classify the severity of congestive heart failure (CHF) and to monitor the effect of treatment. The New York Heart Association classification (NYHA) is widely used (Table 5.2).

Investigations for all patients with heart failure (see Fig. 5.3)

ECG
Although there are no specific changes in CHF, a completely normal ECG should encourage you to reconsider the diagnosis. Look for AF or other tachy- or bradyarrhythmias, conduction system defects, evidence of previous MI, or ongoing ischemia.

CXR
See Figure 5.4. A normal CXR and ECG make the diagnosis of heart failure very unlikely.

Echocardiogram
This is the key investigation in patients with heart failure. It is used to evaluate resting LV size and function and to rule out valvular heart disease, pericardial disease and myocardial diseases. Absolute values for ejection fraction do not necessarily reflect the clinical severity of heart failure.

Box 5.3 Common signs and symptoms of heart failure

- Dyspnea (exertion or at rest)
- Fatigue
- Paroxysmal nocturnal dyspnea
- Orthopnea
- Palpitations
- Raised JVP
- Third heart sound
- Hepatomegaly
- Peripheral edema
- Chest pain
- Cachexia
- Sleep apnea

Table 5.2 NYHA classification of heart failure

Class I	No limitation of physical activity
Class II	Slight limitation of physical activity—symptoms with ordinary levels of exertion (e.g., walking up stairs)
Class III	Marked limitation of physical activity—symptoms with minimal levels of exertion (e.g., dressing)
Class IV	Symptoms at rest

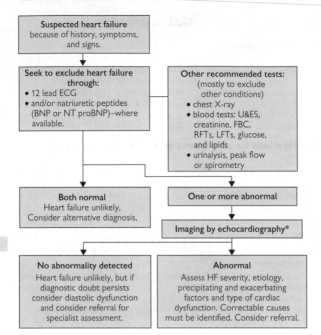

Figure 5.3 Algorithm summarizing recommendations for the diagnosis of heart failure.

Alternative methods of imaging the heart should be considered when a poor image is produced by transthoracic Doppler 2D echocardiography. Alternatives include transesophageal echocardiography (TEE), radionuclide imaging, or cardiac magnetic resonance imaging. BNP, B-type natriuretic peptide; ECG, electrocardiogram; CBC, complete blood count; LFTs, liver function tests; NTproBNP, N-terminal pro-B-type natriuretic peptide; TFTs, thyroid function tests; U&Es, urea and electrolytes.

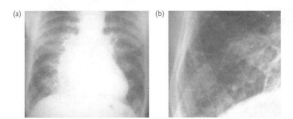

Figure 5.4 CXR findings in heart failure. (a) There is cardiomegaly with prominent upper lobe vessels and alveolar edema ("bat's wing shadowing"). (b) Magnification of right costophrenic angle showing septal lines (Kerley B lines) due to interstitial edema.

Blood tests

These may alert you to possible underlying etiologies for heart failure as well as establishing a baseline prior to initiation of therapy.

- CBC (anemia), Chem7, glucose, liver function tests (LFTs), thyroid function tests (TFTs) (hypo- or hyperthyroidism), uric acid
- BNP has a high negative predictive value if <100 pg/mL.

Investigations for selected patients with heart failure

- Ferritin
- Immunoglobulins and protein electrophoresis
- Viral titers
- BNP: serum levels of natriuretic peptides are frequently elevated in patients with impaired LV function. They appear to have a useful role in identifying patients who merit more extensive investigation of cardiac function.
- Coronary angiography
- Holter monitoring (± QT dispersion, heart rate variability)
- Cardiopulmonary exercise testing or 6-minute walk test
- Pulmonary function tests
- Radionuclide ventriculography
- Stress imaging (for assessment of viable/hibernating myocardium)
- Cardiac magnetic resonance

By using these signs and symptoms as well as initial basic diagnostic tests, one can make the diagnosis of heart failure with reasonable certainty (see Table 5.3).

Table 5.3 Framingham criteria for diagnosis of heart failure*

Major criteria

• Paroxysmal nocturnal dyspnea	• S3 gallop rhythm
• Raised JVP; distended neck veins	• Hepatojugular reflux
• Crackles in lung fields	• Weight loss >4.5 kg in 5 days in response to treatment of heart failure
• Cardiomegaly on CXR	
• Acute pulmonary edema	

Minor criteria

• Bilateral ankle edema	• Pleural effusion
• Nocturnal cough	• Tachycardia rate >120/min
• Dyspnea on ordinary exertion	• Decrease in vital capacity by one-third
• Hepatomegaly	

* This table was published in Ho KL (1993). The epidemiology of heart failure: the Framingham Study. *J Am Coll Cardiol*, 22(Suppl A):6A. Copyright Elsevier 1993.

Management

Management outline
- Establish that the patient has heart failure.
- Ascertain severity of symptoms and presenting features: pulmonary edema, exertional breathlessness, fatigue, peripheral edema.
- Try to determine the etiology of heart failure.
- Identify precipitating and exacerbating factors and any concomitant diseases relevant to heart failure and its management.
- Estimate prognosis.
- Anticipate complications.
- Counsel the patient and relatives.
- Choose appropriate management (e.g., see Fig. 5.5).
- Monitor progress and manage accordingly.

Aims of treatment

1. Prevention of heart failure
- Prevention and/or controlling of diseases leading to cardiac dysfunction and heart failure
- Prevention of progression to heart failure once cardiac dysfunction is established

2. Maintenance or improvement in quality of life

3. Increased duration of life
It is always better to try and prevent heart failure than to treat it once it has developed. This includes management of risk factors for ischemic heart disease, treatment of ischemia and revascularization where appropriate, early reperfusion therapy for acute MI, aggressive management of hypertension, and management of diabetes and valvular heart disease. Stop exacerbating drugs if possible (NSAIDs, steroids, negative inotropes).

Education of the patient and relatives is an important aspect of management of patients with heart failure. Many hospitals now employ heart failure specialist nurses who are able to provide excellent service and should be used whenever possible. Formal cardiac rehabilitation classes may be beneficial. It is important to explain the diagnosis and symptoms, how the treatment will help, the role of self-weighing, and the importance of exercise. Mild to moderate aerobic exercise can increase functional capacity in these patients.

General measures include restriction of dietary salt and water intake, smoking cessation, reducing alcohol intake (stopping completely if alcohol is implicated in the etiology of HF), addressing obesity with a weight-reducing program, and vaccinations (Pneumovax once and influenza yearly).

Patients should also be counseled about their drug therapy. The desired effects and potential side effects need to be explained, as well as the fact that while effects may take some time to become apparent, it is important to stay adherent to the therapy. Self-management of diuretics may be appropriate for some patients. Patients also need to be aware of drug interactions (e.g., with over-the-counter NSAIDs).

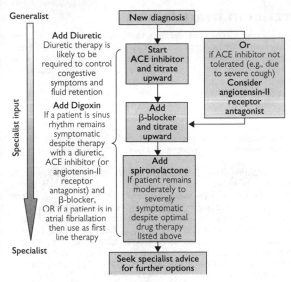

Figure 5.5 Seeking a specialist opinion for patients with heart failure. Reproduced with permission from NICE guidelines. www.nice.org.uk

Diuretics in heart failure

Diuretics are used for the symptomatic treatment of fluid overload (either pulmonary congestion or peripheral edema). With the exception of aldosterone antagonists, there are no randomized, controlled trials that have shown any prognostic benefit. However, they do improve symptoms and may slow the progression of LV remodeling.

Loop diuretics (furosemide, bumetanide, and torsemide) are the most effective. Use the lowest dose that controls symptoms effectively (see Table 5.4).

If there is insufficient response to diuretic, a combination of a loop diuretic and a thiazide diuretic can be used (see Box 5.4). Thiazides reduce magnesium absorption and hypomagnesaemia may occur with prolonged use.

Potassium-sparing diuretics (amiloride and triamterene) used alone do not achieve a net negative Na^+ balance, as Na^+ retention in HF occurs proximal in the tubule. They should be used with caution in conjunction with ACE inhibitors and spironolactone (may result in hyperkalemia).

In "diuretic resistance," the effectiveness of loop diuretics may decrease with worsening HF. This is due to a variety of factors, including reduced bioavailability of oral drug, excessive dietary salt intake, compensatory hypertrophy of the distal tubule increasing Na^+ reabsorption, other drugs (e.g., NSAIDs or COX-2 inhibitors), and reduced renal perfusion pressure by volume depletion.

This can be managed by switching to IV diuretics (perhaps by continuous infusion) and/or adding in a thiazide. In hospitalized patients, treatments such as IV dopamine at low dose and even short-term infusion of nesiritide (human BNP) have been shown to enhance effects of diuretics.

Table 5.4 Diuretics dosages for treating heart failure

Loop diuretics	Initial dose	Maximum dose
Furosemide	20–40 mg qd or bid	Titrate to achieve dry weight (up to 400 mg daily)
Bumetanide	0.5–1 mg qd or bid	Titrate to achieve dry weight (up to 10 mg daily)
Torsemide	10–20 mg qd or bid	Titrate to achieve dry weight (up to 200 mg daily)
Thiazides		
Hydrochlorothiazide	25 mg qd	50–75 mg daily
Metolazone	2.5 mg qd	10 mg daily
Indapamide	2.5 mg qd	2.5 mg daily

Box 5.4 Diuretic therapy for heart failure

Initial diuretic treatment
- Loop diuretics or thiazides.
- Always administered in addition to an ACE inhibitor (or ARB)
- If GFR <30 mL/min, do not use thiazides, except as therapy prescribed synergistically with a loop diuretics (see below).

Inadequate response
- Increase dose of diuretic.
- Combine loop diuretics and thiazides.
- With persistent fluid retention: administer loop diuretics twice daily and consider changing from furosemide to alternatives that are better absorbed (e.g., bumetanide or torsemide).
- In severe chronic heart failure add a thiazide (e.g., metolazone) with frequent measurement of creatinine and electrolytes.

Potassium-sparing diuretics: triamterene, amiloride, spironolactone
- Use only if hypokalemia persists after initiation of therapy with ACE inhibitors and diuretics.
- Start 1-week low-dose administration, check serum potassium and creatinine after 5–7 days, and titrate accordingly. Recheck every 5–7 days until potassium values are stable.

ACE, angiotensin-converting enzyme; CHF, chronic heart failure; GFR, glomerular filtration rate.

Adapted with permission from Swedberg K, et al. (2005). *Eur Heart J* 26(11):1115–1140.

ACE inhibitors for heart failure

Angiotensin-converting enzyme (ACE) inhibitors significantly improve the survival and symptoms and reduce hospitalization of patients with moderate and severe HF and LV systolic dysfunction. ACE inhibitors should be used as first-line therapy for patients with a reduced LV systolic function (ejection fraction [EF] <40%–45%). The absolute benefit is greatest in patients with most severe heart failure.

In the absence of fluid retention, ACE inhibitors should be given first. In patients with fluid retention, diuretics may be added.

Furthermore, the dosage of ACE inhibitors should be up-titrated to the dosages shown to be effective in large, controlled trials in heart failure, and not titrated on the basis of symptomatic improvement alone (see Table 5.5).

Asymptomatic patients with a documented LV systolic dysfunction benefit from long-term ACE inhibitor therapy. Large trials (SOLVD Prevention Study, SAVE, and TRACE) have shown that asymptomatic patients, but with left ventricular dysfunction, will have less development of symptomatic heart failure and hospitalizations for heart failure.

ACE inhibitors may prevent further deterioration of LV function and attenuate further cardiac dilatation. However, they do not consistently reduce cardiac size.

Starting an ACE inhibitor

- Review diuretic dose and avoid excessive diuresis before treatment.
- Consider giving first dose at night to minimize the hypotensive effect.
- Start with a low dose and build up to target levels.
- Stop treatment if there is a substantial deterioration in renal function (see Table 5.6).
- Avoid NSAIDs and potassium-sparing diuretics.
- Check BP and Chem7 1–2 weeks after each dose increment and at 6-month intervals.
- Low BP (systolic <90 mmHg) is acceptable if patient is asymptomatic.

Table 5.5 Which ACE inhibitor and at what dose?

Licensed ACE-I	Starting dose (mg)	Target dose (mg)*
Captopril	6.25 three times daily	50–100 three times daily
Enalapril	2.5 twice daily	10–20 twice daily
Fosinopril	10 once daily	40 once daily
Lisinopril	2.5–5.0 once daily	30–35 once daily
Quinapril	2.5–5.0 once daily	10–20 once daily

*Target dose is based on manufacturer's recommendation rather than large outcome study.

How to use?

- Start with a low dose (see above).
- Seek specialist advice when the patient is on a high dose (e.g., furosemide 80 mg) of a loop diuretic.
- Double dose at not less than 2-week intervals.
- Aim for target dose (see above) or, failing that, the highest tolerated dose.
- Remember, some ACE inhibitor is better than no ACE inhibitor.
- Monitor blood electrolytes (in particular potassium), urea, creatinine, and blood pressure.
- When to stop up-titration/down-titration—see Table 5.6.

Advice to patient?

- Explain expected benefits.
- Treatment is given to improve symptoms, prevent worsening of heart failure, and increase survival.
- Symptoms improve within a few weeks to a few months.
- Advise patients to report principal adverse effects, i.e., dizziness/symptomatic hypotension, cough.

Table 5.6 Problem solving with ACE inhibitors

- Asymptomatic low blood pressure usually does not require any change in therapy.

Symptomatic hypotension

- If there is dizziness, light-headedness, and/or confusion and a low blood pressure, consider discontinuing nitrates, calcium channel blockers,* and other vasodilators.
- If no signs or symptoms of congestion consider reducing diuretic dose.
- If these measures do not solve the problem seek specialist advice.

Cough

- Cough is common in patients with chronic heart failure, some of whom may also have smoking-related lung disease.
- Cough is also a symptom of pulmonary edema, which should be excluded when a new or worsening cough develops.
- ACE inhibitor–induced cough rarely requires treatment discontinuation.
- If the patient develops a troublesome dry cough that interferes with sleep and is likely to be caused by an ACE inhibitor, consider substituting an angiotensin-II receptor antagonist for the ACE inhibitor.

Worsening renal function

- Some rise in urea, creatinine, and K^+ is expected after initiation of an ACE inhibitor; if the increase is small and asymptomatic no action is necessary.
- An increase in creatinine of up to 50% above baseline, or to 200 μmol, whichever is smaller, is acceptable.
- An increase in K^+ to ≤5.9 mmol/L is acceptable.
- If urea, creatinine, or K^+ rise excessively, consider stopping concomitant nephrotoxic drugs (e.g., NSAIDs), nonessential vasodilators (e.g., calcium antagonists, nitrates), and K^+ supplements/retaining agents (triamterene, amiloride), and if there are no signs of congestion, reduce dose of diuretic.
- If greater rises in creatinine of K^+ than those outlined above persist despite adjustment of concomitant medications, the dose of ACE inhibitor should be halved and blood chemistry rechecked; if there is still an unsatisfactory response, specialist advice should be sought.
- If K^+ rises to ≥6.0 mmol/L or creatinine increases by >100% or to above 4 mg/dL, the dose of ACE inhibitor should be stopped and specialist advice sought.
- Blood electrolytes should be monitored closely until K^+ and creatinine concentrations are stable.

Note: it is very rarely necessary to stop an ACE inhibitor, and clinical deterioration is likely if treatment is withdrawn. Ideally, specialist advice should be sought before treatment discontinuation.

*Calcium channel blockers should be discontinued unless absolutely essential, e.g., for angina or hypertension.

Adapted with permission from McMurray et al. (2001). Practical recommendations for the use of ACE Inhibitors, beta-blockers and spironolactone in heart failure: putting guidelines in to practice. *Eur J Heart Failure* 3(4):495–502.

β-Blockers for heart failure

β-Blockers were once contraindicated in patients with heart failure. However, several studies (Carvedilol studies, Merit-HF, COPERNICUS; see Chapter 15) have shown that they are effective in reducing the risk of sudden cardiac death (of the order of 30%).

β-Blockers are recommended for all patients with HF, whether due to ischemic heart disease or not and irrespective of the severity of LV dysfunction (NYHA classes II to IV).

The effect does not appear to be a class effect, and only metoprolol, carvedilol, and bisoprolol can be recommended in HF.

β-Blockers should be initiated under careful physician monitoring, as there may be an initial deterioration in heart failure symptoms. The drugs are started at a low dose and up-titrated to target over a period of weeks or months (see Table 5.7).

Starting a β-blocker (see Table 5.8)
- Patients should be on an ACE inhibitor if possible.
- Heart failure symptoms should be relatively stable before initiation.
- Start with a low dose and titrate up to target every 1–2 weeks if the preceding dose was tolerated.
- Monitor patient for symptoms and signs of HF, bradycardia, and hypotension.
- If symptoms worsen, increase dose of diuretics or ACE inhibitor initially. The β-blocker dose may need to be decreased transiently.
- If patient is hypotensive, reduce dose of vasodilators and reduce dose of β-blockers if necessary.

Table 5.7 Titration scheme for β-blockers

Drug	First dose	Increments	Target dose
Carvedilol	3.125 mg bid	6.25, 12.5, 25, 50	50 mg daily
Bisoprolol	1.25 mg daily	2.5, 3.75, 5, 7.5, 10	10 mg daily
Metoprolol succinate	12.5 mg daily	25, 50, 100, 200	200 mg daily

NB: Carvedilol maximum dosage is 25 mg bid if there is severe heart failure. For patients with mild–moderate heart failure, maximum dosage is 50 mg bid if weight is above 85 kg; otherwise maximum dosage is 25 mg bid.

Table 5.8 β-Blockers

How to use?

- Start with a low dose (see above).
- Double dose at not less than 2-week intervals.
- Aim for target dose (see above) or, failing that, the highest tolerated dose.
- Remember some β-blocker is better than no β-blocker.
- Monitor heart rate, blood pressure, and clinical status (symptoms, signs, especially signs of congestion, body weight).
- Check blood electrolytes, urea, and creatinine 1–2 weeks after initiation and 1–2 weeks after final dose titration.
- When to down-titrate or stop up-titration—see Table 5.9.

Advice to patient

- Explain expected benefits.
- Emphasize that treatment is given as much to prevent worsening of heart failure as to improve symptoms. β-Blockers also increase survival rates.
- If symptomatic improvement occurs, this may develop slowly—over 3 to 6 months or longer.
- Temporary symptomatic deterioration may occur (estimated 20%–30% of cases) during initiation/up-titration phase.
- Advise patient to report deterioration (see Table 5.9) and that deterioration (tiredness, fatigue, breathlessness) can usually be easily managed by adjustment of their medication. Patients should be advised not to stop β-blocker therapy without consulting their physician.
- Patients should be encouraged to weigh themselves daily (after waking, before dressing, after voiding, and before eating) and to consult their doctor if they have persistent weight gain.

Table 5.9 Problem solving with β-blockers

Worsening symptoms or signs (e.g., increasing dyspnea, fatigue, edema, weight gain)

- If marked fatigue (and/or bradycardia, see below), halve dose of β-blocker (if increasing diuretic does not work).
- If increasing congestion, double dose of diuretic and/or halve dose of β-blocker (if increasing diuretic does not work).
- Reassess patient in 1–2 weeks; if not improved seek specialist advice.
- If serious deterioration, halve dose of β-blocker or stop this treatment (see note below) (rarely necessary); seek specialist advice.

Low heart rate

- If <50 beats/min and worsening symptoms, halve dose of β-blocker or, if severe deterioration, stop β-blocker (rarely necessary).
- Consider need to continue treatment with other drugs (if any) that slow the heart (e.g., digoxin, amiodarone, diltiazem) and discontinue if possible.
- Arrange ECG to exclude heart block.
- Seek specialist advice.

Asymptomatic low blood pressure

- This does not usually require any change in therapy.

Symptomatic hypotension

- If low blood pressure causes dizziness, light-headedness, or confusion, consider discontinuing drugs such as nitrates, calcium channel blockers, and other vasodilators.
- If no signs or symptoms of congestion, consider reducing diuretic dose.
- If these measures do not solve the problem seek specialist advice.

Note: β-Blockers should not be stopped suddenly unless absolutely necessary (there is a risk of a "rebound" increase in myocardial ischemia/infarction and arrhythmias). Ideally, specialist advice should be sought before treatment discontinuation.

Adapted with permission from McMurry et al. (2001). Practical recommendations for the use of ACE Inhibitors, beta-blockers and spironolactone in heart failure: putting guidelines in to practice. *Eur J Heart Failure* 3:495–502.

Angiotensin II receptor antagonists for heart failure

Angiotensin II receptor blockers (ARBs) are often used in those patients who do not tolerate an ACE inhibitor because of cough. In patients with heart failure, ARBs are as effective as ACE inhibitors in reducing mortality and morbidity.

One study (ValHeft II) showed that the combination of an ACE inhibitor and valsartan was better than either drug alone. However, this benefit was reversed in patients also taking a β-blocker. This adverse effect was not seen in the CHARM-Added Trial, which used the ARB candesartan.

When combined with ACE inhibitors, ARBs reduce HF hospitalizations.

In patients with heart failure and preserved LV systolic function (i.e., patients with diastolic dysfunction), the ARB candesartan reduces hospitalization for HF.

Aldosterone receptor antagonists in heart failure

Aldosterone levels are not reduced by ACE inhibitors, and these raised levels produce myocardial fibrosis and predispose to arrhythmias.

In the RALES study, spironolactone (an aldosterone receptor antagonist) produced a 30% reduction in total mortality of patients with severe CHF (NYHA classes III and IV) compared with placebo.

Long-term usage of spironolactone is associated with gynecomastia, impotence, and menstrual irregularities. Newer agents have less of these antiandrogenic and progesterone-like effects.

Eplerenone was evaluated in EPHESUS (Eplerenone Post Acute Myocardial Infarction Heart Failure Efficacy and survival Study). Patients with LVEF <40% were randomized to eplerenone or placebo 3–14 days after acute MI. Eplerenone produced a significant (15%) reduction in mortality. Gynecomastia, breast tenderness, and impotence were no different in the two groups.

Starting spironolactone

- Consider whether a patient is in severe heart failure (NYHA III–IV) despite ACE inhibition and diuretics.
- Check serum K^+ (<5·0 mmol/L) and creatinine (<2.8 mg/dL).
- Start 25 mg spironolactone daily (see Table 5.10).
- Check serum K^+ and creatinine after 4–6 days.
- If at any time serum K^+ >5–5.5< mmol/L, reduce dose by 50%. Stop it if serum K^+ >5.5 mmol/L.
- If after 1 month symptoms persist and K^+<5.5 mmol/L, increase to 50 mg daily. Check serum potassium/creatinine after 1 week.
- If endocrine-related side effects of spironolactone are observed, change to eplerenone.

Table 5.10 Which dose of spironolactone?

- 12.5–25 mg daily, although 50 mg may be advised by a specialist if heart failure deteriorates and there is no problem with hyperkalemia.

How to use?

- Start at 25 mg once daily.
- Check blood chemistry at 1, 4, 8, and 12 weeks; 6, 9, and 12 months, and every 6 months thereafter.
- If K$^+$ rises to between 5.5. and 5.9 mmol/L or creatinine rises to 2.3 mg/dL, reduce dose to 25 mg on alternate days and monitor blood chemistry closely.
- If K$^+$ rises to ≥6.0 mmol/L or creatinine to >2.3 mg/dL stop spironolactone and seek specialist advice.

Advice to patient?

- Explain expected benefits
- Treatment is given to improve symptoms, prevent worsening of heart failure, and increase survival rate.
- Symptom improvement occurs within a few weeks to a few months of starting treatment.
- Avoid NSAIDs not prescribed by a physician (self-purchased over-the-counter treatment, e.g., ibuprofen).
- Temporarily stop sprionolactone if there is diarrhea and/or vomiting and contact physician.

Problem solving—worsening renal function/hyperkalemia

- See How to Use? section, above.
- A major concern is hyperkalemia (≥6.0 mmol/L), although this was uncommon in the RALES clinical trial. A potassium level at the higher end of normal range may be desirable in patients with heart failure, particularly if taking digoxin.
- Some low-salt substitutes have a high K$^+$ content.
- Male patients may develop breast discomfort and/or gynecomastia.

Adapted with permission from McMurray et al. (2001). Practical recommendations for the use of ACE inhibitors, beta-blockers and spironolactone in heart failure; putting guidelines into practice. *Eur J Heart Failure* 3:495–502.

Digoxin in heart failure

Digoxin is very useful controlling heart rates in supraventricular arrhythmias, including AF, in patients with chronic HF. Its role in patients with sinus rhythm, however, is less clear.

Two large digoxin withdrawal trials (RADIANCE and PROVED) demonstrated that patients from whom digoxin was withdrawn were more likely to be admitted with worsening HF.

The DIG trial enrolled 6800 patients with classes I to III HF with a mean EF of 28%. This showed that there was no decrease in overall mortality in the group given digoxin. There was a trend to a decrease in mortality due to pump-failure, balanced by a slight increase in non-pump failure related cardiac deaths. Digoxin reduced the number of hospitalizations for HF significantly.

Overall the clinical trials support the use of digoxin in patients in sinus rhythm with mild to moderate HF for symptomatic control. Trough levels should be maintained between 0.5–1.0 ng/mL.

Contraindications are significant bradycardia; heart block, WPW.

Vasodilators in heart failure

Vasodilators are not a particularly effective method to improve the natural history of chronic HF, but are useful for dealing with acute decompensation. They are also useful in patients intolerant of both ACE-I and ARBs.

Nitrates are primarily venodilators, but are potent coronary vasodilators making them useful in ischemic HF. Isosorbide dinitrate is the only nitrate formulation that has been shown to increase exercise tolerance, and in combination with hydralazine, prolongs survival in patients with HF. The addition of hydralazine appears to attenuate nitrate tolerance by acting as a reducing agent.

In V-HeFT-II, enalapril was shown to be superior to hydralazine and isosorbide dinitrate except in African Americans, where the opposite was found: this is still under investigation.

Nesiritide (human brain natriuretic peptide, hBNP) infusion has been shown to improve hemodynamics and clinical status in patients with decompensated HF, and is less arrhythmogenic than dobutamine. It is in trial as a subcutaneous injection for chronic HF.

Neutral endopeptidase inhibitors with or without intrinsic ACE-inhibitor activity are being explored for the treatment of chronic HF as they prevent the inactivation of ANP and BNP; promising small trials have been followed by disappointing results in larger scale studies.

Although all three classes of calcium antagonists are effective arteriolar vasodilators, none produces a sustained improvement in HF. All except amlodipine appear to worsen symptoms.

Phosphodiesterase inhibitors in heart failure

In large-scale placebo-controlled trials, selective type III phosphodiesterase inhibitors (PDEI) are associated with an increase in mortality.

Individual agents like milrinone and enoximone produce sustained inotropic and vasodilator effects when administered intravenously and are useful in the short term in decompensated HF.

Positive inotropic support

Inotropes (e.g., dobutamine) can be used to limit very severe episodes of heart failure or as a bridge to transplantation in end-stage heart failure. While longer term inotropic therapy may improve a patient's quality of life, they also increase mortality and are therefore not recommended.

Antiplatelet agents and anticoagulants

There has been much controversy regarding the use of aspirin in patients with CHF. As a general rule, NSAIDs are avoided because of their fluid-retaining and renotoxic properties. It is also thought that the beneficial effect of ACE inhibitors is reduced by these drugs.

Generally, patients with ischemic heart disease as their underlying etiology should be treated with aspirin.

Formal anticoagulation with warfarin is indicated for patients with heart failure and atrial fibrillation (paroxysmal or persistent). It is also often used in those with demonstrated LV thrombus or patients with very large LV cavities where it is thought that the risk of LV thrombus formation is high. There are, however, no randomized data to support this use.

Miscellaneous drugs for heart failure

Patients with CHF may require drug treatment for systems other than the heart:

- Gout is a common problem. Acute flare-ups should be treated with colchicine followed by allopurinol once the acute event has settled.
- While most calcium channel antagonists are avoided in patients with CHF, amlodipine has a neutral effect on prognosis and can be used for the treatment of hypertension or angina.
- Anemia is frequently seen in CHF patients. Correction of this with IV iron and erythropoietin has been shown to improve symptoms.

Device therapy for heart failure

Clearly, patients fulfilling the standard indications for permanent pace-maker implantation should undergo this procedure. Wherever possible, dual-chamber systems should be implanted to maintain atrioventricular synchrony.

Implantable cardiac defibrillators (ICD)

ICDs are devices capable of recognizing ventricular arrhythmias (VT or VF) and delivering a DC shock to terminate them. They are implanted in the same way as pacemakers.

Several studies have shown that patients with impaired LV function benefit from their implantation. The MADIT II trial showed a 30% improvement in survival in patients with ischemic heart disease and an ejection fraction of <30%.

The SCD-HeFT trial enrolled patients with ischemic and with nonischemic cardiomyopathies with an LVEF <35%. There was a similar reduction in mortality in ischemic and nonischemic cardiomyopathy patients who received an AICD compared with those patients receiving amiodarone.

Cardiac resynchronization (CRT)

Many patients with CHF have bundle branch block (BBB) patterns on their ECG, in particular LBBB. A wide QRS duration is associated with a worse outcome in patients with CHF. LBBB results in delayed depolarization and contraction of the lateral LV free wall, which is thought to contribute to disease progression. Biventricular pacemakers are able to reduce this ventricular dysynchrony by pacing the LV via a cardiac vein.

Current indications for implantation include severe symptoms (NYHA III or IV), a broad QRS complex (>130 ms), and impaired LV function (LVEF <35%). These indications alone, however, do not necessarily predict patients who will benefit from resynchronization. Current research is assessing the value of using noninvasive imaging techniques (tissue Doppler and MRI) to identify true inter- and intraventricular dysynchrony.

Studies in patients with HF undergoing cardiac resynchronization (CRT) have shown an improvement in quality of life, improved exercise capacity (6-minute walk test), and, in one study, improved survival.

Biventricular devices can now be combined with ICDs to further improve the outlook of these patients.

The devices can be difficult to implant, require close and careful follow-up, and are expensive, which has reduced their widespread use.

Surgery for heart failure

Valve surgery

Patients with valve disease as the source of their heart failure should be considered for valve replacement surgery. This is discussed more fully in Chapter 4 on valve disease.

Coronary artery bypass grafting (CABG)

Ischemic heart disease is the most common cause of heart failure in developed countries. In some cases, these patients will have evidence of either stress-induced ischemia or hibernation (muscle that has reduced function due to reduced blood supply but is still viable).

Revascularizing these patients can lead to an improvement in cardiac function.

Transplantation

Cardiac transplantation is reserved for those patients with end-stage heart failure (see Table 5.11). It is a major undertaking for the patient, who must be willing to undergo intensive treatment and be emotionally capable of withstanding the uncertainties that occur before and after transplantation.

There are a number of contraindications, listed below.

Contraindications for heart transplantation
• Persistent alcohol or drug abuse
• Treated cancer with remission and <5 years follow-up
• Systemic disease with multiorgan involvement
• Infection
• Fixed high pulmonary vascular resistance

Despite problems with rejection and complications of immunosuppressive therapy (infection, hypertension, renal failure, malignancy) the 5-year survival is of the order of 70%–80% with many patients returning to work.

Assist devices

Because of the lack of organ donors for cardiac transplantation, much interest has been shown in the development of left ventricular assist devices (LVAD) and mechanical hearts. LVADs are automatic pumps that take over the work of the heart. They have been used as a bridge to transplantation and as a bridge to recovery in those with potentially reversible causes for their heart failure (e.g., post-viral).

The next stage up from these large devices is the implantation of a permanent artificial heart. An example is the Jarvik 2000, which has been successfully been implanted in a relatively small number of patients.

Table 5.11 Heart transplantation guidelines adapted from ESC/AHA guidelines

Indications	Contraindications and cautions
• Patients must be willing and able to withstand the physical and emotional demands of the procedure and its postoperative sequelae. • Objective evidence of limitation, e.g., peak oxygen consumption <10 mL/min/kg on cardiopulmonary exercise test with evidence for anaerobic metabolism* • Patients dependent on intravenous inotropes and mechanical circulatory support	• Present alcohol and/or drug abuse • Chronic mental illness that cannot be adequately controlled • Treated cancer with remission and <5 years follow-up • Systemic disease with multiorgan involvement • Uncontrolled infection • Severe renal failure (creatinine clearance <50 mL/min) or creatinine >2.3 mg/dL, although some centers accept patients on hemodialysis • Fixed high pulmonary vascular resistance (6–8 Wood units and mean transpulmonary gradient >15 mmHg and pulmonary artery systolic pressure >60 mmHg) • Recent thromboembolic complication • Unhealed peptic ulcer • Evidence of significant liver impairment • Other coexisting disease with a poor prognosis

* Patients with significant exercise limitation that have a peak oxygen consumption <55% predicted or between 11 and 15 mL/min/kg also warrant consideration for cardiac transplantation if they have recurrent unstable myocardial ischemia untreatable by other means, or recurrent episodes of congestive heart failure in spite of adherence to optimum medical therapy.

Palliative care for heart failure

The demographic spread of most patients with heart failure means that the hi-tech and expensive therapies outlined earlier are not available and consideration must be made about end-of-life issues. Increased input from specialist palliative care teams will help to allow patients and their relatives live with a chronic and terminal disease and help the patient die with dignity.

Worsening heart failure

When a patient is seen with worsening heart failure, it is important to try and ascertain the cause. The most frequent reasons for symptom deterioration are shown below.

Causes of worsening heart failure

Noncardiac
- Noncompliance (lifestyle changes, medication)
- Newly prescribed drugs (see Table 5.12)
- Renal dysfunction
- Infection
- Pulmonary embolus
- Anemia

Cardiac
- Atrial fibrillation
- Other tachyarryhthmias
- Bradycardia/heart block
- Worsening valve disease
- Myocardial ischemia (including infarction)

Table 5.12 Side effects of drugs for heart failure

Drugs	Complications
Diuretics	*Common:* postural hypotension, gout, urinary urgency *Serious:* electrolyte imbalance (hypokalemia, hypomagnesemia, hyponatremia), arrhythmia
ACE inhibitors	*Common:* cough, hypotension including postural *Serious:* worsening renal function, renal infarction in renal artery stenosis, angioedema
β-Blockers	*Common:* tiredness, bradycardia, coldness *Serious:* asthmatic attack, exacerbation of heart failure, heart block
Spironolactone	*Common:* gynecomastia, tiredness, rashes *Serious:* hyperkalemia, hyponatremia
Digoxin	*Common:* nausea *Serious:* life-threatening arrhythmias
Angiotensin-II receptor antagonists	*Common:* hypotension including postural *Serious:* worsening renal function, renal infarction in renal artery stenosis
Amiodarone	*Common:* photosensitivity, nausea, thyroid dysfunction, sleep disturbance, corneal microdeposits. *Serious:* thyrotoxic storm, proarrhythmia, pulmonary or hepatic fibrosis
Intropes	*Common:* nausea, palpitation *Serious:* arrhythmia, cardiotoxicity

Diastolic heart failure

Approximately one-third of patients with heart failure have diastolic heart failure. This is defined as symptoms and signs of heart failure but with preserved (normal) LV systolic function.

A number of clinical settings are associated with diastolic dysfunction. Most causes of diastolic dysfunction relate to impaired left ventricular diastolic relaxation. The most common underlying diseases are hypertension and ischemia as a result of coronary artery disease. Other causes include aortic stenosis, hypertrophic cardiomyopathy, and infiltrative (such as in cardiac amyloidosis) and restrictive cardiomyopathies.

Pericardial restraint, such as in constrictive pericarditis and cardiac tamponade, impairs ventricular filling. In addition, mitral valve stenosis causing left ventricular outflow obstruction leads to elevated left atrial pressure and, in severe cases, cardiac failure that is solely due to impaired filling.

Pathophysiology

Ventricular relaxation may be impaired. This is an energy-dependent process and is sensitive to hypoxia. Myocardial ischemia can induce diastolic dysfunction via this mechanism. Ischemia may be caused, not only by epicardial coronary artery disease but possibly also by changes in the microvascular coronary supply.

Increased compliance of the left ventricle leads to a stiff chamber and impaired filling. There is evidence that this altered compliance is mediated by an increase in myocardial collagen.

Most conditions causing left ventricular hypertrophy are associated with impairment of diastolic function; however, in conditions where myocardial hypertrophy is not associated with fibrosis, such as chronic anemia, hyperthyroidism, and exercise training, diastolic stiffness is normal.

Clinical assessment

Clinical features of HF may be similar, regardless of whether LV systolic function is impaired or preserved. The clinical presentation should be considered along with assessment of systolic and diastolic function (see Table 5.13).

Table 5.13 Assessment of diastolic heart failure

Diagnostic criteria for diastolic HF	Signs and symptoms of HF plus
Possible diastolic HF	LVEF >50% but not at the time of HF
Probable diastolic HF	LVEF >50% within 72 hr of HF event
Definite diastolic HF	LVEF >50% within 72 hr of HF event, and Abnormal LV relaxation, filling and/or distensibility at cardiac catheterization or by non-invasive imaging

Adapted with permission from Vasan RS, Levy D (2000). *Circulation* 101(17):2118.

Diagnosis

A definitive diagnosis of diastolic heart failure can be made when the rate of relaxation of the LV in diastole is slowed. This physiological abnormality is characteristically associated with the finding of an elevated left ventricular filling pressure in a patient with normal left ventricular volumes and contractility.

Noninvasive methods (e.g., Doppler echocardiography) have been developed to assist in the diagnosis of diastolic dysfunction, but these tests have significant limitations, because cardiac filling patterns are readily altered by nonspecific and transient changes in loading conditions in the heart as well as by aging, changes in heart rate, or the presence of mitral regurgitation.

Every effort should be made to exclude other possible explanations or disorders that may present in a similar manner (see Box 5.5).

Principles of treatment

Unlike LV systolic dysfunction, there is little evidence-based data on how to treat patients with presumed diastolic dysfunction. Causes of diastolic heart failure include ischemia, hypertension, and hypertrophy, which should be identified and treated accordingly.

Current recommendations suggest the use of β-blockers, rate-slowing calcium channel antagonists (verapamil or diltiazem), ACE inhibitors, and diuretics. Management of this group is difficult and should probably be tailored to the individual, with the following in mind:

- Control of systolic and diastolic hypertension
- Control of ventricular rate in patients with atrial fibrillation
- Diuretics to control pulmonary congestion and peripheral edema
- Coronary revascularization in patients with coronary artery disease in whom symptomatic or demonstrable myocardial ischemia is judged to be having an adverse effect on diastolic function
- Restoration of sinus rhythm in patients with atrial fibrillation

---

Box 5.5 Differential diagnoses with HF and preserved LV ejection fraction

- Incorrect diagnosis of HF
- Inaccurate measurement of LVEF
- Primary valvular disease
- Restrictive (infiltrative) cardiomyopathy (e.g., amyloidosis, sarcoidosis, hemochromatosis)
- Pericardial constriction
- Severe hypertension, ischemia
- High-output cardiac failure (anemia, thyrotoxicosis, AV fistulas)
- Chronic pulmonary disease with right HF
- Pulmonary hypertension
- Atrial myxoma

Reprinted with permission from the ACC/AHA Guidelines: Hunt et al. (2005). *Circulation* 112:e154–e235. ©2005, American Heart Association, Inc.

High-output heart failure

In high-output states, the only way that the oxygen demands of the peripheral tissues can be met is by an increase in cardiac output. If there is underlying heart disease, the heart may be unable to chronically augment its output, and HF results.

Causes of high-output states are listed in Box 5.5.

Anemia

When the Hb levels fall below 8 g/dL, the anemia produces a high cardiac output. However, even when severe, anemia rarely causes heart failure or angina in patients with normal hearts. Look for an underlying cardiac problem or valve disease. Try to determine the etiology for the anemia.

Patient should be on bed rest and transfused with packed red blood cells accompanied with IV diuretics.

Systemic arteriovenous fistulas

The increase in cardiac output depends on the size of the fistula. The Branham sign consists of slowing of the heart rate after manual compression of the fistula. It also raises arterial blood pressure. Surgical repair or excision is the ideal treatment.

Pregnancy (see p. 421)

Thyrotoxicosis

Raised levels of thyroxine produce increased heart rate and cardiac contractility, reduction in systemic vascular resistance, and enhanced sympathetic activation. Thyrotoxicosis does not usually precipitate heart failure unless there is reduced cardiac reserve.

Atrial fibrillation occurs in about 10% of patients, exacerbating the HF. Respiratory muscle weakness may contribute to the dyspnea.

Beriberi

Paget's disease

There is a linear relationship between the extent of bone involvement and rise in cardiac output. Involvement of about 15% of the skeleton is required before the rise is seen, and patients may tolerate the early stages well for years.

Concomitant valvular disease or ischemic heart disease results in decompensation. Successful treatment of Paget's disease with bisphosphonates may reverse the rise in cardiac output over several months.

Box 5.5 Causes of high-output states

- Anemia
- Acquired arteriovenous fistula
- Hemangioma
- Hereditary hemorrhagic telangiectasia
- Hepatic hemangioendothelioma
- Pregnancy
- Acromegaly
- Thyrotoxicosis
- Beriberi heart disease
- Paget's disease of the bone
- Fibrous dysplasia
- Polycythemia rubra vera
- Carcinoid syndrome
- Multiple myeloma

Chapter 6

Preventive cardiology

Background

While great strides have been made over the past several decades in the management of symptomatic ischemic heart disease, with dramatic improvements in outcomes from acute coronary syndromes, the identification and modification of atherosclerotic risk factors has also contributed significantly to overall public health.

The field of preventive cardiology focuses on the management of cardiovascular disease risk factors in order to prevent disease occurrence and reduce the incidence of subsequent clinical events in those with established cardiovascular disease. *Primary prevention* involves controlling risk in order to prevent disease, while *secondary prevention* strategies focus on early disease detection and interventions to limit progression of disease.

In this chapter, the pathophysiology of atherosclerosis will be reviewed, which provides the basis for understanding risk factors and how to manage them.

Atherosclerosis: pathophysiology

Atherosclerosis is a disease of the large and medium-sized arteries, characterized by a gradual buildup of fatty plaques within the arterial wall. This may eventually result in a significant narrowing of the vessel lumen, impairing blood flow.

These plaques may also become unstable and thrombose leading to an acute coronary syndrome.

Pathophysiology

The atherogenic process is characterized by dysfunction of the endothelial lining of the vessel, associated with inflammation of the vascular wall. This leads to the buildup of lipids, inflammatory cells, and cellular debris within the intima and subintimal layers of the vessel, resulting in plaque formation and remodeling of the arterial wall.

This process is complex, involving a series of interactions between endothelial and smooth muscle cells, leukocytes and platelets in the vascular wall.

Endothelial dysfunction

The atherosclerotic process appears to be triggered by endothelial cell injury from exposure to stimuli such as tobacco toxins, oxidized low-density lipoprotein (LDL), advanced glycation end products, elevated homocysteine, or infectious agents. This initiates a cascade of events resulting in cellular dysfunction (see Fig. 6.1).

The hallmark of endothelial dysfunction is a change in the balance of production of endothelium-derived vasoactive molecules. There is a *reduced bioavailability of endothelial nitric oxide (NO)*, which possesses important vasodilator, antithrombotic, and antiproliferative properties, in parallel with increased generation of the potent vasoconstrictor agents, endothelin-1 and angiotensin-II, which also promote cell migration and growth. Dysfunctional endothelial cells also express adhesion molecules and secrete chemokines promoting cell migration and adhesion.

Levels of plasminogen activator inhibitor and tissue factor are increased, tissue plasminogen activator and thrombomodulin are reduced, and low NO release results in increased platelet activation and adhesion.

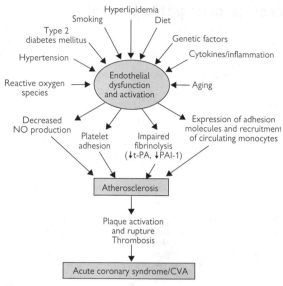

Figure 6.1 Endothelial dysfunction is the underlying process in atherosclerosis, from lesion initiation, progression, through to acute cardiovascular events. Endothelial dysfunction is caused by a variety of genetic factors (and aging), as well as environmental factors that can be modified.

Development of atherosclerotic plaques

Endothelial dysfunction creates a local milieu that facilitates initiation and development of the atherosclerotic plaque (see Fig. 6.2). Circulating leukocytes, predominantly monocytes, are attracted and bind to activated endothelial cells and migrate into the subendothelial layer where they transform into macrophages. Here they act as local "scavenger" cells taking up modified LDL cholesterol, ultimately becoming the characteristic "foam cells" of established atherosclerosis.

The earliest lesions are known as *fatty streaks*, which consist predominantly of lipids and foam cells. These lesions may develop into fibrous plaques, as a consequence of further lipid accumulation accompanied by local migration, proliferation, and fibrous transformation of smooth muscle cells. These cells are responsible for the deposition of extracellular connective tissue matrix, leading to formation of a fibrous cap. This cap overlies a central core consisting of foam cells, extracellular lipid, necrotic cellular debris, and a mixture of other inflammatory cells, including T lymphocytes.

This process is facilitated by ongoing endothelial dysfunction, together with local generation of powerful mitogens such as platelet-derived growth factor (PDGF), transforming growth factor β (TGF-β), and insulin-like growth factor (IGF) from endothelial cells, macrophages, and activated platelets.

Further growth of the plaque initially causes outward remodeling of the vessel wall, thus minimizing the impact on the cross-sectional area of the lumen. However, progressive plaque accumulation results in luminal narrowing and ultimately vessel obstruction (see Fig. 6.2).

Plaque initiation and progression tend to occur more predictably at certain locations of the vascular system. Blood flow through arteries causes local "shear stress," which influences the biology of the underlying endothelium. High laminar shear (from blood flowing quickly through a straight vessel) favors the generation of NO, which helps maintain the functional integrity of the vessel.

In contrast, low shear, or "differential" shear, caused by turbulent flow, results in dysfunction of the underlying endothelium, which facilitates initiation and progression of atherosclerosis. This is a consequence of differential gene activation profiles in response to laminar (athero-protective), as opposed to turbulent (athero-inducing), blood flow, which may explain why plaques are more commonly found at sites of vessel branching or curvature. These sites experience more dramatic and abrupt changes in blood flow velocity.

These shear stress–mediated effects are most marked in the coronary, carotid, renal, and iliofemoral arteries, in which the majority of clinically important atherosclerotic lesions develop.

The vulnerable plaque

Erosion of the endothelial layer, or rupture of the overlying fibrous cap, may expose the highly thrombogenic, lipid-rich core of the plaque to circulating blood. Collagen, tissue factor, and other factors activate platelets and trigger the coagulation cascade, leading to acute thrombosis, which

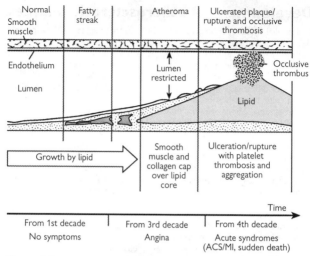

Figure 6.2 Cellular interactions in the development and progression of atherosclerosis. VSMC, vascular smooth muscle cells. Reproduced with permission from Weissberg PL (2000). *Heart* 83(2):247–252.

may rapidly occlude the vessel. Myocardial infarction (MI) can result, usually characterized by ST-segment elevation.

Coronary thrombosis is a dynamic process in vivo and may be reversed, at least in part, by activation of tissue plasminogen activator and proteins C and S of the intrinsic antithrombotic/fibrinolytic system. Acute, subtotal occlusion of a coronary artery typically causes acute non-ST-segment elevation MI (STEMI) or unstable angina.

Atheromatous plaques that have a thin fibrous cap and a large necrotic lipid core and containing a high proportion of inflammatory cells and mediators are particularly predisposed to destabilization or rupture, with consequent thrombosis.

Conversely, plaques with a smaller lipid pool, thicker fibrous caps, and less inflammatory activity are more stable and less prone to rupture.

Several studies have shown that well over half of all MIs are caused by acute destabilization of plaques that were previously not flow limiting (i.e., <50% stenosis), suggesting that the likelihood of an acute coronary event is more closely related to the stability of the plaque rather than the severity of the stenosis.

Epidemiology

Cardiovascular disease, including coronary disease, stroke, and peripheral arterial disease, is the leading cause of death in the United States, accounting for more than 900,000 deaths annually.

At age 40, the lifetime risk of developing coronary disease is 49% for men and 32% for women. Although mortality rates have decreased by approximately 25% over the past 30 years, the rate of decline has slowed since 1990.

Autopsy data have confirmed a decreased prevalence of coronary atherosclerosis in both men and women since the late 1970s. A substantial component of this reduction is the modification of risk factors, particularly decreased smoking and better hypertension treatment.

A concerning trend in recent times is the rising prevalence of obesity and diabetes, particularly among younger people. This trend may explain the declining mortality rate reduction from cardiovascular disease.

Approximately 14 million people in the United States have symptomatic coronary disease. This number is likely an underestimation of the total population disease burden, as many patients are asymptomatic or have silent or clinically unrecognized manifestations of disease.

Much of our understanding of cardiovascular disease risk factors is derived from large epidemiologic studies, including the Framingham Heart Study and the Nurses Health Study.

As we will discuss, the important modifiable risk factors for cardiovascular disease include *smoking, diet, hypertension, dyslipidemias, physical inactivity, obesity,* and *diabetes.* It is important to recognize that many patients with cardiovascular disease have multiple risk factors, each of which requires appropriate management for optimal risk reduction.

Atherosclerosis is a systemic disease

Atherosclerosis in one vascular territory is often associated with disease elsewhere, as the risk factors for coronary disease, stroke, and peripheral vascular disease are similar. It is important to recognize this association, as clinically evident disease in one vascular bed may be a harbinger of silent, and potentially modifiable, disease in another, particularly the coronary arterial system. Cardiac events are the leading cause of mortality in patients with peripheral vascular disease.

For this reason, cerebrovascular disease and peripheral vascular disease are considered coronary disease equivalents. Appropriate preventive strategies and goals should be applied in these patients.

Assessment of atherosclerotic risk

Identification and treatment of risk factors is essential for the prevention of atherosclerotic disease in individuals and society. When multiple risk factors such as dyslipidemia, high blood pressure, and smoking coexist, as is commonly the case, the cardiovascular risk is greatly increased, suggesting a synergistic interaction among these factors.

For example, the absolute risk of a cardiovascular event occurring in a patient with high blood pressure is greatly influenced by their age, sex, lipid profile, presence of diabetes and other factors.

Thus, modern approaches to risk management should involve careful consideration of the combined impact of all important factors operating in the individual that contribute to their risk of atherosclerotic disease.

Global risk assessment

Several risk assessment systems are currently available, derived from large, prospective population cohorts, most commonly the Framingham study (Tables 6.1, 6.2). These systems allow the calculation of the "absolute risk" of having a cardiovascular event (i.e., the probability of having a heart attack or stroke) within the next 10 years, which is derived from patients' risk factor variables (age, sex, cholesterol, HDL, BP, smoking).

Subjects with established coronary disease or stable angina have a 10-year event rate of approximately 20%. Therefore, subjects without clinical disease that have a predicted 10-year likelihood of suffering a cardiovascular event of ≥20% are considered to be at high risk and are candidates for aggressive risk factor management.

Although these conventional scoring systems have the potential to identify most high-risk individuals in Western populations, a significant proportion of events occur in subjects calculated to be at intermediate and low risk. For example, risk is typically underestimated when using conventional methods in young subjects with multiple risk factors, subjects with a family history of premature cardiovascular disease, and certain ethnic groups, including individuals of South Asian racial origin. Identification of subjects with intermediate (10%–20%) conventional risk scores that are actually at high risk remains a major challenge, as these individuals are also likely to benefit from aggressive preventive therapy.

It has been proposed that measurement of C-reactive protein (CRP) levels, ultrasound assessment of carotid artery intima-medial thickness, and coronary artery calcium scoring with CT scanning may improve risk assessment, especially in patients at intermediate risk based on traditional risk factor assessment. These techniques are highly promising and under intense investigation, but their clinical utility and cost have not yet been confirmed in large prospective clinical studies, and they are not currently used in routine clinical practice.

However, in selected asymptomatic patients at intermediate risk based on traditional scoring systems, the use of these techniques may be appropriate if the results will alter the management strategy by reclassifying a patient as low or high risk.

Likewise, routine use of stress testing for coronary artery disease (CAD) screening in asymptomatic subjects is also not currently recommended.

Table 6.1 Framingham risk scoring system for men

Age		Diabetes	
Years	**Points**		**Points**
30–34	−1	No	0
35–39	0	Yes	2
40–44	1	**Smoker**	
45–49	2		**Points**
50–54	3	No	0
55–59	4	Yes	2
60–64	5		
65–69	6		
70–74	7		

LDL-C			HDL-C		
mg/dL	mmol/L	Points	mg/dL	mmol/L	Points
<100	<2.59	−3	<35	<0.90	2
100–129	2.60–3.36	0	35–44	0.91–1.16	1
130–159	3.37–4.14	0	45–49	1.17–1.29	0
160–190	4.50–4.92	1	50–54	1.30–1.55	0
>190	>4.92	2	>60	>1.56	−1

Systolic blood pressure, mmHg	Diastolic <80 mmHg	Diastolic 80–84 mmHg	Diastolic 85–89 mmHg	Diastolic 90–99 mmHg	Diastolic ≥100 mmHg
<120	0	0	1	2	3
120–129	0	0	1	2	3
130–139	1	1	1	2	3
140–159	2	2	2	2	3
≥160	3	3	3	3	3

Coronary heart disease (CHD) risk

Total points	10-year CHD risk (%)	Total points	10-year CHD risk (%)
< 3	1	6	11
−2	2	7	14
−1	2	8	18
0	3	9	22
1	4	10	27
2	5	11	33
3	6	12	40
4	7	13	47
5	9	14	56

Use to calculate the risk of developing clinical coronary heart disease (CHD) in men who do not have known CHD. To calculate the Framingham risk estimate, add points for age, presence of diabetes, smoking status, LDL cholesterol (LDL-C), HDL cholesterol (HDL-C), and blood pressure. Find the total point score on the bottom table to determine the 10-year risk of CHD. Reprinted with permission from Wilson PW, et al. (1998). Prediction of coronary heart disease using risk factor categories. *Circulation* 97:1837–1847.

Table 6.2 Framingham risk scoring system for women

Age		Diabetes	
Years	**Points**		**Points**
30–34	−9	No	0
35–39	−4	Yes	4
40–44	0		Smoker
45–49	3		**Points**
50–54	6	No	0
55–59	7	Yes	2
60–64	8		
65–69	8		
70–74	8		

LDL-C			HDL-C		
mg/dL	**mmol/L**	**Points**	**mg/dL**	**mmol/L**	**Points**
<100	<2.59	−2	<35	<0.90	5
100–129	2.60–3.36	0	35–44	0.91–1.16	2
130–159	3.37–4.14	0	45–49	1.17–1.29	1
160–190	4.50–4.92	2	50–54	1.30–1.55	0
>190	>4.92	2	>60	>1.56	−2

Systolic blood pressure, mmHg	Diastolic <80 mmHg	Diastolic 80–84 mmHg	Diastolic 85–89 mmHg	Diastolic 90–99 mmHg	Diastolic ≥100 mmHg
<120	−3	0	0	2	3
120–129	0	0	0	2	3
130–139	0	0	0	2	3
140–159	2	2	2	2	3
≥160	3	3	3	3	3

Coronary heart disease (CHD) risk

Total points	10-year CHD risk (%)	Total points	10-year CHD risk (%)
<−2	1	8	8
−1	2	9	9
0	2	10	11
1	2	11	13
2	3	12	15
3	3	13	17
4	4	14	20
5	5	15	24
6	6	16	27
7	7	17	32

Use to calculate the risk of developing clinical coronary heart disease (CHD) in men who do not have known CHD. To calculate the Framingham risk estimate, add points for age, presence of diabetes, smoking status, LDL cholesterol (LDL-C), HDL cholesterol (HDL-C), and blood pressure. Find the total point score on the bottom table to determine the 10-year risk of CHD. Reprinted with permission from Wilson PW, et al. (1998). Prediction of coronary heart disease using risk factor categories. *Circulation* 97:1837–1847.

CAD risk equivalents

Patients with atherosclerotic disease in other vascular territories, including peripheral arterial disease, abdominal aortic aneurysms, and carotid disease, are at high risk (10-year risk >20%) and should be managed aggressively in terms of secondary prevention.

Diabetic patients have a similar risk for cardiac events as those with established coronary disease and are therefore high risk (10-year risk >20%) as well.

Risk factors for coronary artery disease

Age

The U.S. population is aging. In the United States, the proportion of the population aged ≥65 years is projected to increase from 12.4% in 2000 to 19.6% in 2030. The number of persons aged ≥65 years is expected to increase from approximately 35 million in 2000 to an estimated 71 million in 2030, and the number of persons aged ≥80 years is expected to increase from 9.3 million in 2000 to 19.5 million in 2030.

Aging is a major risk factor for atherosclerotic disease because of the degenerative process associated with aging and the cumulative impact of the worsening risk factor profile that develops with increasing age.

For men, the reported prevalence increases with age, from 7% at ages 40–49 years to 13% at 50–59 years, 16% at 60–69 years, and 22% at 70–79 years. The corresponding estimates for women are substantially lower than for men: 5%, 8%, 11%, and 14%, respectively.

Although about 45% of myocardial infarctions occur in people under 65 years of age, this condition is more likely to be fatal in older individuals, with 80% of deaths due to MI seen in those over 65.

Gender, menopausal status, and hormone replacement therapy (HRT)

CAD is more common and tends to occur at an earlier age in men than in women. The incidence of CHD in women increases rapidly at menopause and is similar to that seen in men in the population over 65. Although less common, the disease remains the leading cause of death in women. For example, the age-adjusted mortality rates from heart disease are four to six times higher than their mortality rates from breast cancer.

Although cardiovascular risk factors promote disease in both genders, the strength of the association differs. For example, diabetes and low high-density lipoprotein (HDL) cholesterol are stronger risk factors for women than for men.

Female sex hormones probably contribute to the lower risk of atherosclerotic disease in premenopausal women. Additionally, observational studies showed that the risk of ischemic heart disease is reduced by up to 40% in women using HRT. However, HRT users are typically healthier than nonusers, suggesting that these results could be explained by selection bias.

Several large, randomized, controlled trials of HRT in postmenopausal women (WHI, HERS/HERS II, ESPRIT, ERA) with and without atherosclerosis have suggested that HRT does not reduce the risk of cardiovascular events and, in fact, leads to a small but statistically significant increase in morbidity and mortality from cardiovascular disease. The age at entry into these trials has recently brought the broad implications of these data into question.

However, HRT should not be recommended for primary or secondary prevention of atherosclerotic disease in postmenopausal women.

Family history of atherosclerotic disease

CAD is a multifactorial, polygenic disorder, caused by interactions among lifestyle, the environment, and the effects of variations in the genetic sequence of a number of genes (see Table 6.3 and Box 6.1). The family history is considered significant when atherosclerotic disease presents in a first-degree male relative before the age of 55, or before age 65 in a female relative.

A positive family history is associated with a 75% increase in risk in men, and an 84% increase in women. The risk is even greater if both parents are affected.

In the Physician's Health Study, compared to no parental history of an MI, a maternal history, a paternal history, and both maternal and paternal history were associated with a relative risk of cardiovascular disease of 1.71, 1.40, and 1.85 in men and 1.46, 1.15, and 2.05 in women.

In the Framingham Offspring Study, cardiovascular disease in a sibling was associated with a significant increase in cardiovascular disease risk with an adjusted odds ratio of 1.45.

Table 6.3 Risk factors for coronary heart disease

Nonmodifiable risk factors	Modifiable risk factors
• Age	• Smoking
• Male gender	• High blood pressure
• Family history	• Dyslipidemia
• Ethnic origin	• Diabetes mellitus
	• Obesity and the metabolic syndrome
	• Psychological stress
	• High-calorie high-fat diet
	• Physical inactivity

Box 6.1 Emerging risk factors and disease markers

• Inflammation, elevated C-reactive protein
• Fibrinogen, and other factors involved in thromboregulation
• Elevated homocysteine
• Chronic kidney disease, microalbuminuria
• Estrogen deficiency
• Oxidative stress
• Endothelial dysfunction, decreased endothelial progenitor cells
• Asymmetric dimethylarginine
• Hyperuricemia
• Carotid–intimal media thickness
• Collagen vascular disease
• Coronary artery calcium

Ethnic origin

A difference in cardiovascular disease prevalence among various ethnic groups is likely explained by clustering of risk factors in these groups, although a genetic component may be contributing as well.

Between 1970 and 2000, the rate of coronary disease decreased in whites while the rates actually increased for blacks and Hispanics. Differences in the delivery of health care, as well as risk factors, among these groups may explain this trend.

Smoking

Smoking increases the risk of coronary disease by approximately 50%, with mortality from any cardiovascular disease around 60% higher in smokers (and 85% higher in heavy smokers) than in nonsmokers (see Fig. 6.3).

In 2004, approximately 21% of U.S. adults (23% of men, 19% of women) were current smokers. Although the number of smokers has declined substantially over the past 50 years, this trend has slowed in the adolescent population, where smoking prevalence has not declined since 2002.

The incidence of an MI is increased sixfold in women and threefold in men who smoke at least 20 cigarettes per day compared to subjects who never smoked. Second-hand smoke (smoke that has been exhaled by a smoker) also increases the risk of coronary disease by around 25%.

Smoking cessation carries almost immediate benefit and the long-term benefits are greatest in those who stop smoking before the age of 40, such that the survival curve overlaps with nonsmokers. Stopping smoking in middle age is also beneficial. For example, in those aged 30–59 who stop smoking after an MI, the 5-year mortality is 10% compared with 14% in those who continue to smoke.

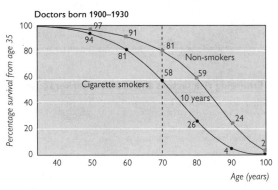

Figure 6.3 Survival from age 35 for continuing cigarette smokers and lifelong nonsmokers among UK male doctors born 1900–1930, with percentages alive at each decade of age. Adapted with permission from Doll R, et al. (2004). *BMJ* 328(7455):1519.

Individuals with established atherosclerosis, as well as those at risk, should be advised to stop smoking. Evidence shows that focused psychosocial support, nicotine replacement therapy, and bupropion are quite effective in smoking cessation, with higher quit rates than those for no intervention.

Obesity

Obesity significantly increases the risk of CAD, with 25%–49% of cases in developed countries attributable to increased body mass index (BMI). Obesity is also associated with a number of other risk factors for atherosclerosis, including hypertension, insulin resistance and glucose intolerance, hypertriglyceridemia, reduced HDL cholesterol, and low levels of adiponectin.

Overweight is defined as a BMI between 25 and 30 kg/m^2, and obesity as a BMI 30 kg/m^2. Central obesity, in which excess fat is localized in the abdomen, can be identified by a high waist-to-hip ratio and confers a particularly high relative risk if the waist circumference is >40 inches in men and >35 inches in women.

The prevalence of obesity is increasing rapidly worldwide. Compared to NHANES data from 1988 to 1994, data from NHANES 1999 to 2000 demonstrates an increase in the prevalence of overweight and obese adults, from 55.9% to 64.5% for overweight and from 22.9% to 30.5% for obese adults.

Of particular concern is the dramatic increase in prevalence of obesity in children, a trend that is likely to exacerbate the problem in adulthood and undo many of the other recent improvements in cardiovascular health.

Overweight and obese individuals also tend to be less physically active and consume unhealthy diets with excess calories, which further contributes to their atherogenic risk. Dietary modification and exercise are thus the first-line interventions in these individuals, together with careful surveillance for and aggressive management of other risk factors and complications of obesity when present.

Bariatric surgery may have a role in selected patients, especially if more conservative weight loss measures fail.

Psychological stress

The burden of risk attributable to psychological stress is difficult to quantify. However, increased stress at work, lack of social support, hostile personality type, anxiety, and depression are consistently associated with increased risk of atherosclerosis and acute coronary events.

The link between psychological stress and atherosclerosis may be both direct, through endothelial damage, and indirect, via exacerbation of traditional risk factors such as smoking and hypertension.

Inflammation

Inflammation is involved in the atherosclerotic process from plaque origination and progression to acute rupture and thrombosis. This inflammatory process directly links known risk factors to the underlying mechanism of disease.

Large studies have shown that low-grade elevation of inflammatory markers, most notably CRP, predicts outcomes from cardiovascular disease and may add to the prognostic information provided by traditional risk factors. It has been suggested that a CRP level below 1 mg/L is associated with low risk, between 1 and 3 mg/L reflects intermediate risk, and a level above 3 mg/L is associated with a high long-term risk of vascular events.

Certain treatments that reduce atherosclerotic risk, particularly statins, have anti-inflammatory effects that may contribute to their clinical benefits. However, the incremental value of CRP as a marker of risk and target of therapy in global risk management remains a controversial topic that requires further investigation, such as the recently completed JUPITER trial, which demonstrated improved outcomes with rosuvastatin in patients with elevated CRP and normal lipids.

Homocysteine

The genetic disease homocystinuria is associated with aggressive, premature atherosclerosis. Additionally, strong epidemiological and mechanistic evidence suggests that even modest increases in homocysteine levels promote atherosclerosis progression. Vascular inflammation and oxidative stress appear to be the responsible mechanisms.

Dietary supplementation with folic acid, alone or in combination with vitamins B_6 and B_{12}, can reduce levels of homocysteine and improve aspects of vascular biology in vivo as well as in vitro. However, large randomized trials (VISP, WENBIT, NORVIT, HOPE-2) of vitamin supplementation to lower homocysteine levels in patients with established cardiovascular disease have found no decrease in cardiovascular events or death. Therefore, folate ± B_6/B_{12} supplementation is not currently recommended for secondary prevention in patients with cardiovascular disease.

Folate supplementation as primary prevention has yet to be examined in a large randomized trial so this use is also not currently recommended.

Antioxidant vitamins

Despite excellent epidemiological and mechanistic evidence that increased oxidative stress is associated with vascular injury, inflammation and increased risk of cardiovascular morbidity and mortality, large randomized controlled trials (HOPE, HPS and GISSI-P) of vitamin A, C, and E supplementation have shown no effect on cardiovascular outcomes in primary or secondary prevention.

Currently, antioxidant vitamin supplementation should not be routinely recommended for prevention of atherosclerotic disease.

Dietary measures

Several dietary measures can reduce the risk of developing cardiovascular disease. Total fat intake should be reduced to below <30% of total calories. Intake of saturated fat and foods high in trans fatty acids should be limited to <7% total calories and replaced with monounsaturated fat (canola and olive oil).

Based on data from the Nurses' Health Study, the risk of coronary heart disease would be reduced by 42% if 5% of energy from saturated fat were replaced by energy from unsaturated fats, and by 53% if 2% of energy from trans fat was replaced by energy from unhydrogenated, unsaturated fat.

Recommended cholesterol intake is <200 mg/day. Dietary salt intake should be reduced and intake of fresh fruits and vegetables increased (5 portions per day). Fish consumption, especially oily fish, should be encouraged, as evidence suggests that at least one fish meal 2–3 times per week can reduce the incidence of heart attack and stroke.

High fiber intake is also associated with a reduced risk of cardiovascular disease.

Physical activity

Observational studies have shown a strong inverse relationship between exercise and risk of coronary disease and death. The effect appears to be graded such that the greater the degree of physical activity, the lower the risk of coronary events. This effect is mediated, at least in part by weight loss, a reduction in blood pressure, and improvements in lipid profile (particularly increased HDL).

Regular, aerobic exercise of moderate intensity should be undertaken ≥3 times per week for at least 30 minutes. Greater frequency and duration of exercise is associated with increasing benefits, both in primary and secondary prevention.

Alcohol

Consumption of small to moderate amounts of alcohol (one or two drinks per day) is associated with a reduced risk of cardiovascular disease, whereas higher levels of alcohol intake, particularly in binges, are associated with an increased risk of disease.

The United States Dietary Guidelines recommend alcohol intake in moderation, if at all (one drink per day for women and up to two drinks per day for men). Any benefit of moderate alcohol consumption must be weighed against the potential risks.

Hypertension

Definition and etiology

There are approximately 60 million adults in the United States with high blood pressure. A continuous relationship exists between increasing blood pressure and cardiovascular risk; therefore it is impossible to define hypertension precisely.

Systolic blood pressure (BP) is at least as powerful a coronary risk factor as the diastolic BP, and isolated systolic hypertension is now established as a major risk for coronary disease and stroke. Both the duration and degree of hypertension are risk factors.

For practical purposes, levels of blood pressure above which the risk increases significantly and treatment can provide significant benefit are used as a working definition of hypertension (see Table 6.4).

According to the Seventh Report of the Joint National Committee on Prevention, Detection, Evaluation, and Treatment of High Blood Pressure (JNC-7), in persons older than 50 years, systolic BP >140 mmHg is a much more important cardiovascular disease risk factor than diastolic BP. Also, the risk of disease increases beginning at 115/75 mmHg and doubles with each increment of 20/10 mmHg.

The average of two readings at each of a number of visits should be used to define a patient's blood pressure. Blood pressure should also ideally be measured in both arms.

The majority of patients (>95%) have *essential (primary) hypertension*, in which an underlying cause for the hypertension is not found. Others have *secondary hypertension*, in which a recognizable etiology is identified (see Box 6.2).

Symptoms and signs

Hypertension is usually asymptomatic, although a patient will occasionally complain of headache. A history of cardiac or neurological symptoms should always be sought. The cardiovascular system should be examined in detail and fundoscopy should be performed to look for retinopathy (see Box 6.3).

Clinical signs of an underlying cause (radiofemoral delay or weak femoral pulses, renal enlargement or bruit, or cushingoid features) and evidence of end-organ damage (heart failure, retinopathy, aortic aneurysm, carotid or femoral bruit) should be sought.

Malignant hypertension is diagnosed when severe hypertension (SBP >200 ± DBP >130 mmHg) is identified together with grade III–IV retinopathy. The patient may have a headache and occasionally visual disturbance. Proteinuria and hematuria are often present. This is a medical emergency requiring immediate treatment to prevent rapid progression to renal failure, heart failure, and/or stroke.

Investigation

All patients presenting with hypertension should have an ECG, fasting glucose, lipid profile, blood urea nitrogen (BUN)/creatinine, and urinalysis for blood and protein.

If secondary hypertension is suspected, further investigation should focus on the possible underlying cause (e.g., urine cortisol, plasma renin-aldosterone levels, renal ultrasound, MRA of renal arteries, and 24-hour urinary catecholamines).

Table 6.4 JNC-7 Blood pressure classification

Category	SBP (mmHg)	DBP (mmHg)
Normal BP	<120 AND	<80
Pre-hypertension	120–139 OR	80–89
Stage 1 hypertension	140–159 OR	90–99
Stage 2 hypertension	≥160 OR	≥100

Box 6.2 Secondary hypertension (<5%)

Renal disease
- Diabetic nephropathy, renovascular disease, glomerulonephritis, vasculitis, chronic pyelonephritis, polycystic kidney disease

Endocrine disease
- Conn's and Cushing's syndromes, pheochromocytoma, acromegaly, hyperthyroidism, hyperparathyroidism

Other
- Aortic coarctation
- Pregnancy-induced hypertension and pre-eclampsia
- Obesity
- Excessive dietary salt or licorice intake
- Drugs (NSAIDs, sympathomimetics, illicit stimulants, oral contraceptives)
- Obstructive sleep apnea

Box 6.3 Grading of hypertensive retinopathy

I. Tortuous arteries, with thickened bright walls ("silver wiring")
II. Arteriovenous nicking (narrowing in a vein where crossed by an artery)
III. Flame hemorrhages and cotton wool spots (small retinal bleeds and exudates)
IV. Papilledema

Treatment of high blood pressure

When to treat

The predicted decrease in mortality from the 5 to 6 mmHg average fall in diastolic blood pressure achieved in the multiple clinical trials performed over the past 30 years is a 40% reduction in stroke mortality and a 25% reduction in coronary mortality. At any blood pressure, the cardiovascular risk is significantly affected by the presence or absence of other risk factors that need to be considered when deciding when and how to treat.

Patients with malignant hypertension or with persistent BP >140/90 mmHg after lifestyle measures should receive drug treatment. Subjects with BP >140/90 mmHg after lifestyle measures who have evidence of end-organ damage (LVH on ECG, proteinuria, or retinopathy) or a calculated 10-year risk of a cardiovascular event ≥20% should also receive drug treatment.

In patients with diabetes, chronic kidney disease, or known cardiovascular disease, antihypertensive therapy is indicated when the systolic pressure is persistently above 130 mmHg and/or the diastolic pressure is above 80 mmHg.

Blood pressure targets

Most patients should have their blood pressure lowered to a target of <140/85 mmHg. Patients with diabetes and chronic kidney disease have been shown to benefit from more aggressive BP reduction (UKPDS and HOT studies) and a target of <130/80 mmHg is more appropriate in this group.

Lifestyle measures

- Minimize dietary salt intake (<2.4 g sodium/day).
- Limit alcohol consumption to 2 drinks/day for men and 1 drink/day for women.
- Regular aerobic exercise (at least 30 minutes, ≥3 times/week).
- Achieve and maintain healthy BMI (20–25 kg/m²).
- Adopt DASH diet.
- Consume at least five portions/day of fresh fruit and vegetables.
- Reduce dietary fat content, especially saturated and trans-fatty acids.
- Stop smoking.

These measures should be followed in all individuals with hypertension, regardless of whether the decision has been made to implement drug therapy. Adopting and maintaining these lifestyle measures is often difficult. Implementation is most successful in a multidisciplinary professional setting when supported by clear written information including individualized strategies and goals.

Choice of drug therapy

Although recommendations for initiating medical therapy in essential hypertension have been proposed, there is no uniform agreement on which antihypertensive agent should be used for initial treatment. A variety of different classes of drugs can be used in this setting, including thiazide diuretics, β-blockers (BB), angiotensin-converting enzyme (ACE) inhibitors, angiotensin II receptor blockers (ARB), and calcium channel blockers (CCB).

Large meta-analyses of blood pressure–lowering trials have clearly shown that the degree of blood pressure lowering is the best determinant of risk reduction. Comparative studies, such as ALL-HAT, have typically shown that there is little evidence favoring one class of drug over another with respect to overall cardiovascular outcome.

Thiazide diuretics are effective and cheap and widely recommended as first-line antihypertensive therapy. Although calcium channel blockers may be less protective than other agents against the development of heart failure, their safety and effectiveness in preventing atherosclerotic events are now confirmed.

Treatment with the angiotensin receptor blocker losartan demonstrated a small advantage, particularly in reducing stroke, compared to β-blocker therapy in high-risk hypertensive patients with left ventricular hypertrophy (LIFE study).

It is useful to review a patient's complete medical history, as other compelling indications for various antihypertensive medications may exist and guide therapeutic decision-making (see Table 6.5).

Table 6.5 Considerations for individualizing antihypertensive therapy

Indication	Antihypertensive drugs
Compelling indications	
Systolic heart failure	ACE inhibitor or ARB, β-blocker, diuretic, aldosterone antagonist
Post-myocardial infarction	ACE inhibitor, β-blocker, aldosterone antagonist
Proteinuric chronic renal failure	ACE inhibitor and/or ARB
High coronary disease risk	Diuretic, ACE inhibitor
Diabetes mellitus	ACE inhibitor
Angina pectoris	β-Blocker, calcium channel blocker
Atrial fibrillation rate control	β-Blocker, nondihydropyridine calcium channel blocker
Favorable effect on comorbid conditions	
Benign prostatic hypertrophy	α-Blocker
Essential tremor	β-Blocker (noncardioselective)
Hyperthyroidism	β-Blocker
Migraine	β-Blocker, calcium channel blocker
Osteoporosis	Thiazide diuretic
Perioperative hypertension	β-Blocker
Raynaud's syndrome	Dihydropyridine calcium channel blocker
Indication	Antihypertensive drugs
Contraindications	
Angioedema	ACE inhibitor
Bronchospastic disease	β-Blocker
Depression	Reserpine
Liver disease	Methyldopa
Pregnancy	ACE inhibitor, ARB
Second- or third-degree heart block	β-blocker, nondihydropyridine calcium channel blocker
Adverse effect on comorbid conditions	
Depression	β-Blocker
Gout	Diuretic
Hyperkalemia	Aldosterone antagonist, ACE inhibitor, ARB
Hyponatremia	Thiazide diuretic
Renovascular disease	ACE inhibitor or ARB

Adapted from Chobanian AV, et al. (2003). *JAMA* 289(19):2560–2571. Copyright 2003 American Medical Association. All rights reserved.

Combining antihypertensive drugs

Many hypertensive patients require more than one drug for optimal blood pressure control. Using a combination of drugs often results in better blood pressure control with fewer side effects than maximizing the dose of an individual agent. This is because most drug combinations use agents that act by different mechanisms and thus tend to have an additive effect.

A low dose of a thiazide diuretic, e.g., increases the antihypertensive effect of all other antihypertensive drugs by minimizing volume expansion. It is also reasonable to administer two drugs as initial therapy in patients with blood pressures more than 20/10 mmHg above their goal. This approach may allow target blood pressures to be reached more efficiently. Fixed-dose combination pills are also available that may improve patient compliance and lower costs.

The JNC-7 report recommends the use of a thiazide diuretic when combination therapy is indicated unless compelling indications exist for the use of other agents (see Fig. 6.4).

The recent ACCOMPLISH trial, however, demonstrated the superior effectiveness of ACE inhibitor + dihydropyridine calcium channel blocker (benazepril + amlodipine) to that of an ACE inhibitor + thiazide combination in reducing cardiovascular events.

Other therapy

The lipid-lowering arm of the ASCOT study was terminated early because of a sizeable reduction in major vascular events seen in patients with hypertension and "average" cholesterol levels treated with atorvastatin 10 mg daily for <4 years.

Statin therapy should be initiated in these high-risk individuals regardless of baseline cholesterol levels. It is also recommended that aspirin 75–162 mg daily be prescribed to hypertensive patients who have evidence of clinical atherosclerotic disease or ≥10% 10-year cardiovascular event risk.

Hypertension Treatment Algorithm

STEP 1: Initiate lifestyle modifications (exercise, low salt diet, weight loss, smoking cessation)

STEP 2: Initiate pharmacotherapy if not at goal BP with consideration of compelling indications (see Table 6.5). Use agents for compelling indications if present

STEP 3: Determine hypertension stage to guide pharmacotherapy
- Stage 1 **HTN:** Use Thiazide-diuretic or may consider ACEI/ARB, or CCB
- Stage 2 **HTN:** 2-drug combination for most:
  - Thiazide diuretic and an ACEI/ARB or CCB or BB

  OR
  - CCB + ACEI/ARB

STEP 4: Add additional medications if needed, preferably a thiazide diurentic, ACEI/ARB, BB, OR CCB

STEP 5: If not at goal BP:
- Optimize doses
- Add additional agents
  Consider further work-up for secondary causes of hypertension
- Consider referral to hypertension specialist

Figure 6.4 Hypertension treatment algorithm.

ACEI, angiotensin-converting enzyme inhibitor; ARB, angiotensin II receptor blocker; BB, β-blocker; BP, blood pressure; CCB, calcium channel blocker. Adapted in part from Chobanian AV, et al. (2003). *JAMA* **289**(19):2560–2571; Jamerson K, et al. (2008). *N Engl J Med* **359**(23):2417–2428.

Lipid management in atherosclerosis

Dyslipidemia and risk of atherosclerosis

Numerous epidemiological studies have confirmed that a direct continuous relationship exists between plasma cholesterol level and risk of coronary artery disease, even within the normal range of cholesterol. Elevated LDL cholesterol levels appear to be the primary determinant of this relationship, but other atherogenic lipoprotein particles, including very low density lipoprotein (VLDL), chylomicron remnants, and Lp(a) also appear to play an important role as well.

LDL, particularly modified LDL, is recognized by the scavenger receptor on the surface of macrophages in the arterial wall, which take up these cholesterol-rich particles and eventually become the foam cells that form the lipid-rich core of atherosclerotic plaques.

Increasing levels of HDL, involved in reverse cholesterol transport from the peripheries to the liver, protect against the development of atherosclerosis. An increased triglyceride level is also now recognized as an independent risk factor for coronary disease.

Emerging data suggest that the nature of the lipoprotein particles plays an important part in their atherogenicity. For example, small, dense LDL particles, as seen in subjects with diabetes, are more readily taken up by macrophages and appear to be more atherogenic than larger, less dense LDL.

Lipids and risk assessment

It is essential to consider the lipid profile together in the context of the other risk factors present by estimating the 10-year cardiovascular risk. Although only total and HDL cholesterol are considered in most risk models, LDL cholesterol and triglyceride levels should also be considered in the assessment of risk (see Table 6.6).

Blood should ideally be sampled after a 12-hour fast, as triglycerides and calculated LDL cholesterol levels are affected by food intake. In general, a fasting lipid profile should be obtained in individuals with known cardiovascular disease and those at increased risk (Box 6.4).

Classification of primary dyslipidemias is provided in Table 6.7. Secondary causes of dyslipidemia are listed in Box 6.5.

Box 6.4 U.S. Preventive Services Task Force (USPSTF) recommendations

- Strongly recommend screening men aged 35 and older for lipid disorders
- Recommend screening men aged 20–35 for lipid disorders if they are at increased risk for coronary heart disease
- No recommendation for or against routine screening for lipid disorders in men aged 20–35, or in women aged 20 and older who are not at increased risk for coronary heart disease

Table 6.6 Adult Treatment Panel III classification of LDL, total, and HDL cholesterol

LDL cholesterol, mg/dL (mmol/L)	
<100 (2.58)	Optimal
100–129 (2.58–3.33)	Near or above optimal
130–159 (3.36–4.11)	Borderline high
160–189 (4.13–4.88)	High
≥190 (4.91)	Very high

Total cholesterol, mg/dL (mmol/L)	
<200 (5.17)	Desirable
200–239 (5.17–6.18)	Borderline high
≥240 (6.20)	High

HDL cholesterol, mg/dL (mmol/L)	
<40 (1.03)	Low
≥60 (1.55)	High

Adapted from Adult Treatment Panel III at http://www.nhlbi.nih.gov/

Table 6.7 WHO/Fredrickson classification of primary dyslipidemias

Phenotype	Elevated particles	Lipid levels
Type I (lipoprotein lipase deficiency or apoCII deficiency)	Chylomicrons	Triglycerides (TG) >99th percentile
Type IIa (familial hypercholesterolemia/ LDL receptor defects) Most common primary dyslipidemia	LDL	Total cholesterol (TC) >90th percentile; depending on type, may also see TG and/ or apolipoprotein B ≥90th percentile
Type IIb (familial combined hyperlipidemia, defective apoprotein B-100)	LDL and VLDL	TC and/or TG ≥90th percentile and apolipoprotein B ≥90th percentile
Type III (dysbetalipoproteinemia)	IDL	TC and TG >90th percentile
Type IV (familial hypertriglyceridemia, familial combined hyperlipidemia)	VLDL	TC >90th percentile, TG >90th percentile, low HDL
Type V	Chylomicrons, VLDL	TG >99th percentile

Box 6.5 Secondary causes of dyslipidemia

- Renal failure*
- Nephrotic syndrome*
- Hypothyroidism*
- Type 2 diabetes and obesity**
- Cholestasis
- Alcohol abuse
- Drugs
  - Antiretroviral protease inhibitors
  - Thiazides
  - Oral contraceptive pill
  - Isotretinoin
  - Steroids

* Cholesterol elevation.

** Minor elevation in cholesterol, but greater increase in atherogenic VLDL, chylomicron remnants, and triglycerides, as well as a fall in HDL.

Lipid-lowering medications

Statins

Atorvastatin, fluvastatin, pravastatin, rosuvastatin, simvastatin

Statins reduce cholesterol levels by inhibiting HMG CoA-reductase, the rate-limiting enzyme in cholesterol biosynthesis. They also increase clearance of circulating LDL by up-regulating LDL-receptor expression, further lowering cholesterol levels.

These agents are extremely effective at lowering cholesterol levels; e.g., the most potent statins, atorvastatin and rosuvastatin, can lower LDL cholesterol levels by >50%. Statin therapy typically results in a small increase in HDL and decrease in triglycerides as well.

A large evidence base has emerged over the past decade that strongly supports the use of statins in primary and secondary prevention of cardiovascular disease. Data from large randomized clinical trials have shown a consistent reduction (25%–30%) in the relative risk of major cardiovascular events with the use of atorvastatin, pravastatin, and simvastatin in both the primary (ASCOT, WOSCOPS, HPS, CARDS) and secondary prevention settings (MIRACL, CARE, LIPID, 4S, HPS).

In the first outcome study comparing two statins, the PROVE-IT study showed that high-dose atorvastatin (80 mg) was more effective than pravastatin (40 mg) at preventing further major cardiovascular events during the first 2–3 years after presentation with an acute coronary syndrome.

Typically recommended evidence-based doses are simvastatin 40 mg, pravastatin 40 mg, and atorvastatin 10–80 mg. Statins should not be prescribed to individuals with porphyria or severe liver or muscle disease. Caution is advised with their use in milder liver dysfunction and in combination with fibrates.

Fibrates

Fenofibrate, gemfibrozil

Fibrates improve the lipid profile by activating peroxisome proliferator-activated receptor α (PPAR-α), resulting in a mild lowering of total and LDL cholesterol, a more significant reduction in triglycerides (by 35%–50%), and increases in HDL (by 15%–25%).

Patients with combined hyperlipidemia or other reasons for a low HDL and/or high triglycerides respond well to fibrates. Although the VA-HIT study showed that gemfibrozil reduced major cardiovascular events in patients with average cholesterol and low HDL levels, subgroup analysis of the Heart Protection Study (HPS) suggested that similar benefits were observed with simvastatin (40 mg) in such individuals.

For most patients with and at risk of cardiovascular events, fibrates are typically recommended as second-line agents in patients intolerant of statins, particularly if they have low HDL or high triglycerides. The likelihood of transaminitis or myopathy is increased if fibrates and statins are used in combination. Thus careful monitoring is recommended when using this combination. The risk is lower with fenofibrate than that with other fibrates.

Anion-exchange resins

Cholestyramine, cholestipol

These agents bind bile salts in the small bowel, which inhibits their reabsorption, resulting in upregulation of the LDL receptor on hepatocytes and increased plasma cholesterol clearance. Although these drugs effectively lower cholesterol levels, many patients experience intolerable GI side effects that limit their widespread use.

These drugs are generally recommended as second- or third-line therapy in subjects with hypercholesterolemia.

Inhibitors of intestinal cholesterol absorption

Ezetimibe

This medication binds to an intestinal transport protein and inhibits cholesterol absorption. LDL cholesterol is reduced by 15%–20%. The dose is 10 mg daily. Ezetimibe is most often used in combination with a statin in those patients who do not achieve their LDL cholesterol target at higher statin doses.

Although it is effective in lowering LDL levels and has been used as monotherapy in statin-intolerant patients, clinical outcome data are currently lacking, so it should not be used as first-line therapy as a substitute for statins.

Niacin

Niacin reduces hepatic VLDL synthesis and inhibits fatty acid release from adipocytes. HDL levels are significantly increased (by 30%–35%), and reduced hepatic synthesis results in a small reduction in LDL.

Although particularly beneficial in mixed dyslipidemias, use of the short-acting formulation is limited by a high incidence of intolerable GI side effects and facial flushing. It may also worsen glucose tolerance in diabetics. The modified-release formulation (niaspan 500–2000 mg daily) is more tolerable, and ongoing outcome studies should confirm the use of this agent in preventing cardiovascular events.

Niacin is particularly useful in patients with low HDL and is often used in combination with statins. Pretreatment with aspirin can minimize flushing, and taking it with food or water can reduce the incidence of GI side effects.

Fish oils

Fish oil supplements containing high concentrations of omega-3 fatty acids are indicated for the treatment of severe hypertriglyceridemia (e.g., Lovaza 4 g/day). They act by reducing VLDL production and in sufficient doses (>3 g/day) can lower serum triglycerides by 50%.

The FDA has limited approval for Lovaza to the treatment of severe hypertriglyceridemia (≥500 mg/dL [≥5.6 mmol/L]) because of concerns that it appears to increase LDL cholesterol levels.

Dietary plant stanols (3 g/day) can reduce LDL cholesterol by up to 15%.

Goals of lipid-lowering therapy

Current Adult Treatment Panel (ATP) guidelines are more aggressive than previous iterations, especially in patients with established coronary disease and those at high risk. This is the result of a better understanding of the cardiovascular risk associated with hyperlipidemia and the benefits of lipid-lowering therapy determined from large randomized trials.

The first step in planning therapy is to ascertain the patient's cardiovascular risk based on presence of risk factors and coronary disease or its equivalent, determine the 10-year risk of events (Framingham score), and categorize the patient as low, moderate, moderately high, or high risk. Each category has recommended LDL goals and guidelines for when to initiate therapy (see Table 6.8).

It is also important to remember the importance of high triglycerides and low HDL when planning therapy. Some recommend focusing therapy on the serum total–to–HDL cholesterol ratio and non–HDL cholesterol levels, especially in patients with hypertriglyceridemia. The goal for non-HDL-C in this circumstance is a concentration that is 30 mg/dL higher than that for LDL (see Table 6.9). An elevated HDL >60 mg/dL is considered a negative risk factor.

Therapeutic lifestyle changes, including exercise, weight loss, and dietary modifications, are the first step in treatment of all patients with dyslipidemia. Moderate weight reduction (10% of body weight) can significantly improve the lipid profile and lower risk. The composition of the optimal diet is controversial, though general recommendations include
- Reduced cholesterol to <200 mg/day and saturated fats (especially trans fats) to <7% total calories
- Increased plant stanols, sterols, and soluble fiber (20–30 g/day)
- Adoption of a Mediterranean diet

Exercise should also be done on a regular basis, although the resulting changes in LDL and HDL cholesterol are modest.

Based on current guidelines, statin therapy should be started in all patients with established clinical atherosclerotic disease, including CAD and cerebrovascular, renovascular, and peripheral arterial disease, and diabetics and those patients with a 10-year cardiac risk of ≥20% (Table 6.10).

Although all of these patients should receive statins (unless contraindicated) regardless of the cholesterol level (HPS, ASCOT, CARDS), it is still important to measure lipid levels to ensure that subjects are responding appropriately to therapy and achieving their guideline-based targets for cholesterol lowering. These targets are based on observations from clinical trials (PROVE-IT, TNT) and cohort studies suggesting that "lower is better" when it comes to cholesterol levels and outcomes. It is also recommended that a second agent (such as niacin, a fibrate, or ezetimibe) be added if the LDL target is not achieved on high-dose high-potency statins (as tolerated), although the data for this are limited.

There is also less outcome-based evidence informing us when to initiate drug therapy for isolated dyslipidemia in the absence of other risk factors. Primary and familial hyperlipidemias should be treated aggressively, particularly if there is a family history of premature CAD.

Table 6.8 NCEP Adult Treatment Panel III LDL goals: 2004 update

Risk category	LDL goal	LDL level at which to initiate therapeutic lifestyle changes	LDL level at which to consider drug therapy
High risk: coronary heart disease (CHD) or CHD risk equivalent (10-year risk >20%)	<100 mg/dL; optional goal of <70 mg/dL in very high risk (see Box 6.6)	≥100 mg/dL	≥100 mg/dL; <100 mg/dL consider drug options
Moderately high risk: 2 or more risk factors (10-year risk 10 to 20%)	<130 mg/dL	≥130 mg/dL	≥130 mg/dL; 100–129 mg/dL consider drug options
Moderate risk: 2 or more risk factors (10-year risk <10%)	<130 mg/dL	≥130 mg/dL	≥160 mg/dL
Lower risk: 0 to 1 risk factor	<160 mg/dL	≥160 mg/dL	≥190 mg/dL; 160–189 mg/dL consider drug options

Adapted from National Cholesterol Education Program (NCEP) Adult Treatment Panel III at http://www.nhlbi.nih.gov/guidelines/cholesterol/

Box 6.6 NCEP definition of very high risk

Established coronary disease *PLUS*:
1. Multiple major risk factors (especially diabetes)

OR

2. Severe and poorly controlled risk factors (especially continued smoking)

OR

3. Multiple risk factors of the metabolic syndrome (especially triglycerides ≥200 plus non-HDL-C ≥130 plus HDL-C <40)

OR

4. Acute coronary syndrome

Table 6.9 Adult Treatment Panel III non-HDL goals

Risk category	Non-HDL cholesterol (mg/dL)
Coronary heart disease (CHD) or equivalent (10- year risk of CHD >20%)	<130
Two or more CHD risk factors and 10-year risk of CHD ≤ 20%	<160
0 to 1 CHD risk factor	<190

Adapted from NCEP Adult Treatment Panel III at http://www.nhlbi.nih.gov/guidelines/cholesterol/

Table 6.10 Suggested treatment goals in patients with cardio-metabolic risk and lipoprotein abnormalities (2008 ACC/ADA Consensus Report)

	Goals		
	LDL (mg/dL)	Non-HDL (mg/dL)	apoB (mg/dL)
Highest-risk patients, including those with 1) known CVD or 2) diabetes plus one or more additional major CVD risk factor	<70	<100	<80
High-risk patients, including those with 1) no diabetes or known clinical CVD but two or more additional major CVD risk factors or 2) diabetes but not other major CVD risk factors	<100	<130	<90

Other major risk factors include smoking, hypertension, and family history of premature CAD.

CAD, coronary artery disease; CVD, cardiovascular disease.

From 2008 ACC/ADA Consensus Report on Lipoprotein Management in Patients with Cardiometabolic Risk.

Diabetes and atherosclerosis

Over 7% of U.S. adults are known to have diabetes mellitus (DM), the vast majority of whom have type 2 diabetes. However, because of the associated microvascular and macrovascular complications, diabetes accounts for nearly 14% of U.S. health care expenditures.

Although diabetes is more common in older individuals, the incidence is increasing at a dramatic rate in all age groups, especially young adults, driven by the increased prevalence of obesity.

Macrovascular complications are the leading cause of death in patients with diabetes (see Fig. 6.5). The National Cholesterol Education Program (NCEP) report considers type 2 diabetes a coronary disease equivalent, placing these patients in the highest risk category. This classification is based on the observation that type 2 diabetics without a prior MI are at the same risk for MI and cardiac mortality as nondiabetics who had a prior MI.

In the Framingham Heart Study, presence of diabetes doubled the age-adjusted risk for cardiovascular disease in men and tripled it in women.

Mechanisms responsible for increased CV risk in DM

Diabetics have a greater burden of atherogenic risk factors than that of nondiabetics. These include obesity, low HDL, high triglycerides (VLDL and remnant particles), increased small, dense LDL, hypertension, low-grade inflammation, a procoagulant state (increased PAI-1, and platelet activation), increased oxidative stress, and increased levels of harmful advanced glycation end products.

Coronary atherosclerotic plaques in diabetics contain a greater amount of lipid-rich atheroma and more macrophage infiltration, which may increase risk of rupture and thrombosis. Conventional risk factors only

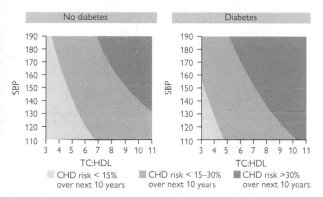

Figure 6.5 Effect of type 2 DM on CHD risk (nonsmoker, age 60 years). Adapted with permission from the British Cardiac Society, British Hyperlipidaemia Society, British Hypertension Society, British Diabetic Association. *Heart* 1998; 80(Suppl. 2):S1–S29.

account for a relatively small proportion (<25%) of the increased risk observed in diabetes.

Not only are diabetic subjects more likely to suffer a major vascular event, they are also more likely to die from this event than if they did not have diabetes. The atherosclerotic process tends to be more diffuse in diabetics, often affecting multiple vascular territories, and diabetics presenting with acute coronary syndrome are much more likely to have multivessel coronary disease. The burden of diffuse coronary disease also makes percutaneous and surgical revascularization more technically challenging and risky (see Figure 6.6).

Outcome is better when diabetics with multivessel coronary disease undergo CABG rather than percutaneous coronary revascularization (RITA, BARI). However, data from large studies suggest that outcome after PCI in diabetics is improved by use of drug-eluting stents as well as abciximab, a platelet glycoprotein IIb/IIIa antagonist.

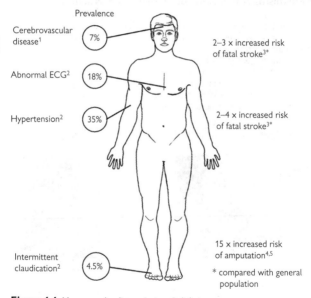

Prevalence

Cerebrovascular disease[1]   7%

2–3 × increased risk of fatal stroke[3]*

Abnormal ECG[2]   18%

Hypertension[2]   35%

2–4 × increased risk of fatal stroke[3]*

15 × increased risk of amputation[4,5]

Intermittent claudication[2]   4.5%

* compared with general population

Figure 6.6 Macrovascular disease in type 2 diabetes.
1. Wingard DL, et al. (1993). *Diabetes Care* 16:1022–1025. 2. UKPDS 6 (1990). *Diabetes Res* 13:1–11. 3. Balkau B, et al. (1997) *Lancet* 350:1680. 4. King's Fund. Counting the Cost. BDA, 1996. 5. Most RS, Sinnock P (1983). *Diabetes Care* 6:67–91.

Visceral neuropathy is responsible for silent MI and reduced heart rate variability. Diabetic nephropathy further contributes to cardiac risk by increasing blood pressure and causing deterioration in the lipid profile.

Recommendations for risk reduction in diabetes

Blood glucose should be aggressively controlled by means of diet and exercise coupled with appropriate hypoglycemic drug therapy. Target HbA1c is ≤7%. However, intense blood sugar control is better at reducing progression of microvascular disease and neuropathy than prevention of macrovascular events (UKPDS study).

Aggressive blood pressure (UKPDS, HOT studies) and lipid management (CARDS, ASCOT, HPS, ALLIANCE, SPARCL) has a greater impact on prevention of coronary disease and stroke than tight glucose control and reduces progression of nephropathy.

Cardiovascular risk in diabetics is similar to that seen in patients with established coronary disease; therefore, appropriate preventive strategies employing guideline-based therapies are recommended (see Table 6.11).

Table 6.11 Therapeutic recommendations for CV prevention in diabetes

Measure	Target
Aggressive lifestyle ± oral hypoglycemic therapy	HbA1c ≤7%
Statin therapy (regardless of baseline lipid levels)	LDL <100 mg/dL
Aggressive blood pressure control	<130/<80 mmHg
Aspirin	

ACE inhibitor or ARB is used in most patients, especially if there is evidence of nephropathy.

The metabolic syndrome

The *metabolic syndrome* describes a frequently observed cluster of adverse risk factors within an individual. It has also been referred to as *syndrome X* and the *insulin resistance syndrome*. The syndrome is characterized by visceral obesity, insulin resistance, moderate hypertension, dyslipidemia (low HDL and high triglycerides with average cholesterol levels), and low-grade inflammation.

Several definitions of this syndrome have been proposed, but the NCEP ATP-III diagnostic criteria (Table 6.12) are the most practical and widely used, as well as being a robust predictor of vascular risk.

The prevalence of this syndrome is increasing in parallel with the increase in numbers of obese and overweight individuals. It has been described in a high proportion of American children and adolescents. Thus, the metabolic syndrome is projected to contribute substantially to the societal burden of atherosclerotic disease in the next few decades.

Unless effective interventions to slow, and hopefully reverse, this trend are delivered at a population level, much of the progress that has been made in the fight against coronary disease is likely to be overturned.

Mechanisms of increased risk

Visceral obesity causes insulin resistance, which is associated with increase in blood glucose and abnormalities in the lipid profile. Increased levels of inflammatory cytokines such as TNF-α, some of which are produced by adipocytes, cause endothelial dysfunction that increases vascular tone and blood pressure, as well as promoting local pro-atherosclerotic changes in the vascular wall (see Fig. 6.7).

Increased leptin and reduced adiponectin levels influence insulin sensitivity, as well as some of the adverse metabolic consequences of obesity, but their incremental clinical value remains a subject of investigation. It has been proposed that the degree of insulin resistance is less important than the impact of other risk factors, including lipids, blood pressure, inflammation and pro-thrombotic factors, but these factors also remain under investigation.

Table 6.12 ATP-III criteria for diagnosis of the metabolic syndrome

Variable	Threshold
Waist circumference	>40" Men
	>35" Women
Fasting glucose	>100 mg/dL
Blood pressure	>130/>85 mmHg
HDL cholesterol	<40 mg/dL in men
	<50 mg/dL in women
Triglycerides	>150 mg/dL

Three out of five criteria must be satisfied for firm diagnosis. Drug treatment for hyperglycemia, hypertension, low HDL, and elevated triglycerides satisfies the criteria for these variables.

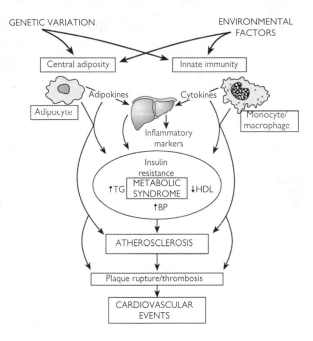

Figure 6.7 Pathophysiology of atherosclerotic cardiovascular disease in the metabolic syndrome. Central adiposity and innate immunity play key roles in the development of insulin resistance, chronic inflammation, and metabolic syndrome features through the effects of adipokines (e.g., leptin, adiponectin, resistin) and cytokines (e.g., tumor necrosis factor-α, interleukin-6) on liver, skeletal muscle, and immune cells. In addition, monocyte/macrophage and adipocyte-derived factors may have direct atherothrombotic effects that promote the occurrence of atherosclerotic cardiovascular events. Common genetic variants and environmental factors may impact the development of atherosclerosis at multiple levels through influences on central adiposity, innate immunity, glucose and lipoprotein metabolism, and vascular function. Reproduced with permission from Reilly MP, Rader D (2003). *Circulation* 108(13):1546–1551.

Metabolic syndrome: management

The treatment of patients with the metabolic syndrome is essentially the same as treatment of the individual variables. Weight loss and exercise are the cornerstones of management, and cardiovascular risk factors should be further treated if they persist despite lifestyle modifications.

Management of insulin resistance with insulin-sensitizing drugs (metformin, and thiazolidenediones; see Fig. 6.8) has theoretical benefits but is currently under investigation, as the ability of such an approach to improve outcomes compared to weight reduction and exercise alone is not yet well supported by clinical trials.

As far as management of the dyslipidemia is concerned, treatment with a statin is clearly indicated if the 10-year cardiac risk is ≥20%, or if LDL cholesterol is elevated as per the ATP-III guidelines.

The nature of the risk factor profile in the metabolic syndrome frequently results in the underestimation of 10-year risk, but at present no studies are currently available to support use of specific evidence-based drug therapy in this syndrome. Most, if not all, of these patients should also take a daily aspirin for primary prevention.

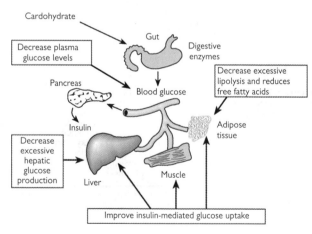

Figure 6.8 Glitazones decrease insulin resistance at target tissues.

Aspirin for primary prevention

The Physician's Health Study (PHS) was the first reported trial of aspirin in the primary prevention of cardiovascular disease. The study was stopped early because of a statistically significant 44% reduction in first MI.

The decision to prescribe aspirin for primary prevention should be an individual clinical judgment that weighs the benefit of reducing risk of a first MI, the risk factor profile of the patient, and the adverse effects of long-term administration, specifically gastrointestinal bleeding. An important consideration is that, when aspirin is used for primary prevention, the absolute benefit is much smaller than that for secondary prevention, while the risk of major gastrointestinal bleeding is the same.

The United States Preventive Services Task Force recommends aspirin for all apparently healthy men and women whose 10-year risk of a first CHD event is 6% or greater. The American Heart Association uses a 10% or greater cut-off risk for which the benefits of aspirin are likely to outweigh the risks of chronic administration.

Current data suggest that aspirin is underutilized, both for primary and secondary prevention. Approximately 40% of adults over age 40 in the United States have the metabolic syndrome and a 10-year risk of a first cardiac event of 16% to 18%. Thus, wider use of aspirin in such patients seems warranted.

A single daily dose of 81 mg aspirin is appropriate for primary prevention.

Diseases of the myocardium and pericardium

Myocardial diseases

Classification

Heart muscle diseases include a diverse range of cardiomyopathies and myocarditides. They are classified according to the predominant patho-physiological process (Box 7.1).

Arrhythmogenic right ventricular cardiomyopathy (dysplasia) has been included in its own right and a few conditions remain unclassified because they do not easily fit into any of these categories (systolic dysfunction with minimal dilatation, fibroelastosis, ventricular non-compaction, and mito-chondrial disease).

Specific cardiomyopathies are heart muscle diseases associated with specific cardiac or systemic disorders and include conditions previously excluded from this classification (Box 7.2).

Myocarditis is an inflammatory process involving myocytes, interstitium, and vascular components. It can be caused by a large number of infectious agents.

Box 7.1 WHO/ISFC classification of cardiomyopathies

- Dilated cardiomyopathy
- Hypertrophic cardiomyopathy
- Restrictive cardiomyopathy
- Arrhythmogenic right ventricular cardiomyopathy (dysplasia)

WHO, World Health Organization; ISFC, International Society and Federation Cardiology.

Box 7.2 Specific cardiomyopathies

- Ischemic
- Valvular
- Hypertensive
- Alcohol
- Metabolic
- Nutritional
- General system disease
- Muscular dystrophies
- Neuromuscular disorders
- Sensitivity and toxic reactions
- Peripartum

Dilated cardiomyopathy

Dilated cardiomyopathy (DCM) is characterized by cardiac chamber enlargement and impaired systolic dysfunction, although diastolic dysfunction is almost always also present. The syndrome of heart failure (HF) often ensues. The prevalence is 5–8 per 100,000, and it is 3 times more frequent in blacks and males than whites and females.

The etiology of DCM is presented in Box 7.3.

Symptoms

Clinical presentation can be abrupt with acute pulmonary edema but more often patients present with symptoms of heart failure such as breathlessness, in particular exertional dyspnea, orthopnea, paroxysmal nocturnal dyspnea, and fatigue.

Arrhythmias (e.g. AF, particularly with high alcohol intake) are also common and patients are at risk for VT and sudden cardiac death (SCD).

Diagnosis

Diagnosis is established by physical examination, electrocardiography, chest X-ray, and echocardiography (see also Box 7.4).

- *ECG* may show evidence of LVH, previous myocardial infarction (MI), or arrhythmias. A sinus tachycardia is common with nonspecific T-wave changes and poor R wave in anterior chest leads.
- *Chest X-ray* may show an enlarged cardiac size and pulmonary edema.
- *Echocardiography* allows accurate assessment of cardiac chamber sizes as well as LV systolic and diastolic function and valvular function. There is usually biventricular dilatation with poor septal motion. There may be mural thrombus in either or both ventricles. Often a small pericardial collection is found. Ejection fraction and fractional shortening are low. Dilatation of the ventricles results in mitral and tricuspid regurgitation.
- *Exercise testing* with or without measurement of maximum ventilatory oxygen consumption is useful to assess functional capacity.
- *Ambulatory ECG* monitoring is essential to assess for the presence of prognostically significant ventricular arrhythmias.
- *Cardiac catheterization* should be performed with caution in all patients with a dilated cardiomyopathy to do the following:
  - Exclude significant coronary disease
  - Assess severity of mitral regurgitation and pulmonary artery pressures
  - Ventricular biopsy: not routinely performed

Treatment

Management of DCM focuses on relieving symptoms and improving prognosis. Therapies are designed to correct the maladaptive neurohormonal abnormalities involving the sympathetic system and renin–angiotensin–aldosterone axis. The management of heart failure is discussed in Chapter 5.

Box 7.3 Etiology of dilated cardiomyopathy

Although originally considered to be idiopathic, experimental and clinical data now suggest that genetic, viral, and autoimmune factors play a role in its pathophysiology.

Several genetic mutations have been identified as the causative problem in familial DCM, while certain viruses have been shown to cause sporadic cases of DCM.

The following list is not exhaustive and there is some overlap with specific cardiomyopathies.

• Inherited (may account for >25% of cases)
• Myocarditis (infective, autoimmune, toxic)
• Metabolic (hemochromatosis, thyrotoxicosis).
• Nutritional (vitamin deficiencies—thiamine [beriberi])
• Persistent tachycardia (tachycardia-induced cardiomyopathy)

DCM is essentially a diagnosis of exclusion, and potentially reversible causes, including coronary artery disease, valvular heart disease and adult congenital heart disease, should be sought. Careful attention should be paid to dietary history and alcohol consumption, as some reversibility is possible with modification of these factors.

Box 7.4 Additional investigations for DCM

• Renal function
• Liver function tests
• Serum ferritin, iron, transferrin
• Thyroid function
• Viral serology
• Infective screen (HIV, hepatitis C, enteroviruses)
• Autoantibodies

Hypertrophic cardiomyopathy

Hypertrophic cardiomyopathy (HCM) is characterized by maladaptive left ventricular hypertrophy (LVH) inappropriate for the degree of afterload. Prevalence is thought to be 1–2 per 1000.

The hypertrophy is classically localized to the proximal interventricular septum, resulting in a dynamic outflow tract obstruction in association with systolic anterior motion (SAM) of the mitral valve leaflets (present in 35% of patients).

However, there is considerable phenotypic variability and the hypertrophy can be concentric, apical, or mid-cavitary, resulting in an intracavitary gradient (often in association with an apical aneurysm). In addition, genetic studies have demonstrated that affected family members may have little or no cardiac hypertrophy despite the presence of a disease causing mutation (variable penetrance). The reason for this marked phenotypic variability is poorly understood but is almost certainly multifactorial.

HCM has also been associated with accessory atrioventricular pathways and conduction abnormalities in certain families.

Etiology

HCM is an autosomal dominant inherited cardiac condition. However, there is marked allelic and nonallelic heterogeneity with multiple mutations (more than 450) in at least 20 genes now identified as causing the disease. Most of these mutations are in genes encoding proteins of the sarcomere.

In contrast to mutations causing DCM, mutations frequently affect sarcomeric proteins involved in force generation as opposed to force transmission. This is, however, not consistent and some genes have different mutations causing both HCM *and* DCM. Other mutations have been found in genes encoding nonsarcomeric proteins.

Histologically there is myofibrillar disarray and extensive fibrosis. Small intramural arterioles are also hypertrophied. The findings may be patchy but are concentrated in the septum.

Subvalvular obstruction occurs between the anterior leaflet of the mitral valve and the hypertrophied septum. The mitral valve apparatus moves anteriorly in systole (a combination of malaligned papillary muscles and Venturi effect of a high-velocity jet in the outflow tract). The valve becomes thickened and mitral regurgitation occurs.

Obstruction of the LV outflow tract is not always present. It is possible to have asymmetric septal hypertrophy (ASH) alone. Occasionally there is obstruction more evident toward the apex rather than at the outflow tract.

Symptoms

Patients often are asymptomatic and are increasingly picked up incidentally from the wider use and availability of echocardiography or as part of family screening after identification of an affected family member. Symptoms, when they do occur, may include the following:

- Fatigue and breathlessness due to impaired diastolic filling and decreased cardiac output. Atrial transport is very important for maintaining cardiac output; symptoms typically get much worse with AF.

- Chest pain (angina) can result from increased cardiac work secondary to the LVH, a relative blood supply–demand mismatch and plugging of intramural arterioles. High diastolic pressures increase the diastolic wall stress and impair diastolic coronary blood flow.
- Atrial and ventricular arrhythmias are common and can result in palpitations, presyncope and syncope, or even sudden death.
- Presyncope and syncope can also occur due to increased outflow tract obstruction during exercise, at times of relative intravascular dehydration, or from certain maneuvers (i.e., Valsalva)
- Approximately 10%–15% of patients may eventually develop left ventricular dilatation and failure.

Sudden cardiac death

The risk of SCD in these patients is extremely difficult to determine because of the marked phenotypic variability, and most risk factors have low sensitivity and specificity. The annual incidence of SCD across the entire population with HCM is about 1%.

Markers of risk for SCD in HCM

- Early age at diagnosis
- History of syncope
- Family history of SCD
- LV wall thickness >30 mm
- Nonsustained VT on ambulatory ECG monitoring
- Abnormal blood pressure response to exercise
- High-risk genetic mutations

Diagnosis

The diagnosis is established by physical examination, electrocardiography, and echocardiography. Close attention must be paid to family history and family members should be offered screening.

A genetic diagnosis can now be made in select individuals who have a definite family history of HCM. Despite the marked genetic heterogeneity, a genetic diagnosis may be established in 70% of patients with inherited HCM, allowing accurate screening of other family members.

Physical examination (see Fig. 7.1)

Evidence of LVH may present with a forceful apical impulse and an S_4 heart sound. Outflow tract obstruction is evident by a double apical impulse and ejection systolic murmur beginning in mid-systole, which may be augmented by provocation by maneuvers such as Valsalva or standing.

A pansystolic murmur due to mitral regurgitation resulting from systolic anterior movement of the mitral valve may also be present.

Investigations

- **ECG** is rarely normal but usually shows voltage criteria for LVH with associated repolarization abnormalities. Features include
  - LVH with ST and T wave change
  - Deep Q waves in inferior and lateral leads (septal hypertrophy)
  - Pre-excitation and WPW syndrome
  - Ventricular ectopics

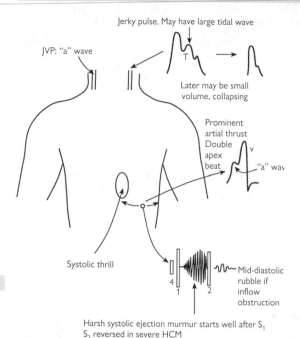

Jerky pulse. May have large tidal wave

JVP: "a" wave

Later may be small volume, collapsing

Prominent artial thrust
Double apex beat
"a" wave

Systolic thrill

Mid-diastolic rubble if inflow obstruction

Harsh systolic ejection murmur starts well after S_1
S_2 reversed in severe HCM

Figure 7.1 Clinical signs of hypertrophic cardiomyopathy. Reproduced with permission from Swanton RH (2003). *Cardiology Pocket Consultant*, 5th ed. Copyright Wiley-Blackwell 2003.

- **Echocardiography** is essential for diagnosis with accurate measurement of chamber sizes and wall thicknesses. It also facilitates demonstration of outflow tract or intracavitary gradients. Features include the following:
  - ASH: grossly thickened septum compared with posterior LV wall, with reduced septal motion
  - Small LV cavity with hypercontractile posterior wall
  - Mid-systolic aortic valve closure or fluttering of the aortic valve leaflet tips
  - SAM: systolic anterior movement of the mitral valve apparatus. There may be contact between the anterior mitral leaflet and septum in systole.
  - Reduced diastolic closure rate of the anterior mitral valve leaflet
- **Cardiac MRI** may be helpful in borderline cases.

Other investigations may help in risk stratification, although no one investigation accurately predicts those at risk of SCD and negative tests do not exclude the risk of SCD.

- **Ambulatory ECG** monitoring—atrial and ventricular arrhythmias.
- **Exercise testing**—functional capacity and blood pressure response to exercise.
- **Cardiac catheterization**—coronary anatomy and intracavitary and outflow tract gradients.
- **Electrophysiology testing**—VT studies have no proven role in risk assessment but EP studies may be useful to assess suspected accessory AV pathways.
- **Genetic testing**—only useful for screening family members if causative gene in proband can be identified.

Treatment

Approximately half of sudden deaths in HCM occur during or shortly after strenuous exercise, thus patients should be advised against competitive sports. Unfortunately, this also means that a significant proportion die unexpectedly without any obvious precipitant.

Treatment of symptoms usually consists of the following.

β-Blockers

β-Blockers reduce myocardial oxygen demand and improve diastolic filling, reducing chest pain and improving breathlessness. They are the mainstay of therapy for angina, dyspnea, and syncope. Large doses may be required.

Calcium channel antagonists

Calcium channel antagonists (verapamil and diltiazem) are useful as they are negative inotropes (reducing outflow tract obstruction) and reduce heart rate during exercise. Use diltiazem cautiously with β-blockers. Avoid verapamil in patients on β-blockers.

Disopyramide

Disopyramide is a negative inotrope antiarrhythmic agent that has been shown to reduce outflow tract gradients. Unfortunately, its use is limited by anticholinergic side effects.

Antiarrhythmics

Other antiarrhythmic drugs such as amiodarone and sotalol are useful for controlling supraventricular arrhythmias but have not been shown to reduce the risk of SCD from ventricular arrhythmias. AF should be cardioverted as soon as possible (using amiodarone to improve chances of success).

Nonpharmacological treatments

Surgical septal myotomy–myectomy (Morrow procedure) directly debulks the proximal septum. This procedure is recommended in patients with severely symptomatic heart failure (NYHA Class III or IV) or who have recurrent syncope despite medical therapy and is the preferred debulking procedure over alcohol septal ablation.

There is a risk of high-degree AV block requiring permanent pacing (about 5%) and long-term complications include aortic regurgitation. Cardiac transplantation may be necessary in patients who develop left ventricular dilatation and systolic heart failure.

Alcohol septal ablation involves injecting alcohol into the first or second septal perforator artery. This causes a localized infarct of the hypertrophied proximal septum, reducing LVOT gradient (see Table 7.1 for assessment of LVOT obstruction). However, a significant number of patients (10%–15%) require permanent pacing afterward from AV block, and theoretically there is increased risk of ventricular arrhythmias due to creation of further arrhythmic substrate.

Dual-chamber pacing with short AV delay may be used in patients with significant obstruction and symptoms refractory to drug therapy and who are not candidates for surgical septal myectomy. By ensuring ventricular pre-excitation, LV contraction is desynchronized, reducing LVOT gradients. Maintaining RV capture especially during exercise is difficult and shortening the AV delay too much impairs diastolic filling.

Implantable cardioverter defibrillators (ICDs) should be considered in patients who have survived a cardiac arrest or who have presented with hemodynamically unstable VT. Although not currently recommended in all HCM patients, the utility of ICDs, even for primary prevention of SCD, is increasingly appreciated.

Table 7.1 Dynamic maneuvers to assess LVOT obstruction

Decreased LVOT obstruction (murmur softer and shorter)	Increased LVOT obstruction (murmur louder and longer)
↑ *LV volume*	↓ *LV volume*
Squatting	Sudden standing
Handgrip	Valsalva (during)
Passive leg elevation	Sublingual GTN
Valsalva (after release)	Hypovolemia
Mueller maneuver (deep inspiration against a closed glottis)	Dehydration
↓ *Contractility*	↑ *Contractility*
β-Blockers (acute IV)	β-Agonists (e.g., isoprenaline)
↑ *Afterload*	↓ *Afterload*
Phenylephrine	α-Blockade
Handgrip	

Restrictive cardiomyopathy

Restrictive cardiomyopathy is a rare condition characterized by impaired diastolic function due to reduced ventricular compliance. It is very important to distinguish restrictive cardiomyopathy from constrictive pericarditis as the latter can be treated surgically by stripping the pericardium from the myocardium.

Etiology

The etiology of truly idiopathic cases remains obscure. A few cases are familial and tend to be associated with skeletal muscle disease. Other cases are associated with systemic diseases, infiltration, or endomyocardial fibrosis (see Box 7.5).

Symptoms

Patients often have severely limited exercise tolerance because of an inability to increase cardiac output as the stroke volume is relatively fixed. They are also limited by breathlessness and have evidence of right heart failure (peripheral edema).

Diagnosis

Physical examination

In addition to signs of HF, a loud S_3, S_4, or both may be present. There also may be prominent *x* and *y* descents of the JVP and venous pressure may increase on inspiration (Kussmaul sign). The apex beat will be palpable in contrast to constrictive pericarditis.

Investigations

- **ECG** may show P-mitrale or -pulmonale, reduced precordial QRS voltages, and atrial arrhythmias.
- **Echocardiography** may be normal or at least demonstrate normal systolic function. Alternatively, systolic function may be reduced in advanced cases. Infiltration may be evident by hypertrophied ventricles and thickened intra-atrial septum and the myocardium may appear speckled. Biatrial enlargement may also be present. A restrictive mitral inflow pattern is seen on Doppler tracing.
- **Laboratory test** are aimed at determining causes of infiltration. Left and right heart catheterization may be necessary to help exclude constrictive pericarditis (difference in LVEDP and RVEDP >7 mmHg at end expiration makes constriction unlikely).
- **CT and MRI** scanning are useful to look at pericardial disease.

Treatment

Treatment is aimed at the symptoms of HF and the underlying condition. Rate control in atrial fibrillation is important, as reducing ventricular filling times will have significant impact.

Box 7.5 Causes of restrictive cardiomyopathy

Myocardial

Noninfiltrative
- Idiopathic
- Scleroderma

Infiltrative
- Amyloid
- Sarcoid

Storage diseases
- Lysosomal storage diseases (Gaucher's, Hurler's, Fabry)
- Glycogen storage disease
- Hemochromatosis

Endomyocardial
- Endomyocardial fibrosis
- Hypereosinophilic syndrome
- Metastatic malignancies
- Carcinoid
- Iatrogenic (radiation, anthracyclines)

Arrhythmogenic right ventricular cardiomyopathy

Arrhythmogenic right ventricular cardiomyopathy (ARVC) is a disease in which the normal right ventricular myocardium is replaced by a fibro-fatty infiltrate. It was originally termed a dysplasia, reflecting the idea that it was somehow a developmental defect, but further understanding has led to the appreciation that it is a continuing process and has subsequently been reclassified as a cardiomyopathy.

It can progress to right ventricular dilatation and failure, and in some cases there may also be left ventricular involvement.

Etiology

Half of cases are familial with an autosomal dominant pattern of inheritance. Disease-causing genes have not been found, but several loci have been mapped to chromosomes 1, 2, 3, 10, and 14. An autosomal recessive variant, which is characterized by ARVC, palmoplantar keratosis, and wooly hair (Naxos disease), has been mapped to chromosome 17.

Symptoms

Patients are usually asymptomatic and presentation is usually in the form of ventricular arrhythmias with typical LBBB pattern indicating probable origin from the right ventricle. Therefore, otherwise healthy young individuals can present with cardiac arrest or SCD. Other patients present in later life with symptoms of HF with or without ventricular arrhythmias and are misdiagnosed as having DCM.

Diagnosis

Diagnosis of affected individuals can be very difficult, especially during family screening, as standard noninvasive investigations have poor sensitivity. Only a minority may have classic findings of typical right ventricular arrhythmias with LBBB pattern, abnormal depolarization/repolarization abnormalities, particularly on right precordial ECG leads, and evidence of structural abnormalities of the right ventricle.

Right ventricular free wall abnormalities are best characterized by MRI, but this too has limitations. Therefore, patients with suspected ARVC but negative investigations may need repeated studies.

There are no established or proven specific risk factors for SCD. Markers of increased risk include young age at diagnosis, malignant family history, syncope, right ventricular dysfunction and left ventricular involvement, and presence of VT on ambulatory monitoring.

Therefore, baseline investigations in addition to a carefully taken history should include the following:
- 12 lead and signal-averaged ECG
- 24-hour ambulatory ECG monitoring
- Exercise testing
- Echocardiogram (± MRI scan)

Treatment

There are no established best treatment options for patients with ARVC, and, as the disease is progressive, antiarrhythmic options are used for symptomatic benefit in patients with hemodynamically well-tolerated ventricular arrhythmias.

Patients who have developed RV and LV dysfunction can be managed with standard treatments for HF. In severe cases, transplantation may be an option.

Antiarrhythmics

β-Blockers alone or in combination with class I and III antiarrhythmics are the most effective in reducing symptomatic but well-tolerated ventricular arrhythmias. Sotalol and amiodarone have been shown to be most effective.

Patients with more sustained ventricular arrhythmias may have drug therapy guided by their response during programmed electrical stimulation, but this has no proven benefit in reducing the risk of SCD.

Radiofrequency ablation

A small subset of patients with drug-refractory arrhythmias who are felt to have fairly localized disease may be amenable to electrophysiological mapping and radiofrequency ablation. However, it must be remembered that ARVC is a progressive disease; this can only be viewed as a palliative procedure.

Implantable cardioverter defibrillators

In patients with life-threatening or drug-refractory ventricular arrhythmias and widespread disease, ICDs probably offer the best protective measure against SCD.

Ischemic cardiomyopathy

This is a condition in which coronary artery disease (CAD) causes a picture that is often indistinguishable from DCM with or without a preceding history of angina or myocardial infarction. Often the degree of dysfunction is inconsistent with the extent of CAD.

It is important to recognize patients with hibernating myocardium, as they will benefit from revascularization.

Valvular cardiomyopathy

Patients with valvular heart disease will develop a cardiomyopathy dependent on the predominant valvular lesion. Often significant improvement in cardiac function can be seen after correction of the valve disease.

Hypertensive cardiomyopathy

Hypertension causes LVH in response to increased afterload, which is compensatory and protective to a point. However, there are ultimately detrimental effects on systolic and diastolic ventricular function.

Hypertension also leads to accelerated atherosclerosis and ischemic heart disease. Hypertensive cardiomyopathy is the most common form of HF outside the Western world.

Alcoholic cardiomyopathy

Chronic alcohol excess is the most common cause of DCM in the Western world. Proposed mechanisms include 1) direct toxic effect, 2) concomitant nutritional deficiencies (especially thiamine), and 3) rarely toxic effects of additives (cobalt).

Unlike other forms of DCM, abstinence from alcohol early in the disease process may stop progression or even result in significant improvement in cardiac function.

Metabolic cardiomyopathy

Various abnormalities in metabolism can result in cardiomyopathy. Lysosomal and glycogen storage diseases can cause a form of restrictive cardiomyopathy. Hemochromatosis also causes restrictive cardiomyopathy by unknown mechanisms.

Acquired errors of metabolism such as acromegaly result in biventricular hypertrophy. Diabetes mellitus can cause cardiomyopathy with systolic and/or diastolic dysfunction even in the absence of significant epicardial CAD.

Takotsubo cardiomyopathy ("broken heart syndrome")

Takotsubo cardiomyopathy is a stress-induced cardiomyopathy whose presentation mimics an ST-elevation MI without evidence of significant epicardial coronary artery disease on angiogram. Its hallmark is apical ballooning on left ventriculography (in a minority of patients there may be mid-ventricular ballooning instead).

Originally described in Japan, it is becoming a more widely recognized syndrome. In series evaluating acute coronary syndromes, it accounts for about 1%–2% of cases. The syndrome is much more common in women than in men and in a review of 7 series, postmenopausal women accounted for 82%–100% of the reported cases.

Pathogenesis

Takotsubo cardiomyopathy is typically triggered by acute medical illness or by an extreme emotional stressor. Although the exact pathophysiology is not known, it is hypothesized that the underlying mechanism may include catecholamine excess resulting in microvascular spasm and resultant myocardial stunning, myocarditis, or coronary artery vasospasm.

Clinical presentation

Patients typically present with sudden onset of substernal chest pain following an extreme emotional stressor or critical illness. Occasionally patients will present with heart failure symptoms or in shock.

The initial ECG typically reveals ST elevations (Box 7.6). Cardiac biomarkers are often elevated. The degree of elevation is often mild and not consistent with degree of LV dysfunction or hemodynamic compromise.

Echocardiography reveals apical akinesis or dyskinesis. By definition, angiograms do not reveal any significant epicardial coronary disease.

Acute complications include tachy- and bradyarrhythmias, pulmonary edema, hypotension/shock, and transient LVOT obstruction.

Treatment and prognosis

Stress-induced cardiomyopathy is typically a transient phenomenon and has a good prognosis. Patients who survive the acute episode typically have normalization of their left ventricular function within 4 weeks.

Treatment is therefore supportive. It is reasonable to initiate standard heart failure therapy with β-blockers, ACE-I, and diuretics if needed.

Box 7.6 Diagnostic criteria of Takotsubo cardiomyopathy

- Transient akinesis or dyskinesis of the apical and midventricular segments in association with regional wall motion abnormalities that extend beyond the distribution of a single epicardial vessel
- Absence on angiography of obstructive coronary artery disease or evidence of acute plaque rupture
- New ST-segment elevation or T-wave inversion on ECG
- Absence of recent significant head trauma, intracranial bleeding, pheochromocytoma, myocarditis, or hypertrophic cardiomyopathy

General system disease

Systemic lupus erythematosus (SLE) can cause heart disease in many ways. Approximately 10% of patients with SLE have evidence of myocarditis. Patients with associated antiphospholipid antibody syndrome have increased risk of valvular abnormalities and DCM due to thrombotic occlusions of the microcirculation without vasculitis. They also have increased atherogenesis.

Pulmonary hypertension due to pulmonary vasculitis is an uncommon cause of cardiomyopathy in patients with rheumatoid arthritis.

Nutritional cardiomyopathy

Thiamine is an important coenzyme in the hexose monophosphate shunt. Infants breast-fed in areas with diets deficient in thiamine develop mainly right ventricular failure between 1 and 4 months of age. Prompt correction of the vitamin deficiency results in rapid improvement in the cardiac abnormalities without long-term consequence.

Protein-calorie malnutrition (Marasmus, Kwashiorkor) results in thinning and atrophy of muscle fibers and, ultimately, DCM. Careful treatment may result in marked improvement over several months provided the patient survives the initial period.

Muscular dystrophies

The large number of muscular dystrophies can be associated with either DCM or HCM, and this can be the most common cause of death in these patients. Myotonic dystrophy is associated with AV conduction abnormalities and arrhythmias rather than cardiomyopathy.

All patients need careful long-term follow-up.

Neuromuscular disorders

Cardiac involvement in Friedreich's ataxia is relatively common although usually asymptomatic. It is most commonly associated with HCM, which is distinct from the genetic variety by lack of myofibrillar disarray and malignant ventricular arrhythmias. Rarely, it is associated with DCM.

Sensitivity or toxic reactions

A large number of noninfectious agents can damage the myocardium. The damage can be acute with evidence of an inflammatory reaction, or there may be no inflammation and necrosis, as in hypersensitivity reactions.

Other agents lead to chronic changes with progressive fibrosis and an ultimate picture similar to DCM. Numerous chemical and industrial agents can cause myocardial damage, as can radiation and excessive heat.

Peripartum

Peripartum cardiomyopathy is a form of DCM. Symptoms occur in the third trimester and the diagnosis is made in the peripartum period. Approximately half of patients will show complete or near-complete resolution over the first 6 months postpartum. Of the remainder, some will continue to deteriorate and die or require transplantation, while others will continue to experience chronic HF.

Its diagnosis is established by excluding other causes of DCM; the cause is unknown (also see Chapter 10).

Myocarditis

Myocarditis is the process whereby the myocardium becomes inflamed by one of a large range of infectious agents. Unfortunately, the infectious agent is rarely identified. Numerous bacteria, viruses, spirochetes, fungi, parasites, and rickettsia can cause myocarditis (see Table 7.2).

Etiology

Damage can result from a number of mechanisms, including direct toxic effect on the myocyte, production of a toxin (e.g., diphtheria), and immunologically mediated cell damage. Histological findings depend on a number of factors, including the infectious agent, stage of disease, and the mechanism of damage.

Damage can be focal or diffuse and is randomly distributed throughout the myocardium.

Symptoms

The clinical consequences of the damage can range from asymptomatic subclinical infection to rapidly progressive and ultimately fatal HF. Long-term consequences are also variable.

Patients who were initially asymptomatic can present after a prolonged latency period with DCM or have complete recovery. Patients who present early, even with fulminant HF, can also have complete recovery. Patients with nonfulminant presentations can gradually deteriorate and recover gradually.

Diagnosis

The diagnosis is often established by identifying the associated systemic illness. Isolation of the infectious agent is rarely achieved, although clearly supportive of the diagnosis if positive. Endomyocardial biopsy can be useful in confirming the diagnosis but is frequently negative.

Treatment

Management of patients with myocarditis is largely supportive. Physical activity should be restricted, as in animal models exercise was found to be detrimental to cardiac function.

Standard management of HF and eradication of the infectious agent are the mainstay of treatment. Symptomatic arrhythmias should be controlled and β-blockers may be cardioprotective.

Trials of immunosuppressive therapy in patients with myocarditis have been largely disappointing. The use of steroids in acutely ill patients could be considered, but any benefit is unproven.

Table 7.2 Causes of myocarditis

Viral (usually mild and self-limiting)	Spirochetal
Enterovirus (Coxsackie B) most common in Western countries	Lyme disease—about 10% of patients have cardiac involvement
CMV	Leptospirosis
Dengue	Syphilis—direct involvement of myocardium with gummae is rare
Hepatitis	**Protozoal**
EBV	*Trypanosoma cruzi* causes Chagas disease—significant public health problem in S. America. HF may present 20 years after initial infection
Influenza	
Varicella	
HIV	
Rickettsial	**Fungal**
Q fever rarely causes myocarditis	This is rare (typically occurs in patients with concomitant malignant disease or who are otherwise immunosuppressed)
Rocky Mountain spotted fever	
Scrub typhus	*Actinomyces, Aspergillus, Candida, Cryptococcus, Histoplasma*
Bacterial	**Toxic/metabolic**
Diptheria—myocarditis occurs in up to 20% of diptheria infections	Anthracyclines
	Cocaine
Meningococcus	Catecholamines
Mycoplasma	Carbon monoxide
Whipple's disease	Hypocalcemia
	Hypersensitivity—eosinophilic infiltration

Pericardial diseases

Etiology

The pericardium may be involved in the large number of disease processes listed in Table 7.3. In some patients, pericardial disease is the primary disease process dominating the clinical picture, whereas in others it is a manifestation of a systemic disease.

The most common causes are idiopathic (or viral), uremic, neoplastic, tuberculous pericarditis, and acute myocardial infarction. The spectrum of pericardial disease is determined by the age and social circumstances of the patient.

In an elderly North American and Western European population, the most common causes are malignancy, followed by uremia and myocardial infarction. In less privileged communities and in developing countries, tuberculosis is still the predominant cause of pericardial disease.

Table 7.3 Etiology of pericardial diseases

Infections	*Bacterial:* Mycobacterium tuberculosis, Staphylococcus, Pneumococcus, Meningococcus, Mycoplasma
	Viral: Coxsackie, CMV, ECHO, EBV, influenza, HIV, mumps, parvo B19, rubella, varicella
	Fungal: Histoplasmosis, blastomycosis
	Parasitic: Amoebiasis
Autoimmune and hypersensitivity diseases	*Collagen vascular diseases:* systemic lupus erythematosus, polyarteritis nodosa, scleroderma, dermatomyositis
	Type 2 autoimmune disorders: rheumatic fever, autoreactive pericarditis, postmyocardial infarction, and postpericardiotomy syndromes
	Drug-induced: hydralazine, procainamide, penicillin, phenylbutazone
	Other autoimmune disorders: rheumatoid arthritis, ankylosing spondylitis
Pericardial Involvement by disease in surrounding organs	*Heart:* acute myocardial infarction, myocarditis
	Lung: pulmonary infarction, pneumonia
Malignant disease	*Primary:* mesothelioma, sarcoma, fibroma, lipoma
	Secondary: lung carcinoma, breast carcinoma, melanoma, lymphoma, leukemia
Bleeding into the pericardium	*Trauma:* penetrating and nonpenetrating
	Dissecting aortic aneurysm
	Hemorrhagic diathesis: leukemia, scurvy
	Anticoagulants: warfarin
Metabolic disorders	Uremia, dialysis-related, myxedema, gout
Miscellaneous	Acute idiopathic pericarditis, radiation, sarcoidosis, amyloidosis, familial Mediterranean fever

Syndromes of pericardial disease

Pericardial reaction to the various disease processes is limited. The following five clinical and pathological forms of pericarditis can thus be distinguished:

1. Acute pericarditis without effusion
2. Pericardial effusion with or without tamponade
3. Constrictive pericarditis
4. Effusive–constrictive pericarditis
5. Calcific pericarditis without constriction

Acute pericarditis without effusion

("Dry" pericarditis)

Etiology

Any of the causes listed in Table 7.3 may cause dry pericarditis. The clinical syndrome is commonly seen in acute viral pericarditis or after myocardial infarction.

Pathology

There is a fibrinous exudate with an inflammatory reaction involving the visceral and parietal pericardium. The epicardium is also involved and this accounts for the ECG changes seen and the rise in cardiac enzymes (e.g., troponin I).

Symptoms

Sharp, stabbing, central chest pain is common, with radiation to the shoulders and upper arm. It is relieved by sitting up and leaning forward and is aggravated by lying down. It may be accentuated by inspiration, cough, swallowing, or movement of the trunk.

Fever, night sweats, and other constitutional symptoms may be present, depending on the underlying cause.

Signs

A pericardial friction rub is frequently heard. This is a superficial, scratchy, grating sound that is best heard in the second to fourth intercostal spaces when pressure is exerted on the diaphragm of the stethoscope. Positioning the patient leaning forward and listening in held inspiration may bring it out.

The rub is classically described as being triphasic. Usually at least two components are heard because of atrial systole and ventricular systole. Occasionally a third component attributed to rapid ventricular filling is heard.

ECG

The patient is usually in sinus rhythm, but atrial fibrillation may occur. In the early stages there is widespread ST-segment elevation with concavity directed upward, and PR segment deviation opposite the polarity of the P wave. After a few days the ST segments followed by PR segments return to normal, and T waves become inverted.

CXR

The cardiac shadow is not enlarged in dry pericarditis.

Differential diagnosis

Acute pericarditis must be differentiated from myocardial infarction, spontaneous pneumothorax, and pleurisy.

Diagnosis

Diagnosis of acute pericarditis is based on typical symptoms of chest pain, pericardial rub, and/or characteristic ECG changes.

Management

Treat the underlying cause. Good pain relief can be achieved by the use of nonsteroidal anti-inflammatory drugs (NSAIDs).

Pericardial effusion ± tamponade

Etiology

Any of the causes listed in Table 7.3 may cause pericardial effusion. Large effusions are common with neoplastic, TB, uremic pericarditis, and myxedema.

Pathology

In addition to fibrinous inflammation, there is significant fluid exudation. The pericardial fluid may be serous, serosanguineous, hemorrhagic, or purulent depending on the underlying cause.

Hemorrhagic effusion is common in tuberculosis or neoplasia. Brownish fluid with an anchovy sauce appearance of the pus is highly suggestive of amoebic pericarditis.

Clinical features

Clinical presentation varies depending on the rate of accumulation of fluid, the amount of fluid that accumulates, and the stage at which the patient is first seen.

Symptoms

Chest pain may be typically pericardial (as described under Dry Pericarditis), or it may be dull and heavy from distension of the pericardium.

Dyspnea is common, and orthopnea may occur later in the course of the disease. Cough may be present from compression of surrounding structures.

Any constitutional symptoms depend on the cause of the disease.

Signs

Typically, precordial dullness extends beyond the apex beat (which may be impalpable), and dullness is present to the right of the sternum. Dullness and bronchial breathing (Ewart's sign) at the left base posteriorly due to compression of the left lower lobe bronchus may be found.

Cardiac tamponade should be considered in a patient with hypotension, raised JVP, and quiet heart sounds (Beck's triad). The primary defect in cardiac tamponade is interference with diastolic filling of the heart.

Other clinical features of cardiac tamponade are presence of tachycardia, pulsus paradoxus (fall in systolic blood pressure on inspiration of >10 mmHg or inspiratory fall in systolic blood pressure that exceeds half the pulse pressure), elevated JVP with brisk x descents and absent y descents, dyspnea or tachypnea with clear lungs, and hepatomegaly.

Investigations

ECG

Sinus tachycardia and generalized low-voltage QRS complexes with non-specific ST segment and T-wave changes are found. Electrical alternans, involving the QRS complex, suggests the presence of a massive pericardial effusion. Total electrical alternans (P-QRS-T), which is uncommon, is pathognomonic of cardiac tamponade.

CXR
This commonly shows a large globular heart usually with clear lung fields.

Echocardiography
This is diagnostic, showing an echo-free zone surrounding the heart. The fluid may not be evenly distributed. Signs of tamponade on echocardiogram include the following:
• Diastolic collapse of the right ventricle (most specific)
• Diastolic collapse of the right atrium
• Excessive respiratory variation of the mitral inflow (>25%)
• Plethoric, noncollapsible inferior vena cava (IVC)

The following features are more common in patients with marked inflammatory or malignant causes of pericardial effusion:
• Soft tissue density masses
• Thickening of the visceral pericardium
• Presence of fibrinous strands

The hallmark of benign, idiopathic effusion is a clear echo-free space, whereas malignancy, bacterial infection, and hemorrhagic effusions are more likely to have solid components or stranding.

Cardiac catheterization
This modality can be used to establish the diagnosis and severity of tamponade but is rarely necessary. The important findings are
1. Equilibration of mean right atrial, right ventricular end-diastolic, and mean capillary wedge pressure,
2. Rapid *x* descent on the right atrial pressure waveform, and
3. Pulsus paradoxus.

Differential diagnosis
This includes myocardial infarction and pulmonary embolism.

Management
• When an effusion does not cause hemodynamic impairment and the cause is known (e.g., uremia, myxedema), then no further investigations are necessary and the treatment consists of treating the underlying cause.
• If the cause is not known, then pericardiocentesis must be considered. Aspiration of the fluid helps to establish the nature of the effusion.
• Cardiac tamponade is a life-threatening condition. Urgent pericardial aspiration is necessary (See Pericardiocentesis, p. 698). Surgical drainage is indicated for hemopericardium or purulent pericarditis.

Constrictive pericarditis

Etiology

Constrictive pericarditis is usually due to tuberculosis. Other causes are mediastinal irradiation, purulent pericarditis, previous trauma (surgical or nonsurgical) with infection of the pericardial space, and, very rarely, viral pericarditis.

Pathology

The pericardium becomes a dense mass of fibrous tissue that may be calcified. This results in encasement of the heart within a nonexpansile pericardium.

Clinical features

Symptoms include dyspnea, edema, and abdominal swelling due to ascites and hepatomegaly.

Signs include small volume pulse and pulsus paradoxus. JVP is always elevated, usually very high with prominent *x* and *y* descents. A diastolic knock is usually felt at the left sternal border due to the sudden halting of the ventricles during diastolic filling. Apex beat may be impalpable. Heart sounds are usually soft, and an early third sound coincident with the diastolic knock is usually heard.

In the pulmonary area there is sudden instantaneous widened splitting of the second sound that occurs following the first heartbeat of inspiration (Vogelpoel–Beck sign). The liver is commonly grossly enlarged, ascites is marked, and peripheral edema is present.

Investigations

- *ECG* is abnormal in virtually every case, but changes are nonspecific (i.e., generalized low-voltage QRS complexes, and widespread flattening and inversion of T waves). Atrial fibrillation is common in the chronic form.
- *CXR:* Normal or near-normal cardiac size in the presence of marked venous distension or heart failure is suggestive of constrictive pericarditis or restrictive cardiomyopathy. Pericardial calcification is diagnostic; its incidence varies from 5% to 70% of cases in different series.
- *Echocardiography:* Pericardial thickening may be present. A restrictive mitral filling pattern on Doppler, with respiratory variation of >25% over the atrioventricular valves.
- *CT and MRI scans* demonstrate pericardial thickening (>5 mm).
- *Cardiac catheterization* demonstrates elevation and equalization of filling pressures. In the typical case, the difference in filling pressures between the right ventricle and left ventricle does not exceed 6 mmHg. The right atrial waveform shows rapid *x* and *y* descents, and the mean pressure does not decrease normally with inspiration or may show Kussmaul's sign.

Management

Constrictive pericarditis is treated by surgical removal of the fibrous constrictive tissue (pericardiectomy).

Effusive–constrictive pericarditis

Etiology

This is characteristically encountered in active TB pericarditis where there are signs of both pericardial effusion or tamponade and constriction. It may also occur in neoplastic, radiation, and septic pericarditis.

Clinical presentation

Symptoms are usually those of constriction. Examination reveals pulsus paradoxus and raised JVP with prominent x and y descents. The CXR shows an enlarged cardiac silhouette like that of pericardial effusion.

Diagnosis

The clue to diagnosis is persistent signs of constriction following adequate pericardial drainage.

Management

Treatment is of the underlying cause and pericardial drainage if indicated. Pericardiectomy is indicated should hemodynamics not improve.

Calcific pericarditis without constriction

This condition is usually discovered during routine radiological examination, which demonstrates pericardial calcification. There are no symptoms and signs of constriction and the cause is usually unknown.

Viral pericarditis

Clinical presentation

Most patients present with a history of upper respiratory tract infection within the preceding 3 weeks. The viruses most frequently responsible include coxsackie B, echo, mumps, influenza, and varicella.

Pericardial pain, fever, and malaise are typical. The physical examination reveals a pericardial friction rub and/or characteristic changes of acute pericarditis on ECG.

Course

In most patients the illness resolves spontaneously in 1–2 weeks. In some patients, the illness recurs on at least one occasion in the next few weeks or months, and in 20% of patients there are multiple recurrences in the ensuing months or years (benign relapsing pericarditis).

Diagnosis

It is important to search for an underlying disease (see Table 7.3) that may require specific therapy. In most cases of suspected viral pericarditis, special studies for etiologic agents are not necessary because of the low diagnostic yield of viral studies and lack of specific therapy for viral disease.

Management

- NSAIDs are effective in most patients with viral pericarditis. There are no data from randomized controlled trials to guide treatment for relapsing patients who do not respond to NSAIDs.
- Corticosteroids (prednisone 1–1.5 mg/kg for at least 1 month) provide symptomatic relief in most patients; symptoms recur in many patients when the prednisone dose is reduced.
- Colchicine (2 mg/day for 1–2 days, followed by 1 mg/day) may be effective when NSAIDs and corticosteroids fail to prevent relapses.
- If patients do not respond adequately, azathioprine (75–100 mg/day) or cyclophosphamide may be added.
- Pericardiectomy is indicated only in frequent and highly symptomatic recurrences resistant to medical therapy. However, postpericardiectomy recurrences may occur, possibly due to incomplete resection of the pericardium.

Tuberculous pericarditis

Tuberculous (TB) pericarditis is uncommon in the developed world, but is very common in developing countries. The incidence appears to be increasing in sub-Saharan Africa in parallel with the HIV/AIDS epidemic.

The disease presents in three forms: constrictive pericarditis, effusive-constrictive pericarditis, and pericardial effusion.

TB constrictive pericarditis

Clinical presentation

Most cases have an active inflammatory fibrocaseous tissue surrounding the heart and involve visceral and parietal pericardium.

The clinical presentation is highly variable. Patients range from being asymptomatic to showing severe signs and symptoms of constriction. The diagnosis is often missed on cursory clinical and echocardiographic examination.

It is uncommon to find concomitant pulmonary TB, and pericardial calcification is found in <5% of cases.

Treatment

The initial management of patients with noncalcific TB constrictive pericarditis is with anti-TB therapy. Since the process is an active fibro-caseous condition, resolution of constriction occurs in 15%–20% of patients with medical management over 3–4 months.

Pericardiectomy is recommended if no improvement has occurred after 6 weeks of anti-TB treatment or unsatisfactory improvement after several months of treatment.

By contrast, calcific TB pericarditis is treated by early pericardiectomy and anti-TB chemotherapy.

TB effusive–constrictive pericarditis

Features

This mixed form is a common presentation of TB pericarditis. There is increased pericardial pressure due to effusion in the presence of visceral constriction.

The echocardiogram shows porridge-like exudation with loculation of the fluid.

Treatment

Treatment of this condition is by standard four-drug therapy. The role of adjuvant steroids is not known.

The mortality is about 10%, and about 30% of cases will come to pericardiectomy over 2 years of follow-up.

TB pericardial effusion

Pathology

Pericardial effusion is the most common mode of presentation with or without tamponade. The effusion is bloodstained in over 95% of cases, and may even resemble venous blood.

The absence of parenchymatous lung disease and the presence of hilar lymphadenopathy in many of these patients suggest a direct spread from a TB hilar node to the pericardium.

Clinical presentation

Systemic symptoms are variable. Typical pericardial pain is uncommon and the classic ECG features of pericarditis are not seen.

CXR shows an enlarged globular heart, small pleural effusions on one or both sides, and evidence of pulmonary tuberculosis in only 30% of cases. The echocardiogram shows features of pericardial effusion, typically associated with soft tissue density masses, thickening of the visceral pericardium, and fibrinous strands.

Diagnosis

A *definite diagnosis* of TB pericardial effusion is based on demonstration of tubercle bacilli in the pericardial fluid or on histological section of the pericardium. Pericardial fluid should be sent for microscopy (to identify acid-fast bacilli [AFB]) and culture of tubercle bacilli. The chances of a positive culture are improved by bedside inoculation of the fluid into double-strength Kirschner culture medium. Pericardial biopsy and drainage offer the advantage of a histological diagnosis and early complete drainage of the pericardium. This can be performed via the subxiphisternal approach under local anesthesia.

A *probable diagnosis* is made when there is proof of TB elsewhere in a patient with unexplained pericardial effusion. Palpation in the supraclavicular fossa will frequently reveal enlarged lymph nodes, which should be biopsied. AFB-positive sputum will only be found in about 10% of cases. Tuberculin skin testing is of little value in endemic and nonendemic areas. It is not known whether the enzyme-linked immunospot (ELISPOT) test that detects T cells specific for *M tuberculosis* antigen will perform better in TB pericarditis than the tuberculin skin test.

Several tests have been developed for the rapid diagnosis of TB in the pericardial fluid. Polymerase chain reaction (PCR) can identify DNA of *M. tuberculosis* rapidly from only 1 µL of pericardial fluid (sensitivity 75%, specificity 100%). An adenosine deaminase (ADA) level >40 U/L has a sensitivity of 83% and a specificity of 78%. A high interferon-γ level is also a highly sensitive (92%) and specific (100%) marker of pericardial TB.

Treatment

Treatment is by means of standard four-drug anti-TB chemotherapy for 6 months. Overall mortality is about 8%.

Repeat pericardiocentesis is required in about 15% of patients, and during a 2-year follow-up period, about 10% of patients will require surgical pericardiectomy.

While some clinicians favor the addition of steroids to conventional therapy, their role in improving survival is not clearly established, particularly in the context of HIV infection.

Uremic pericarditis

Pathology

Uremia produces a fibrinous, often hemorrhagic inflammation that may lead to tamponade, and constriction in some cases.

Management

Symptomatic pericarditis that occurs before the initiation of dialysis will respond to repeated peritoneal or hemodialysis. Heparin-free hemodialysis should be used to avoid hemopericardium.

Many patients who develop pericardial effusion while on dialysis (dialysis-associated pericarditis) will respond to intensification of the dialysis regime. Those who do not respond will require drainage by either subxyphoid pericardiotomy or pericardial window.

Pericardiocentesis is associated with a high risk of intrapericardial hemorrhage.

Neoplastic pericardial disease

Etiology

This condition is usually secondary to malignancy of the bronchus, breast, or kidney. Primary tumors of the pericardium are rare and usually result from mesothelioma following asbestos exposure.

Diagnosis

Metastases may produce a large hemorrhagic effusion or severe constriction when tumor encases the heart. Malignant cells may be found in 85% of cases of aspirated pericardial fluid.

Tumor markers such as carcinoembryonic antigen (CEA), α-fetoprotein (AFP), and carbohydrate antigens (e.g., CA 125) have been used in the diagnosis of malignant effusion.

The differentiation of TB and neoplastic effusion is virtually absolute with low ADA and high CEA levels.

Management

This depends on the type and stage of malignancy, condition of the patient, and presence of cardiac compression. Pericardiocentesis is effective in relieving neoplastic cardiac tamponade in the vast majority of cases.

Commonly, neoplastic pericardial disease is a preterminal event. Palliation for recurrent tamponade can be obtained by subxyphoid surgical pericardiotomy (which can be performed under local anesthesia) or by percutaneous balloon pericardiotomy to create a pleuropericardial window to allow fluid drainage into the pleural space in patients with large malignant pericardial effusions and a limited life expectancy.

Partial pericardiectomy (pericardial window) through a left thoracotomy should be reserved for patients who have a better prognosis and are likely to respond to chemotherapy or radiation.

Intrapericardial instillation of cytostatic/sclerosing agents has also been used to prevent recurrences of large pericardial effusion. Tetracycline as a sclerosing agent controls malignant pericardial effusion in up to 85% of cases, but side effects, such as fever, chest pain, and atrial arrhythmias, and constriction in long-term survivors, are common.

Myxedematous effusion

Clinical presentation

Effusion with high protein content is common in untreated myxedema. Myxedema must always be excluded in a patient with chronic, asymptomatic, pericardial effusion associated with bradycardia, low voltage of the QRS complexes, and a history of radiation-induced thyroid dysfunction. Cardiac tamponade does not occur.

Diagnosis

This is based on serum levels of thyroxine and thyroid-stimulating hormone.

Treatment

Treatment with thyroid hormone causes resolution of the pericardial effusion.

Nontuberculous bacterial (purulent) pericarditis

Predisposing conditions

These include immunosuppression (e.g., immunosuppressive drugs, lymphoma, or HIV/AIDS), pre-existing pericardial effusion, cardiac surgery, and chest trauma.

In children, pharyngitis, pneumonia, otitis media, endocarditis, and arthritis are found.

Precipitating factors

These include cardiac surgery, pericardial aspiration, extension of aortic root endocarditis into the pericardial sac, or hematogenous spread from a septic focus such as osteomyelitis or pneumonia.

Causative organisms

In adults these are *Staphylococcus aureus*, gram-negative bacilli, and anaerobes. In children they are *Haemophilus, Staphylococcus aureus*, and *N. meningitides*.

Clinical presentation

This is rare in adults. It presents as an acute, fulminating infectious illness and is fatal if not treated. The most important reason for this poor outlook is failure to suspect the condition in debilitated patients with overwhelming systemic infection.

Diagnosis

Pericardiocentesis shows purulent fluid, with high white cell count, low glucose, positive Gram stain for the organism, and positive pericardial fluid and blood culture.

Treatment

Complete pericardial drainage is preferable through a subxyphoid pericardiotomy, and systemic antibiotic therapy should be given. The mortality rate is 40% even with appropriate management.

Radiation pericarditis

Clinical features

This condition usually follows treatment for lymphoma and breast cancer. Incidence of pericarditis depends on how much of the heart is included in the field of radiation, the dose, the duration of treatment, and age of the patient. Radiation is a common cause of effusive–constrictive pericarditis and also may result in myocarditis and premature coronary atherosclerosis.

Clinical evidence of pericarditis may occur during, or shortly after treatment, but is more usually delayed for approximately 1 year. The presentation is one of pericarditis with some effusion. In about 50% of cases there is evidence of tamponade, which requires drainage.

Management

Up to 20% of patients will require pericardiectomy because of severe constriction. The operative mortality is high (21%) and the postoperative 5-year survival is very low (1%), mostly due to underlying myocardial fibrosis and severe thickening of the visceral pericardium.

Drug- or toxin-induced pericarditis

Etiology

Pericardial reactions to drugs and toxins are rare. Pericarditis may develop as part of the lupus erythematosus-like syndrome (hydralazine, INH, procainamide, methyldopa, reserpine), hypersensitivity reaction (cromolyn sodium, penicillins, streptomycin), serum sickness, or envenomation (scorpion fish sting).

Management

This consists of removal of the causative agent and symptomatic treatment.

Postcardiotomy syndrome

Clinical presentation

The syndrome occurs in approximately 30% of patients undergoing any form of cardiac surgery. It is more common in patients receiving aminocaproic acid during the operation.

After a latent period of 2–3 weeks, there is fever, pericarditis, pleuritis, and pneumonitis with a marked tendency to relapse. "Dry" pericarditis or pericarditis with effusion may occur. The illness is self-limited and varies in intensity and duration, but usually lasts only 2–4 weeks.

Treatment

Give NSAIDs and analgesics such as aspirin or colchicine. Steroids (oral or intrapericardial) induce prompt relief of symptoms but should be reserved for severely affected patients, since relapse may occur when they are discontinued and dependency may result.

Anticoagulants should be avoided because of risk of hemopericardium.

Postinfarction pericarditis

Clinical presentation

Two forms of postinfarction pericarditis may be distinguished:
1. The usual early form of pericarditis occurs within a week in at least 20% of patients with transmural MI. It is a result of pericardial irritation by adjacent infarcted myocardium.
2. Less commonly, a delayed autoimmune reaction may produce pericarditis 2 weeks to a few months after the infarct (Dressler syndrome). The delayed form behaves very similarly to the postcardiotomy syndrome.

Treatment

Ibuprofen is said to increase coronary flow, and is the NSAID of choice. Aspirin, up to 650 mg every 4 hours for 2–5 days, has also been used successfully. Occasionally steroids may be required for relapse, but should be avoided as they may delay myocardial healing. Anticoagulants should be avoided because of the risk of hemopericardium.

Rheumatic fever

This is an important cause of pericarditis worldwide, almost invariably associated with severe pancarditis and valvular involvement. Rheumatic pericardial effusion is usually clear, straw-colored, and sterile. Cardiac tamponade is rare and the fluid usually reabsorbs rapidly in response to salicylates or steroid therapy. Chronic constrictive pericarditis is never rheumatic in origin but adherent pericardium with flecks of calcification is not uncommon.

Autoimmune pericarditis

Pericarditis may be the presenting feature of systemic lupus erythematosus (SLE) or complicate scleroderma and polyarteritis nodosa. Dry or effusive pericarditis may occur; and it is important to exclude these disorders in patients presenting with idiopathic benign pericarditis. Generally, other signs and symptoms of these collagen vascular diseases will be present.

Granulomatous pericarditis is a complication of rheumatoid arthritis and ankylosing spondylitis, leading to effusion and occasionally constriction. Aortitis and aortic insufficiency may be associated and occasionally there is invasion of the interventricular septum, producing heart block.

Traumatic pericarditis

This produces two forms of pericarditis. One is a direct result of trauma with hemorrhage into the pericardial cavity and formation of hemopericardium. If associated myocardial or valvular injury is absent, complete recovery is the rule, although chronic constriction may develop.

The second type is a form of recurrent pericarditis associated with the postcardiotomy and post-MI syndromes, which may also result in chronic constriction.

Fungal pericarditis

Clinical presentation

Fungal pericarditis occurs as a rare opportunistic infection in immunocompromised patients (e.g., immunosuppressive therapy, HIV/AIDS). It is caused by endemic fungi (*Histoplasma*, *Coccidioides*), nonendemic opportunistic fungi (candida, *Aspergillus*, *Blastomyces*), and semi-fungi (*Norcadia*, *Actinomycosis*).

Diagnosis

Fungal pericarditis may resemble TB pericarditis. Fungal staining and culture of aspirated pericardial fluid and pericardial biopsy are necessary to make the distinction.

Treatment

Antifungal treatment with fluconazole, ketoconazole, itraconazole, amphotericin B, or amphotericin B lipid complex is indicated. NSAIDs are used for symptomatic relief.

Sulfonamides are the drug of choice for *Norcadiosis*, and a combination of three antibiotics including penicillin should be given for *Actinomycosis*.

Amoebic pericarditis

Pathology

Amoebiasis (caused by *Entamoeba histolytica*) occurs mainly in endemic areas and in travelers from them (in whom the syndrome may appear years later). Pericardial complications are rare, but when they do occur, they carry a high mortality, especially with delayed or missed diagnosis.

The usual cause of amoebic pericarditis is extension from an amoebic liver abscess in the left lobe. Rarely, spread may also occur from the right lobe or disease may reach the pericardium from an amoebic lung abscess.

Clinical presentation

There are two modes of presentation:
1. **Hepatic presentation:** an abscess near the pericardium, which has not yet ruptured, can cause a pericardial friction rub, a nonpurulent pericardial effusion, and ECG/CXR signs of pericarditis.
2. **Cardiac presentation:** perforation of a liver abscess into the pericardium results in a purulent pericarditis. The onset can be acute, with shock and death within a short time, or the onset may be gradual with signs of tamponade as a result of the pericardial fluid.

Diagnosis

Diagnosis is difficult but should be suspected if, in a patient with a purulent pericarditis and signs of cardiac failure, tenderness of the liver in the epigastrium is much more marked than the rest of the palpable liver. A high and immobile left hemidiaphragm detected by fluoroscopy or CT scan is also suggestive.

Definite diagnosis is by pericardiocentesis (which typically shows brownish fluid; the pus may simulate anchovy sauce) and serological testing for antibodies resulting from invasive amoebiasis (fluorescent antibody test or amoebic enzyme immunoassay or amoebic gel diffusion test).

Treatment

With hepatic presentation the pericardial disease resolves with successful treatment of the liver abscess.

With cardiac presentation, treat with pericardial drainage and metronidazole. Constrictive pericarditis is an occasional complication.

Constrictive pericarditis vs. restrictive myocardial disease

It is difficult to separate constrictive pericarditis from restrictive myocardial disease. The distinction is vital, because pericardiectomy is one of the most satisfying operations in terms of cure. Points of differentiation are as presented in Table 7.4.

An exploratory thoracotomy is justified if all of these tests fail to make a distinction between the two entities.

Table 7.4 Comparison of constrictive pericarditis and restrictive myocardial disease

	Constriction	Restriction
Clinical	History of prior pericardial disease, prior pericardial trauma, prior cardiac surgery	• Murmur of MR and TR • Known infiltrative myocardial disease
ECG	Normal	Left axis deviation, LVH, Q waves, LBBB
CXR	Pericardial calcification	No pericardial calcification
Echocardiogram	• Septal bounce • Tissue Doppler Ea >8 cm/sec • Normal LV systolic function	• LVH • "Speckled" appearance of myocardium • LV dysfunction • Tissue Doppler Ea <8 cm/sec
CT or MRI	Pericardium ≥3 mm	Normal pericardium
Endomyocardial biopsy	Normal myocardium	Evidence of infiltrative disease (i.e., amyloid, hemochromatosis)
Right heart catheterization (RHC)	• Dip and plateau • Ventricular interdependence (RVSP increases with inspiration, LVSP decreases with inspiration) • PAS <50 mmHg	• ± Dip and plateau • >6 mmHg difference between LVEDP and RVEDP • PAS >50 mmHg

Pericardial fluid analysis

Analyses of pericardial effusion can establish the diagnosis of viral, bacterial, TB, fungal, amoebic, and malignant pericarditis. The appearance of the pericardial fluid should be noted. The tests should be ordered according to the clinical presentation of the patient.

However, the following routine samples are useful:
- Biochemistry sample for protein and LDH estimation to distinguish between and exudate and a transudate
- Microbiology specimen for microscopy, culture, and sensitivity testing
- Cytology specimen

The following tests are requested for the diagnosis of the specific forms of pericarditis:
- Viral pericarditis—PCR for cardiotropic viruses
- Purulent pericarditis—Gram stain, at least 3 blood cultures of pericardial fluid for aerobes and anaerobes and blood cultures
- TB pericarditis—staining for AFB; bedside inoculation of pericardial fluid into double-strength Kirschner transport medium and culture; ADA level
- Fungal pericarditis—microscopy and culture
- Amoebic pericarditis—brownish pericardial fluid with anchovy sauce appearance of pus
- Malignant effusion—cytology and tumor markers (e.g., CEA)

Pericardiocentesis

See Chapter 1.

Further reading

Akashi YJ, Goldstein DS, Barbaro G, Ueyama T (2008). Takotsubo cardiomyopathy: a new form of acute, reversible heart failure. *Circulation* 118(25):2754–2762.

Dote K, Sato H, Ishihara M (1991). Myocardial stunning due to simultaneous coronary spasms: a review of 5 cases. *J Cardiol* 21(2):203–214.

Kuowski V, Kaiser A, von Hof K, et al. (2007). Apical and midventricular transient left ventricular dysfunction syndrome (tako-tsubo cardiomyopathy): frequency, mechanisms, and prognosis. *Chest* 132(3):809–816.

Nishimura RA, Holmes DR Jr (2004). Clinical practice. Hypertrophic obstructive cardiomyopathy. *N Engl J Med* 350(13):1320–1327.

Watkins H, McKenna WJ (2005). The prognostic impact of septal myectomy in obstructive hypertrophic cardiomyopathy. *J Am Coll Cardiol* 46:477.

Wigle ED, Rakowski H, Kimball BP, Williams WG (1995). Hypertrophic cardiomyopathy. Clinical spectrum and treatment. *Circulation* 92(7):1680–1692.

Congenital heart disease

Introduction

Congenital heart disease (CHD) is one of the most common congenital defects, occurring in approximately 0.6%–0.8% of newborns. Advances in therapy have led to a dramatic improvement in outcome such that over 85% of infants, even with complex CHD, are expected to reach adolescence and early adulthood.

As a result of the success of pediatric cardiology and surgery, the number of adults with CHD is greater than the number of pediatric cases. In addition, there are patients with structural or valvular CHD who may present late during adulthood.

As of 2000 there were roughly 485,000 American adults with moderate to very complex CHD and 300,000 with simple forms of CHD.[1] Many of those with CHD have had palliative or reparative rather than corrective surgery and will require further cardiac operations and procedures.

Role of specialist CHD centers

- Initial assessment of adults with known or suspected CHD
- Surgical and nonsurgical interventions, e.g., transcatheter closure ASD
- Continuing care of patients with moderate and complex CHD
- Advice and ongoing support for noncardiac surgery, pregnancy, and other medical illnesses
- Training new specialists and evidence-based clinical decision-making
- Provide feedback of late results to refine early treatment

Pediatric to adult care transition

A smooth transition from the pediatric to the adult CHD specialist is essential (Box 8.1). This should be tailored to the individual patient with built-in flexibility (see Table 8.1). Transfer to the adult service should occur at around 18 years of age.

Patient education about diagnosis and specific health behavior, including contraception and pregnancy planning, and the need for further care and follow-up should be included. Patient pamphlets that include detailed diagrams of the individual cardiac defect, prior repair if any, and relevant information on topics such as exercise and need for antibiotic prophylaxis should be prepared for each patient.

Treat adult CHD patients with respect (see Box 8.2 for various types of disease). Many problems or errors arise from arrogance or ignorance. The patients may often know more about their condition and its management than the emergency medical team they consult. Therefore, be patient and listen. Patients are often accompanied by the parent(s) even well into their late teens or second or third decade. They can prove a great source of information and help; keep them on your side. **Get to know your local adult CHD center**.

Box 8.1

No patient with CHD should reach adulthood without a clear management plan.

Table 8.1 Disease complexity and hierarchy of care for adults with CHD

Level 1

Exclusive care by specialist service, e.g., Eisenmenger syndrome, Fontan repairs, transposition of the great arteries, any condition with atresia in the name, Marfan's syndrome

Level 2

Shared care with interested adult cardiologist, e.g., coarctation of the aorta, atrial septal defect, tetralogy of Fallot

Level 3

Ongoing management by general adult cardiology service, e.g., mild pulmonary valve stenosis, postoperative atrial, or ventricular septal defect

Information sources on adult congenital heart disease: **1.** Deanfield J, et al. (2003). Management of grown up congenital heart disease. European Society of Cardiology task force report. *Eur Heart J* 24;1035–1084. **2.** British Cardiac Society (2002). Current needs and provision of service for adolescents and adults in the United Kingdom 2002. *Heart* 88(Suppl I):1–14. **3.** Connelly MS, Webb GD, Somerville J, et al. (1998). Canadian Consensus Conference on Adult Congenital Heart Disease. *Can J Cardiol* 14:395–452.

Box 8.2 Congenital heart disease in adults

Acyanotic lesions

- Atrial septal defect
- Ventricular septal defect
- Complete atrioventricular septal defect
- Pulmonary stenosis
- Left ventricular outflow tract obstruction
- Coarctation of the aorta
- Anomalous pulmonary venous drainage
- Ebstein's anomaly of the tricuspid valve

Cyanotic lesions

- Transposition of the great arteries
- Tetralogy of Fallot
- Fontan patients
- Congenitally corrected transposition of the great arteries
- Severe Ebstein's anomaly of the tricuspid valve

Assessment of patients with CHD

History
- Family history of CHD
- Exposure to teratogens or toxins during pregnancy
- CHD suspected during pregnancy or at birth (ask the mother!!)
- History of prolonged childhood illnesses
- Prior interventions
  - Any previous hospitalizations for catheter or surgical-based interventions
  - Names of previous pediatric cardiologists and surgeons as well as hospital in which surgery, if any, was performed
- Dental hygiene

Current symptoms
- Shortness of breath on exertion?
- Ability to climb stairs, hills, walk on the flat, and distance covered?
- Shortness of breath while lying down?
- Chest pain?
  - Precipitating and relieving factors?
  - Any associated symptoms?
- Syncopal episodes?
- Palpitations?
  - Onset, duration
  - Associated presyncope or chest pain?
  - Ask patient to tap out rate and rhythm of palpitations.
- Assess functional capacity.

General evaluation (see also Box 8.3)
- Chart the patient's height, weight, and blood pressure (both arms!) against standard reference charts.
- Does the patient have an obvious syndrome?
  - Down syndrome (1/3 associated with CHD, especially atrioventricular septal defect)
  - Williams syndrome (supravalvar aortic and pulmonary stenosis)
  - Noonan's syndrome (dysplastic pulmonary valvular stenosis, hypertrophic cardiomyopathy)
  - Turner's syndrome (coarctation of the aorta/aortic valve stenosis)
- Is the patient anemic or jaundiced?
- Are there any features to suggest infective endocarditis?
- Is there evidence of poor oral hygiene with dental caries or infected gums?
- Any tattoos or body piercing?
- Are there scars consistent with prior surgical intervention(s)?
- Are distal pulses delayed, absent, or reduced in amplitude and, if so, in what distribution?
- Liver size and pulsatility are barometers of right-sided pressures, filling and function
- Clubbing

Box 8.3 Systematic approach to auscultation of patient with CHD

1. Listen to the heart sounds. Do not assume heart will be left sided

First heart sound

- The first heart sound is usually heard as a single sound, but since mitral closure is loudest, it is best heard at the apex.
- A loud first heart sounds may be heard in mitral stenosis or sometimes with an atrial septal defect (ASD).
- Soft first heart sounds are a feature of poor myocardial contractility or a long PR interval.

Second heart sound

- Fixed splitting in the presence of a significant ASD and is best appreciated in the high or mid left sternal border
- Accentuated in the presence of pulmonary hypertension
- Widely split following repair of tetralogy of Fallot, the second heart sound reflects the right bundle branch block (RBBB), characteristic of the postoperative ECG.

2. Check for systolic and diastolic murmurs.
(Draw an imaginary line between the nipples).

Murmurs loudest above nipple line

- Systolic ejection.
- Arise from the right or left ventricular outflow tract.
- If associated with a carotid or suprasternal thrill, usually from the left ventricular outflow tract.
- If an ejection click is heard, the murmur is valvular in origin.
- Ejection click of aortic valve stenosis is best heard at the apex.
- Ejection systolic murmur best heard in the interscapular region and associated with a left thoracotomy may indicate turbulence across a prior coarctation repair.

Murmurs loudest below nipple line

- Pansystolic and arise from mitral/tricuspid regurgitation or from a ventricular septal defect (VSD).
- A "to and fro" murmur best heard at the upper left sternal edge following cardiac surgery usually results from combined right ventricular outflow tract obstruction and pulmonary regurgitation.
- The mid-systolic click and systolic murmur of mitral valve prolapse is best heard with the patient standing up.
- A continuous murmur arises from a patent ductus, systemic to pulmonary shunt, or arteriovenous fistulas.

Box 8.4

Measure height, weight, blood pressure (both arms!), and oxygen saturation in all patients. 12 lead ECG is essential at every visit.

Electrocardiogram

- Rate and rhythm: consider atrial flutter with variable block if constant rate of 120 or 150/min—this is easily confused with sinus rhythm. Atrial tachycardias are especially common after all forms of atrial surgery, e.g., intra-atrial repair for transposition of the great arteries.
- Look for signs of chamber enlargement—atrial or ventricular hypertrophy.
- Assess for presence or absence of BBB.
- Measure duration of QRS in all postoperative patients with tetralogy of Fallot: QRS duration >180 ms is associated with a higher risk of arrhythmias, right heart dilatation, and late sudden death.
- If tachycardia is suspected, record 12 lead ECG during administration of IV adenosine or other diagnostic or therapeutic interventions.

Role of exercise testing

- Assess heart rate and blood pressure (BP) response to exercise (blunted response in important aortic valve stenosis).
- Compare upper and lower limb BP following coarctation repair.
- Monitor oxygen saturation by pulse oximetry to improve risk stratification in cyanosed patients.
- Improves counseling and planning for pregnancy.
- Formal cardiopulmonary exercise testing is reserved for deciding on retiming of surgical or catheter-based intervention.
- Can help distinguish limitation due to lack of aerobic fitness and assess maximal effort.
- May be useful to identify arrhythmias and chronotropic incompetence.

Chest X-ray

- Inexpensive, readily available, and invaluable investigation in CHD.
- Identify right–left orientation to assess cardiac and visceral positions.
- Assessment of the bronchial branching permits diagnosis of isomeric cardiac defects, e.g., symmetric morphological right bronchi characteristic of right atrial isomerism (usually associated with complex CHD—common right atria, a common atrioventricular orifice, a great artery arising form one ventricular chamber, and total anomalous pulmonary venous connection).
- Identify situs inversus (mirror-image anatomy with liver on the left and stomach bubble on the right with cardiac apex in right chest). Consider Kartagener syndrome. Discordance between position of the apex and visceral situs is usually associated with CHD.
- Record cardiothoracic ratio. Look for rib notching related to collateral blood supply in severe coarctation of the aorta. Assess pulmonary vasculature (see Box 8.5).

See Box 8.6 for use of other imaging modalities in assessing CHD.

Box 8.5 CXR assessment of pulmonary vasculature in patients with CHD

Increased vascularity
- Left-to-right shunt (ASD, VSD)
- Pulmonary edema
- Obstructed pulmonary venous drainage

Decreased vascularity
- Right ventricular outflow obstruction, e.g., isolated severe pulmonary stenosis, following tetralogy repair
- Pulmonary hypertension

Unilateral increased pulmonary vascular markings
- Consider ipsilateral systemic to pulmonary arterial shunt
- Overperfused major arterial pulmonary collateral artery
- Obstructed pulmonary venous drainage, e.g., following Mustard or Senning intra-atrial repair for transposition of the great arteries

Box 8.6 Imaging modalities in CHD

Echocardiography
- This is the most useful investigation in CHD, but only when directed by detailed history taking and clinical examination.
- This should be performed by an experienced examiner with detailed knowledge of all aspects of CHD.
- There is no substitute for sequential data, and a protocol for regular, standardized analysis is required.
- Imaging in adults may be limited by poor windows.

Magnetic resonance imaging
- MRI is ideal for assessment of extracardiac pulmonary arterial and venous trees.
- It provides accurate quantification of valvar regurgitation, e.g., assessment of pulmonary regurgitation and right ventricular function following repair of tetralogy of Fallot.
- Its utility is limited by the presence of implantable pacemakers and defibrillators and is generally only available at academic medical centers or centers equipped to treat CHD.

Cardiac catheterization
- This can aid in quantifying shunts and obtaining accurate hemodynamic data.
- It can facilitate percutaneous transcatheter procedures such as occlusion of atrial septal defects.
- With an aging population, many patients with CHD need to undergo coronary angiography, as combined surgical procedures may be required.

Specific signs in patients with CHD

Inspection

Cyanosis or clubbing

Oxygen saturation should always be measured by pulse oximetry. Central cyanosis is an indication of arterial desaturation and is noted when >5 g/dL of reduced hemoglobin is circulating. Thus it is dependent in part on the total hemoglobin concentration and may be missing in a patient with significant desaturation but who is anemic.

Differential cyanosis implies flow of deoxygenated blood from the pulmonary trunk into the aorta distal to the left subclavian artery, e.g., non-restrictive patent ductus arteriosus with pulmonary vascular disease and right-to-left shunt.

Previous operation scars

Lift patient's arms and look for evidence of thoracotomy scars. Is the apex beat displaced or even in the right chest? Assess comorbidity, e.g., scoliosis and respiratory dysfunction related to prior lateral thoracotomy.

Jugular venous pulse

This can give information about conduction defects and arrhythmias, waveform, and pressure. Increased resistance to atrial filling results in an exaggerated a-wave, which may occur in isolated severe pulmonary stenosis or in tricuspid atresia.

Episodic "cannon" waves occur in cases of heart block when the atrium contracts against a closed tricuspid valve.

A prominent v-wave is characteristic of tricuspid regurgitation.

Palpation

- Feel all the pulses, including the femorals. Coarctation of the aorta is a clinical diagnosis.
- Check the blood pressure in upper and lower limbs, palpating the posterior tibial artery with the cuff inflated around the calf.
- Bounding pulses are characteristic of severe aortic regurgitation, patent ductus, or presence of a surgical systemic to pulmonary arterial shunt (Blalock–Taussig).
- An increase in right brachial pulse may reflect the Coanda effect of supravalvar stenosis in patients with Williams syndrome. Thrills may be felt in the femoral vessels, reflecting arteriovenous malformation following prior cardiac catheterization.
- Check the position of the apex beat. Also, check that the liver and stomach are in the correct position. Situs inversus with the apex in the right chest is the mirror image of normal. 95% of patients with mirror-image dextrocardia have no coexisting congenital cardiac disease. Situs solitus with apex in the right chest is invariably associated with CHD, often complex and unpredictable.
- A parasternal heave represents right ventricular overactivity, which is most marked when there is both pressure and volume overload of the chamber, such as following repair of tetralogy of Fallot.
- A palpable second sound in the upper left intercostal space is detected when pulmonary hypertension is present.

Surgical operations for CHD

Congenital heart disease surgery in adolescents and adults should only be undertaken in specialist centers. There are three categories of patients:
1. Patients who have not undergone prior operations.
2. Patients who have undergone previous palliative operations.
3. Patients who have undergone previous reparative procedures.

Re-do sternotomy, preservation of myocardial performance, attention to pulmonary bed vascular abnormalities, and aortopulmonary collaterals require careful prior planning and close cooperation among the surgeon, cardiac anesthesiologist, cardiologist, and intensive care team.

Blalock–Taussig shunt

A systemic to pulmonary arterial shunt using a subclavian arterial conduit (Classical) or Gore-Tex® tube (Modified) is used to increase pulmonary blood flow and improve oxygenation in cyanotic CHD. This is a palliative procedure that has superseded earlier operations such as the Waterston shunt (ascending aorta to right pulmonary artery) or Pott's shunt (descending aorta to left pulmonary artery). A catheter-based approach is now frequently used.

Coarctation of the aorta

This is relieved by either a subclavian conduit approach or direct end-to-end anastomosis. Occasionally, a bypass graft is required in adult patients, from the ascending to descending aorta.

Glenn shunt

The superior vena cava is anastomosed to the ipsilateral pulmonary artery as a means of improving oxygenation in infants or young children. This procedure is usually confined to patients with "single" ventricles and univentricular circulations.

In its classical form, the right pulmonary artery was detached from the main pulmonary artery. The bidirectional Glenn shunt was fashioned such that blood from the superior vena cava entered both pulmonary arteries.

Tetralogy of Fallot (Fig. 8.1)

This condition requires closure of the ventricular septal defect with a patch of pericardium or Goretex® and relief of right ventricular outflow tract obstruction by transannular patching, valvectomy, or placing a homograft or conduit between the right ventricle and pulmonary artery.

Rastelli operation

This is usually undertaken in patients with complex CHD, e.g., transposition of the great arteries with large ventricular septal defect. The VSD is closed by a large patch in such a way as to connect the left ventricle to the aorta, and a conduit or homograft connects the right ventricle to the pulmonary artery (see Fig. 8.2).

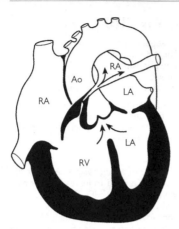

Figure 8.1 Tetralogy of Fallot.

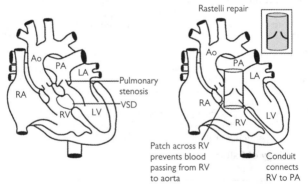

Figure 8.2 Rastelli operation. Ao, aorta; LA, left atrium; LV, left ventricle; PA, pulmonary artery; RA, right atrium; RV, right ventricle; VSD, venrtricular septal defect.

Ross procedure

This is an alternative to aortic valve replacement, which may be attractive to younger patients, especially females. The diseased aortic valve is removed with the coronary arteries detached. The patient's own pulmonary valve is resected and placed in the aortic position with the coronaries reattached. A homograft is placed between the right ventricle and the pulmonary artery.

However, this procedure is currently out of favor with poor outcomes in long-term follow-up.

Fontan operation

This represents the definitive palliation for patients with effectively univentricular circulations such as mitral or tricuspid atresia. Blood from the superior and inferior vena cavae is directed to the pulmonary arteries without the benefit of a subpulmonary ventricle. Oxygenated blood returns to the systemic ventricle and is then pumped to the aorta.

Mustard and Senning operations

These were life-saving innovations for treatment of patients with transposition of the great arteries. They involved intra-atrial redirection of oxygenated and deoxygenated blood to the systemic and pulmonary systems, respectively (see Fig. 8.3). The right ventricle served as the systemic subaortic ventricle. They have been largely abandoned because of late problems with arrhythmias, pathway obstruction, and ventricular failure.

Arterial switch

This has largely superseded the Mustard and Senning procedures. The aorta and pulmonary artery are relocated to their "normal" positions with reanastomosis of the coronary arteries to the neo-aorta.

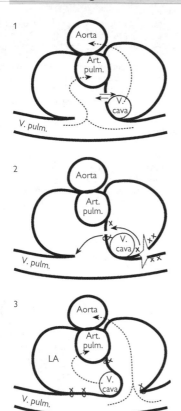

Figure 8.3 Senning operation. This figure was published in *Annals of Thoracic Surgery*, 77(6):2250–2258. Atrial switch operation: past, present, and future. Copyright Elsevier 2004.

Percutaneous transcatheter interventions for CHD

Balloon atrial septostomy

This life-saving intervention is used in neonates with transposition of the great arteries. An atrial communication is created by tearing a hole in the atrial septum using a balloon catheter. This can be performed at the bedside under echocardiographic control or in the catheterization laboratory with both echocardiographic and angiographic guidance.

Pulmonary valvuloplasty

This is the procedure of choice for patients of all ages with pulmonary valvar stenosis. It is less successful if the valve is dysplastic (Noonan's syndrome). The pulmonary valve annulus is measured by echocardiography or angiography and a balloon (100%–120% diameter) is used. It is one of the most effective transcatheter interventions.

Aortic valvuloplasty

This intervention has limited use in adults. If the aortic valve is pliable but not calcified, balloon dilatation may defer the need for definitive surgery, but usually at the expense of aortic regurgitation. The balloon size should not exceed the size of the aorta at the site of the valve attachment. An anterograde approach via a trans-septal puncture is advised to reduce the incidence of valve damage.

Atrial septal defect

Most secundum atrial septal defects are amenable to percutaneous closure. The Amplatzer® septal occluding device is made of Nitinol (a nickel titanium alloy with inherent shape memory) and comprises two discs with a self-centering waist. The device is balloon sized under transesophageal echocardiographic (TEE) guidance. Defects up to 40 mm in size can be closed providing there are sufficient rims (>5 mm) to the pulmonary veins and the attachment of the mitral valve.

This is not suitable for any atrial defects other than those of the secundum variety, i.e., sinus venosus defects or partial atrioventricular septal defects. Procedural complications are rare in expert hands. Antiplatelet agents are administered for 3–6 months until the device has completely endothelialized.

Transient headaches are common in the weeks following closure, but serious complications are rare. These include transient ischemic episodes or stroke, atrial arrhythmias, and embolization of the device.

Concomitant electrophysiological procedures may need to be undertaken in patients with significant atrial arrhythmias.

Ventricular septal defects

Indications for closing defects in adults are limited. Occasionally, small defects can produce volume overload of the left ventricle over time and require closure. Such defects may be amenable to transcatheter occlusion using the Amplatzer® perimembranous or muscular occluding devices.

This should only be undertaken in specialist centers. Complete heart block and device embolization have been described.

Coarctation of the aorta

Surgical correction in the adult is a major challenge with its associated risk of paraplegia. Both native and re-coarctation of the aorta can now be successfully treated by transcatheter balloon dilatation and stenting. Covered stents may be required for native coarctation to reduce the incidence of dissection and rupture. Remember that the aorta in these patients is especially friable and that an aortopathy commonly coexists.

MRI is invaluable in patient selection and for selecting stent size. This intervention should only be undertaken in specialist centers where expert surgical help is readily available. Balloon dilatation of previous patch aortoplasty carries the highest risk of aortic rupture.

Lifelong surveillance is necessary to detect aneurysm formation.

Patent ductus arteriosus

This may occasionally present in later life. If it is small or medium sized with no pulmonary hypertension, it usually can be successfully occluded with a variety of transcatheter occluding devices or coils.

Pulmonary valve implantation

Percutaneous transcatheter implantation of a bovine jugular venous valve mounted within a platinum-iridium stent into the right ventricular outflow tract is now possible. If it stands the test of time, this procedure will revolutionize our approach to management of patients with pulmonary regurgitation following right heart congenital surgery, offering a nonsurgical approach.

It may not be long before an implantable valve that can be used in the systemic circulation becomes widely available.

Specific management issues

Complications of cyanotic CHD

Chronic hypoxemia results in an increased red cell mass and total blood volume. This compensatory mechanism may initially enhance oxygen delivery; however, symptoms of hyperviscosity may develop.

- Symptoms of hyperviscosity include headaches, visual disturbances (blurred or double vision), impaired alertness, fatigue, parasthesia, tinnitus, myalgia, muscle weakness, and restless legs. Transient ischemic events or stroke may also occur.
- Measure hemoglobin and red cell indices; most patients have a compensated erythropoesis with a stable hemoglobin.
- Therapeutic phlebotomy should be reserved for symptomatic patients, e.g., with hemoglobin >20 g/dL or hematocrit >65%. Symptoms may be relieved by removal of 500 mL (maximum) of blood with concomitant fluid replacement of dextrose or saline. Phlebotomy should be performed no more than 2 times per year, as it increases the risk of stroke by causing iron deficiency. Intravenous line filters should always be used.

Iron deficiency in a polycythemic patient should be treated with cautious iron supplementation. Recheck hemoglobin 8–10 days later. Overaggressive treatment can result in further increases in hematocrit.

Skin

Severe acne is common in cyanotic CHD. It can act as a source of infection and endocarditis. Treat it aggressively.

Gallstones

These are common in cyanotic patients. Bilirubin is a product of hemoglobin breakdown. Suspect them if a patient presents with severe abdominal pain and discomfort.

Renal function

- Reduced glomerular filtration rate
- Increased levels of creatinine
- Abnormalities in clearance of uric acid frequently accompany chronic cyanosis and gout may result.
- Use contrast in angiography with caution and always prehydrate and premedicate the patient.

Noncardiac surgery

This should be undertaken in specialist centers and care delivered by a multidisciplinary team. Local anesthesia should be used, if possible; otherwise a cardiac anesthesiologist with experience in congenital heart disease should be consulted.

Consider preoperative phlebotomy if hemoglobin >20 g/dL or hematocrit >65%.

Endocarditis prophylaxis and air line filters should be employed.

Pregnancy

Box 8.7

The majority of women with CHD can tolerate pregnancy.

Maternal congenital heart disease is now the major cause of maternal cardiac death in developed countries. All patients need specialist counseling **before** embarking on pregnancy. Cardiologists are generally ill prepared to give such advice; pediatric cardiologists less so!

All young women of child-bearing age should undergo a detailed clinical and hemodynamic assessment that should include a formal exercise test and detailed echocardiography with emphasis on systemic ventricular function.

All women with complex CHD should be closely monitored in specialist centers where delivery should take place. Multidisciplinary input is essential.

Pregnancy is contraindicated in some CHD patients (see Box 8.8).

Attention to medications
1. Anticoagulation (warfarin embryopathy) must be balanced against the need for effective maternal anticoagulation in the setting of indications such as arrhythmias or prosthetic valves.
2. ARBs and ACE inhibitors are contraindicated in pregnancy.
3. Assess the need for and choice of antiarrhythmic drug (e.g., chance for amiodarone-induced fetal thyroid dysfunction).

Arrhythmia

Arrhythmia is an important cause of morbidity and mortality and a major cause for hospitalization of CHD patients. It may lead to significant hemodynamic deterioration and is poorly tolerated.

It may be due to the following:
- Underlying cardiac defect, e.g., atrial isomerism
- Part of natural history, e.g., hemodynamic changes such as chamber enlargement or scarring
- Residual postoperative abnormalities

Box 8.8 Women with CHD in whom pregnancy is contraindicated

- Pulmonary hypertension
  - E.g., Eisenmenger syndrome (50% maternal and fetal mortality; maternal death may occur up to 2 weeks postpartum)
- Heart failure secondary to failing Fontan circulation
- Women with severe cyanosis and polycythemia
  - If saturation is <80% at rest and hemoglobin is >18 g/dL, there is a greater incidence of miscarriage and intrauterine growth retardation.

Management

Specialist advice is essential. New presentation demands a complete hemodynamic reassessment including electrophysiological investigation. Correction of any underlying postoperative hemodynamic abnormality may be one of the most important therapeutic interventions.

- Record a 12 lead ECG.
- Administer intravenous adenosine while recording the ECG. The mode of termination of the tachyarrhythmia may give very useful information on its etiology, e.g., pre-excitation.
- Urgent direct current cardioversion may be required if hemodynamic compromise is present. Ideally, transesophageal echocardiography should rule out intracardiac thrombus. If the patient is on warfarin, always check the INR as well as the serum electrolytes prior to cardioversion.

Atrial septal defect

Atrial septal defect (ASD) is one of the most common lesions presenting for the first time in adult life. It is often missed, as clinical signs of fixed splitting of the second heart sound can be difficult to appreciate. It may present for the first time with new-onset atrial flutter or fibrillation.

Consider the need for electrophysiological interventions, e.g., the Maze procedure for atrial fibrillation. Shunting tends to increase with aging as the left ventricle stiffens. Closure is indicated in all symptomatic patients; few are truly asymptomatic when assessed by cardiopulmonary testing! There is no upper age limit. The vast majority of secundum defects are amenable to transcatheter closure.

Pulmonary hypertension needs to be excluded.

Atrial arrhythmias are one of the common late medical problems. All other types such as sinus venosus defect (defect in upper atrial septum associated with overriding of the superior vena cava and anomalous right pulmonary venous drainage) and partial atrioventricular septal defect require surgical closure. A sinus venosus defect represents a major surgical challenge involving redirection of anomalous pulmonary vein(s).

Risk of endocarditis is very low. Antibiotic prophylaxis is not indicated except for the 6 months post-repair with a prosthetic device or material.

Ventricular septal defect

The majority of cases are small, as larger defects are usually repaired in childhood.

Eisenmenger syndrome (pulmonary vascular disease and hypertension associated with reverse, right-to-left shunting via intracardiac communication—VSD, ASD, PDA) is becoming increasingly rare. VSD should be closed if there is significant shunt, previous endocarditis, development of aortic regurgitation, or right ventricular outflow tract obstruction.

It is always important to demonstrate reversibility of pulmonary hypertension prior to intervention. This may be amenable to surgical or transcatheter closure.

Ventricular arrhythmias may occur late during follow-up.

Antibiotic prophylaxis is indicated for 6 months post-repair or if a residual defect exists adjacent to the prosthetic material.

Atrioventricular septal/canal defect (endocardial cushion defect)

This is a common defect in patients with Down syndrome. If unoperated, pulmonary vascular disease (Eisenmenger syndrome) develops. Left atrioventricular valve regurgitation and stenosis are the major determinants of need for further interventions. Valve replacement may be necessary.

Endocarditis prophylaxis is recommended if there is a prosthetic valve, cyanosis, or a defect adjacent to the prosthetic material or for 6 months post-repair.

Pulmonary stenosis

This may present for first time in adult life. This can be successfully treated by balloon valvuloplasty, which should be undertaken if the valve gradient exceeds 30 mmHg on Doppler echocardiography.

Surgery is reserved for calcified and dysplastic valves. The outlook is excellent. The risk of endocarditis is low.

Left ventricular outflow tract (LVOT) obstruction

Aortic valve stenosis is especially common in association with a bicuspid valve. This is a complex lesion and an aortopathy is commonly present. There is a risk of aortic dilation and dissection. The degree of stenosis or regurgitation may increase over time. Effort intolerance, chest pain, or syncope, especially with exertion, need to be taken seriously and intervention considered.

It may occasionally be amenable to balloon valvuloplasty but more commonly requires surgical intervention. Aortic valve replacement (lifelong anticoagulation) or homograft insertion or Ross operation (which requires no anticoagulation but potentially further interventions and is critically operator dependent) can be offered.

Subaortic stenosis is uncommon (no ejection click) and requires surgical resection if severe or if the patient is symptomatic. Recurrence is possible. Supravalvar stenosis is commonly seen in patients with Williams syndrome. It may be associated with multiple stenoses in the origins of the coronary arteries and the aortic arch arterial branches.

Reconstructive surgery is complex.

Coarctation of the aorta

Most patients seen in adult clinics will have already undergone surgery. Some may present for the first time with hypertension. Always feel the femoral pulses! Consider Turner's syndrome in female patients.

Coarctation of the aorta is a complex lesion usually associated with a bicuspid aortic valve (ejection click at the apex) and aortopathy. During follow-up, upper (right arm) and lower limb blood pressure should be recorded and evidence of left ventricular hypertrophy on ECG and echocardiography should be noted.

Re-coarctation may occur over time and should be suspected if there are reduced femoral pulses or radiofemoral delay on examination. Doppler echocardiography can help by revealing an increased systolic velocity signal with forward flow through the site of re-coarctation during diastole. MRI with three-dimensional reconstruction is the imaging modality of choice.

Transcatheter balloon dilatation and stenting is feasible in many patients, thus avoiding the risks of thoracic aortic surgery.

Lifelong surveillance is necessary to rule out aneurysm formation or recurrence. Antibiotic prophylaxis is indicated for 6 months post-repair of if there is a defect associated with the prosthetic material.

Anomalous pulmonary venous drainage

Many patients will undergo surgery in early childhood. This may occur in association with Scimitar syndrome. If the patient is symptomatic (shortness of breath, arrhythmia) and there is evidence of right heart volume overload, e.g., on the cross-sectional echocardiogram or MRI, consider surgery. There is a low risk of endocarditis.

Transposition of the great arteries

The aorta arises from the right ventricle and the pulmonary artery from the left ventricle. It is the most common cyanotic cardiac lesion presenting in the first few days of life. In the absence of mixing at the cardiac or great artery level, this condition is uniformly lethal.

The majority of adult survivors have undergone intra-atrial repair by Mustard or Senning procedure. These produced excellent early survival but significant late morbidity and mortality. Common late problems are sinus node dysfunction, atrial arrhythmias (flutter/fibrillation), venous baffle narrowing, and right ventricular failure with tricuspid regurgitation.

Arrhythmias are poorly tolerated, and prompt restoration to sinus rhythm is essential. Baffle stenosis can be relieved by transcatheter balloon dilatation and stenting.

Ventricular failure requires intensive medical therapy but may ultimately necessitate cardiac transplantation. Patients who have undergone the arterial switch procedure are now reaching early adulthood. Problems with coronary arterial stenoses at the site of reanastomosis to the neo-aorta have been identified in some.

Antibiotic prophylaxis is required prior to repair and post-repair if there is a defect adjacent to the prosthetic material or for 6 months.

Tetralogy of Fallot

Tetralogy of Fallot (TOF) comprises a large nonrestrictive VSD, overriding aorta, right ventricular outflow tract (RVOT) obstruction, and right ventricular hypertrophy. This is the most common cyanotic cardiac lesion presenting outside the neonatal period. If it presents with critical cyanosis in the neonatal period, the patient may undergo a palliative Blalock–Taussig shunt prior to complete repair in early childhood.

Many centers now opt for definitive repair even in the first few months of life. The vast majority of adults will have undergone some form of repair with surgical closure of the septal defect and relief of the RVOT obstruction.

Arrhythmias are an almost inevitable consequence of surgery (scarring, ventriculotomy, and pulmonary regurgitation). Late arrhythmias (both atrial and ventricular) and sudden death occur.

Pulmonary regurgitation, ignored for many years as a benign condition, is now known to be one of the most important causes of morbidity and mortality in patients following RVOT surgery. The QRS duration >180 ms on the ECG has been used as a marker for patients at risk of arrhythmia and late sudden death. Patients should be assessed with exercise testing and MRI.

A percutaneous approach to pulmonary valve implantation is now available using a bovine jugular venous valve mounted within a platinum-iridium stent and is suitable for patients with severe pulmonary regurgitation and outflow tracts <20 mm in size.

Branch pulmonary arterial stenoses should be treated aggressively by catheter intervention. Surgical insertion of a homograft valve is currently performed with perioperative mortality <1% in specialist centers. The majority of such conduits need replacing within a 10-year period, i.e., the need for multiple reoperations. Aortic regurgitation may also occur.

Endocarditis prophylaxis is indicated in all patients prior to repair and post-repair if there is a prosthetic valve, a defect adjacent to the repair, or for 6 months.

Fontan patients

This is the definitive palliation for patients born with "single ventricle" physiology in which all the systemic venous return is directed back to the lungs without the benefit of a subpulmonary ventricle, e.g., mitral, tricuspid, pulmonary, or aortic atresia.

It produces excellent early and mid-term survival but late failure occurs even in the most carefully selected candidates. The late problems comprise atrial arrhythmias, sinus node dysfunction and heart block, atrioventricular valve regurgitation, ventricular failure, venous obstruction, and protein-losing enteropathy (<50% 5-year survival).

The failing Fontan is a major challenge; transplantation or conversion to a more streamlined modification with concomitant arrhythmia surgery should be considered. All patients need endocarditis prophylaxis.

Congenitally corrected transposition of the great arteries

Cyanosis is present if there is an associated ventricular septal defect (VSD) and pulmonary stenosis (PS) or if there is pulmonary vascular disease with VSD and no PS. This is a rare lesion with normal survival in some if the lesion is isolated. There is ongoing risk of complete heart block (2% per year).

Atrioventricular valve regurgitation in association with systemic right ventricular failure is a major long-term problem, leading to decreased survival.

Ebstein's anomaly of the tricuspid valve

This condition is associated with apical displacement of the tricuspid valve and is often associated with ASD. Cyanosis occurs via right to left shunt at the atrial level. A wide spectrum of presentations occurs depending on the severity of tricuspid valve regurgitation and associated anomalies.

In infancy this presents with heart failure and cyanosis, and prognosis is poor. In the older child or young adult, the murmur may be an incidental finding, and mild forms can be asymptomatic.

Atrial arrhythmias are common and associated with pre-excitation (accessory pathways). Intervention is warranted if the condition is symptomatic with heart failure and severe tricuspid regurgitation or arrhythmias.

Tricuspid valve replacement or repair can be offered. Interatrial communications causing cyanosis or paradoxical emboli can be closed percutaneously if hemodynamic assessment permits.

Extracardiac complications

Polycythemia

Chronic hypoxia stimulates erythropoietin production and erythrocytosis. The ideal Hb level is ~17–18 g/dL. Some centers advocate phlebotomy to control the hematocrit and prevent hyperviscosity syndrome.

Follow local guidelines. Generally, consider phlebotomy only with moderate or severe symptoms of hyperviscosity and hematocrit >65%.

Remove 500 mL of blood over 30–45 minutes and replace volume simultaneously with 500–1000 mL saline or salt-free dextran (if there is heart failure). Avoid abrupt changes in circulating volume.

If hyperviscosity symptoms are the result of acute dehydration or iron deficiency, phlebotomy is not required and the patient must be rehydrated and/or treated cautiously with iron.

Renal disease and gout

Hypoxia affects glomerular and tubular function, resulting in proteinuria, reduced urate excretion, increased urate reabsorption, and reduced creatinine clearance. Overt renal failure is uncommon.

Try to avoid dehydration and use of diuretics or radiographic contrast. Asymptomatic hyperuricemia does not need treatment. Colchicine and steroids are first-line agents for treatment of acute gout. NSAIDs should be avoided.

Sepsis

Patients are more prone to infection. Skin acne is common with poor healing of scars. Dental hygiene is very important because of the risk of endocarditis. Any site of sepsis may result in cerebral abscesses from metastatic infection or septic emboli.

Thrombosis and bleeding

Causes are multifactorial and due to a combination of abnormal platelet function, coagulation abnormalities, and polycythemia. PT and aPTT values may be elevated and secondary to a fall in factors V, VII, VIII, and X. Both arterial ± venous thromboses and hemorrhagic complications (e.g., petechiae, epistaxis, and hemoptysis) can occur.

Dehydration or oral contraceptives are risk factors for thrombotic events. Spontaneous bleeding is generally self-limited. In the context of severe bleeding general measures are effective, including platelet transfusion, fresh frozen plasma (FFP), cryoprecipitate, and vitamin K.

Aspirin and other NSAIDs should generally be avoided to decrease chances of spontaneous bruising and bleeding.

Primary pulmonary problems include infection, infarction, and hemorrhage from ruptured arterioles or capillaries

Stroke can be either thrombotic or hemorrhagic. Arterial thrombosis, embolic events (paradoxical emboli in right-to-left shunt) and injudicious phlebotomy lead to spontaneous thrombosis. Hemostatic problems, especially when combined with NSAIDs or formal anticoagulation, can lead to hemorrhagic stroke. Any injured brain tissue is also a nidus for intracranial infection or abscess formation.

Complications secondary to drugs, investigations, surgery

Avoid abrupt changes in blood pressure or systemic resistance. Contrast agents may provoke systemic vasodilatation and cause acute decompensation. They may also precipitate renal failure.

Before noncardiac surgery, try to optimize hematocrit and hemostasis by controlled phlebotomy and replacement with dextran. High-flow oxygen is important before and after surgery.

Use extreme caution with IV lines. Consider filters in IVs.

Arthralgia

Arthralgia is mainly due to hypertrophic osteoarthropathy. In patients with right-to-left shunt, megakaryocytes bypass the pulmonary circulation and become trapped in systemic vascular beds, promoting new bone formation.

Hemoptysis

Hemoptysis is common. Most episodes are self-limited and precipitated by infection. Differentiation from pulmonary embolism may be difficult. Try to keep the patient calm and ensure adequate BP control. Give high-flow oxygen by mask. If there is clinical suspicion of infection (fever, sputum production, leukocytosis, raised CRP, etc.) start broad-spectrum antibiotics. A VQ scan may help in the diagnosis of pulmonary embolism but is often equivocal.

Avoid use of aspirin and NSAIDs, as these exacerbate the intrinsic platelet abnormalities. There is anecdotal evidence for the use of low-dose IV heparin, Dextran 40 (500 mL IV infusion q4–6h), acrid (Arvin® reduces plasma fibrinogen by cleaving fibrin), or low-dose warfarin therapy for reducing thrombotic tendency in these patients. Severe pulmonary hemorrhage may respond to aprotinin or tranexamic acid.

Breathlessness

This may be due to pulmonary edema or hypoxia (increased shunt) secondary to chest infection or pulmonary infarction. Do not give large doses of diuretics or nitrates, as this will drop systemic pressures and may precipitate acute collapse. Compare chest X-ray to previous films to assess if there is radiological evidence of pulmonary edema.

JVP in patients with cyanotic CHD is typically high and should not be used as a sole marker of heart failure. Patients need higher filling pressure to maintain pulmonary blood flow. Give high-flow oxygen by mask.

Start antibiotics with clinical suspicion of infection. Give oral diuretics if there is evidence of pulmonary edema or severe right heart failure. Monitor hematocrit and renal function closely for signs of overdiuresis.

Effort syncope should prompt a search for arrhythmias, in particular VT (Holter monitor/EPS), severe valve disease, or signs of overt heart failure. Treat as appropriate.

Chest pain

Chest pain may be secondary to pulmonary embolism or infarction (spontaneous thrombosis), pneumonia, ischemic heart disease, or musculoskeletal causes. It requires careful evaluation with conventional diagnostic modalities as already described.

Arrhythmias

The cardiac conduction system

Cardiac action potential

The intracellular resting potential of the cardiac myocyte is electrically negative with a resting transmembrane voltage between −50 and −95 mV. The transmembrane gradient is due to the relative distribution of the ions K^+, Na^+, Cl^-, and Ca^{2+} across the cell membrane.

During phase 4 of the action potential, the voltage slowly increases until a threshold of −70 to −65 mV is reached, which opens voltage-gated Na^+ channels and triggers depolarization via an influx of Na^+ ions. The resulting voltage changes are propagated to adjacent cells via gap junctions between myocytes, such that a wavefront of electrical activation is propagated.

At least 10 distinct ion channels modulate the voltage changes that occur in the action potential (Fig. 9.1).

Automaticity

Automaticity is the unique ability of myocytes to spontaneously depolarize. It is attributed to the influx of positive ions during diastole (phase 4). At potentials more negative than −60 mV ion channels open, allowing in a slow influx of cations. In the sinoatrial node (SAN) the slow influx of Ca^{2+} allows it to depolarize more rapidly and thus suppress other potential pacemaker sites.

Sinoatrial node

The SAN is normally the dominant pacemaker site in the heart and sits high in the lateral right atrium (RA) just inferior to the superior vena cava (SVC) (Fig. 9.2). It is 1–2 cm long, 2–3 mm wide, and <1 mm from the epicardial surface. The impulses generated in the SAN are conducted out of the sinus node to depolarize the surrounding RA.

The SAN is richly innervated with both adrenergic and cholinergic receptors, which alter the rate of depolarization and therefore heart rate. Electrical impulses spread out from the SAN to the rest of the RA and left atrium (LA) via specialized interatrial connections including Bachmann's bundle.

Atrioventricular node

The atrioventricular node (AVN) is found in the RA anterior to the ostium of the coronary sinus and directly above the insertion of the septal leaflet of the tricuspid valve. It is normally the only electrical connection between the atrium and ventricle.

Electrical impulses transmitted through the AVN subsequently traverse the His bundle, which, like the SAN, is also densely innervated with sympathetic and parasympathetic fibers.

His–Purkinje system

The electrical impulse conducts rapidly through the His bundle into the upper part of the interventricular septum where it divides into two branches. The right bundle branch continues down the right side of the septum to the apex of the right ventricle and the base of the anterior papillary muscle. The left bundle branch further splits into two fascicles, anterior and posterior.

The terminal Purkinje fibers connect with the ends of the bundle branches, forming an interweaving network on the endocardial surface so that a cardiac impulse is transmitted almost simultaneously to the entire right and left ventricles.

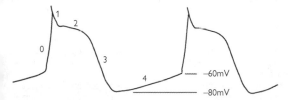

Figure 9.1 The cardiac action potential. The action potential has five parts:
0 Rapid influx of Na, causing fast depolarization
1 Rapid early repolarization due to efflux of Na⁺
2 Plateau phase where repolarization is slowed by an influx of Ca^{2+}
3 Repolarization due to the efflux of K⁺
4 Diastole with a steady-state resting transmembrane voltage and diastolic depolarization in pacemaker cells

The plateau phase distinguishes the cardiac from neuronal action potential. The release of Ca^{2+} during phase 3 triggers mechanical contraction of the cell.

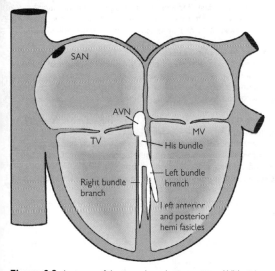

Figure 9.2 Anatomy of the normal conduction system. AVN, atrioventricular node; MV, mitral valve; SAN, sinoatrial node; TV, tricuspid valve.

Bradyarrhythmias: general approach

Ask specifically about previous cardiac disease, palpitations, fainting or blackouts (syncope), dizziness, chest pain, symptoms of heart failure (shortness of breath, edema, exercise intolerance, orthopnea, nocturnal dyspnea), and recent use of drugs.

Examine carefully, noting the BP, JVP waveform and height (?cannon waves), heart rate, sounds and murmurs, and signs of heart failure.

Investigations

- *12 lead ECG and rhythm strip:* Look specifically for the relationship between P waves and QRS complex. A long rhythm strip is sometimes necessary to detect complete heart block if atrial and ventricular rates are similar.
- *Blood tests:* CBC, chemistries including glucose (urgently), Cr, K+, Ca^{2+}, Mg^{2+} (especially if on diuretics), biochemical markers of cardiac injury.
- *Chest X-ray:* heart size; evidence of pulmonary edema.
- *24-hour ambulatory monitor (Holter/event monitor)* provides information about ambient heart rates, intermittent or infrequent arrhythmia and associated symptoms if present.
- *Event monitors,* which patients may have for a month at a time, may be useful to identify even less frequent events.

Management

Hemodynamically unstable patients

- Give **oxygen** via facemask if the patient is hypoxic on room air.
- **Keep NPO** until definitive therapy has been started to reduce the risk of aspiration in case of cardiac arrest or when the patient lies supine for temporary wire insertion.
- Secure peripheral venous access.
- Bradyarrhythmias causing **severe hemodynamic compromise** (cardiac arrest, asystole, SBP <90 mmHg, severe pulmonary edema, evidence of end-organ damage including renal or cerebral hypoperfusion) require immediate treatment often including temporary pacing (technique is described on p. 692).
- Give **atropine 0.5–1 mg IV** (Min-I-Jet®) bolus; repeat if necessary up to a maximum 3 mg.
- Give **isoproterenol 0.02–0.06 mg IV** if there is a delay in pacing and the patient remains unstable. Set up an infusion (1 mg in 100 mL bag normal saline starting at 2–10 µg/min titrating to HR).
- Set up **external pacing system** if available, and arrange for initiation of transvenous pacing (see Box 9.1).
- Bradycardia in shock is a poor prognostic sign. Look for a source of blood loss and begin aggressive resuscitation with fluids and inotropes.

Hemodynamically stable patients

- Admit to cardiac care unit (CCU) or step-down unit when appropriate with continuous ECG monitoring.
- Keep atropine drawn up and ready in case of acute deterioration.
- Evaluate if the patient requires a temporary wire immediately.
- It may be valuable to have appropriate central venous access (internal jugular vein or femoral) in place in case of the need for emergency temporary wire insertion or aggressive resuscitation.

Box 9.1 External cardiac pacing

In emergencies, external cardiac pacing may be used but is often painful for the patient (if conscious) and should be viewed as a temporary measure until transvenous pacing can be initiated.

External cardiac pacing is useful in patients who have received thrombolysis for an acute myocardial infarction (MI) when the risks of perforation and bleeding from transvenous pacing are high.

Hemodynamically stable patients with anterior MI and bifasicular block may be managed simply by application of the external pacing electrodes and having the pulse generator ready if necessary.

Familiarize yourself with the machine in your hospital as soon as possible—a cardiac arrest is not the time to read the manual.

Sinus bradycardia

The sinoatrial node discharges <60/min. P waves are normal in appearance. It is often normal in sleep and in athletes and healthy young adults.

Causes

- Young athletic individual
- Drugs (β-blockers, calcium channel blockers, digoxin, morphine, amiodarone, lithium, propafenone, clonidine)
- Increased vagal tone
  - Vasovagal syncope
  - Nausea or vomiting
  - Carotid sinus hypersensitivity
  - Acute MI (especially inferior)
  - Nasal or endotracheal suctioning
- Hypothyroidism
- Hypothermia
- Ischemia or infarction of the sinus node
- Chronic degeneration of sinus or AV nodes or atria
- Cholestatic jaundice
- Raised intracranial pressure
- Cervical and mediastinal tumors

Management

If hypotensive or presyncopal

- Atropine 0.5 mg IV bolus repeating as necessary.
- Isoproterenol infusion 2–10 µg/min.
- Theophylline infusion 0.2–0.7 mg/kg/hr.
- Temporary pacing.
- Avoid and correct precipitants.
- Stop drugs that may suppress the sinus or AV nodes.

Long-term treatment

- If all possible underlying causes have been removed and symptomatic bradycardia remains, refer for permanent pacing.
- Consider Holter monitoring in patients with possible episodic bradycardia. R-R intervals >2.5 seconds may require permanent pacing, especially if associated with symptoms.

Sinus pause

The SAN fails to generate impulses (sinus arrest) or the impulses are not conducted to the atria (SA exit block). The PP interval with sinus pause does not equal a multiple of the basic sinus interval (PP). A single dropped P wave with a PP interval that is a multiple of the basic PP interval suggests exit block. A period of absent P waves suggests sinus arrest.

Causes include excess vagal tone, acute myocarditis, MI, aging (fibrosis), stroke, digoxin toxicity, and antiarrhythmic drugs.

Sick sinus syndrome

This syndrome encompasses a number of sinus node problems: 1) persistent, inappropriate sinus bradycardia not caused by drugs; 2) sinus arrest or exit block; 3) SAN and AV conduction disturbances; 3) paroxysms of atrial, supraventricular, or junctional tachyarrythmias alternating with slow atrial or ventricular rates. It is usually diagnosed by ambulatory cardiac monitoring.

Atrioventricular block

AV block occurs when an impulse from the atria is conducted with delay or not conducted at all to the ventricle. This can occur at the level of the AVN (nodal) or His–Purkinje system (infranodal).

Common causes are ischemic heart disease, conduction system fibrosis (aging), calcific aortic stenosis, congenital, cardiomyopathy, hypothermia, hypothyroidism, trauma, radiotherapy, infection, connective tissue disease, sarcoidosis, tick-born diseases, and anti-arrhythmic drugs (see Box 9.2). AV block is classified as follows.

First-degree AV block

Every impulse conducts to the ventricle but the conduction time is prolonged. Every P wave is followed by a QRS but with a prolonged PR interval (>200 ms). If the QRS width is normal on ECG, then the delay is usually in the AV node. If the QRS shows aberration (RBBB or LBBB), then the delay may be in the AV node or His–Purkinje system.

Second-degree AV block

Some, but not all, atrial impulses are conducted to the ventricle.

Mobitz type 1 (Wenckebach)

ECG shows a regularly irregular rhythm with grouped beating and progressive prolongation of the PR interval until the P wave is not conducted. The PR interval following the dropped P wave is the shortest in the sequence. The RR interval is therefore irregular.

This block is characteristic of normal AVN physiology and generally is a stable rhythm that does not progress to advanced AVN block.

Mobitz type 2

ECG shows a stable PR interval with periodic block of the atrial impulse at a ratio of 2:1, 3:1, or 4:1. Block is predominantly below the AVN at the His bundle and there is often an aberrant pattern to the QRS complex.

Type 2 block is an unstable rhythm that often predates the development of complete AV block.

Third-degree AV block (complete heart block)

There is no conduction of atrial impulses to the ventricle. The ECG shows no relationship between P and QRS complexes (dissociation).

Generally, a ventricular pacemaker originating just below the site of the block takes over. A narrow QRS usually indicates block in the AVN and the His bundle is the pacemaker, which is faster and more stable than more distal sites. A wide QRS indicates infranodal block and a distal, slower ventricular pacemaker.

Distal block carries a worse prognosis and a greater risk of sudden asystole.

Box 9.2 Causes of atrioventricular block

- Acute myocardial infraction or ischemia
- Drugs (β-blockers, digitalis, Ca^{2+}-blockers)
- Conduction system fibrosis (Lev and Lenegre syndromes)
- Increased vagal tone
- Trauma or following cardiac surgery
- Hypothyroidism (rarely thyrotoxicosis)
- Hypothermia
- Hyperkalemia and other electrolyte abnormalities
- Hypoxia
- Infiltrative diseases (amyloidosis)
- Valvular disease (aortic stenosis, incompetence, endocarditis)
- Myocarditis (diphtheria, rheumatic fever, viral, Chagas' disease, tick-borne)
- Associated with neuromuscular disease, i.e., myotonic dystrophy.
- Collagen vascular disease (SLE, rheumatoid arthritis, scleroderma)
- Cardiomyopathies (hemochromotosis, amyloidosis)
- Granulomatous disease (sarcoid)
- Congenital heart block
- Congenital heart disease (ASD, Ebstein's, PDA, L-transposition)

Bundle branch block

Bundle branch block (BBB) is due to disease in the His–Purkinje system resulting in conduction delay that manifests as a prolonged QRS on surface ECG (QRS >120 ms). Common causes are conduction system fibrosis (aging), ischemic heart disease, hypertension, cardiomyopathies, cardiac surgery, and infiltrative diseases (see Box 9.3).

LBBB: left ventricular depolarization is delayed, giving large notched R waves in leads I and V6 and an inverted-M pattern in V1. Block confined to the anterior or posterior fascicles of the left bundle gives left-axis or right-axis deviation, respectively, on the ECG. BBB leads to asynchronous contraction of the left and right ventricles, which worsens function.

RBBB: right ventricular depolarization is delayed, giving an RSR pattern in V1 and a prominent S wave in I and V6. This can be a normal variant but more commonly is due to causes listed in Box 9.3 as well as atrial septal-defect (ASD), pulmonary embolism (PE), and cor pulmonale.

Bifascicular block = RBBB + left anterior hemiblock (left-axis deviation on ECG), RBBB + left posterior hemiblock (right-axis deviation on ECG) or LBBB. All of these may progress to complete AV block.

Trifascicular block = bifascicular block + first-degree AV block.

Management

Interventricular conduction disturbances alone do not require temporary pacing. However, when associated with hemodynamic disturbance or progression to higher levels of block (even if intermittent), a transvenous pacing wire must be considered.

The need for longer term pacing is dependent on the persistence of symptoms and underlying cause. Consult a cardiologist.

Box 9.3 Common causes of bundle branch block

- Ischemic heart disease
- Hypertensive heart disease
- Valve disease (especially aortic stenosis)
- Conduction system fibrosis (Lev and Lenegre syndromes)
- Myocarditis or endocarditis
- Cardiomyopathies
- Infiltrative diseases (amyloidosis, sarcoidosis)
- Cor pulmonale (RBBB) (acute or chronic)
- Trauma or postcardiac surgery
- Neuromuscular disorders (myotonic dystrophy)
  Polymyositis

Tachyarrhythmias: general approach

Tachyarrhythmias may present with significant symptoms, syncope, and hemodynamic compromise. The approach to patients depends on
1. The effect of the rhythm on the patient
2. The diagnosis from the ECG and rhythm strips
3 Any underlying cardiac abnormality or identifiable precipitant (Box 9.4)

Effect of tachyarrhythmia on the patient

Patients with signs of severe hemodynamic compromise
- Impending cardiac arrest with an unstable rhythm
- Shock—systolic BP <90 mmHg
- Severe pulmonary edema
- Altered mental status

Treat immediately with synchronized external cardioversion for SVT, VT or unsynchronized external defibrillation for VF.

Patients with mild to moderate hemodynamic compromise
- Mild pulmonary edema
- Low cardiac output with cool extremities and oliguria
- Angina at rest during tachycardia

Try to record an ECG and long rhythm strip before giving pharmacological agents and/or defibrillation or intervention. This will be invaluable for long-term management. If the patient deteriorates, treat as above.

Diagnosing the arrhythmia

The main distinctions to make are the following (see also Box 9.5):
- Tachy- (>100/min) vs. brady- (<60/min) arrhythmia
- Narrow (≤120 ms or 3 small sq.) vs. broad QRS complex (Box 9.6)
- Regular vs. irregular rhythm

Box 9.4 Common precipitating factors

Underlying cardiac disease
- Ischemic heart disease
- Acute or recent MI
- Angina
- Mitral valve disease
- LV aneurysm
- Congenital heart disease
- Conduction system disease
- Pre excitation (short PR interval)
- Long QT (congenital or acquired).

Drugs
- Antiarrhythmics
- Sympathomimetics (β_2 agonists, cocaine)
- Antidepressants (tricyclic)
- Adenylate cyclase inhibitors (aminophylline, caffeine)
- Alcohol

Metabolic abnormalities
- ↑ or ↓ K^+
- ↑ or ↓ Ca^{2+}
- ↓ Mg^{2+}
- ↓ P_aO_2
- ↑ P_aCO_2
- Acidosis

Endocrine abnormalities
- Thyrotoxicosis
- Pheochromocytoma

Miscellaneous
- Febrile illness
- Emotional stress
- Smoking
- Fatigue

Box 9.5 Investigations for patients with tachyarrhythmias

12 Lead ECG and rhythm strip	• Reguiar vs. irregular rhythm • Narrow vs. broad QRS complex • Relation of P waves to QRS
Blood tests	• CBC, chemistries including Cr, glucose (urgently) • Ca^{2+}, Mg^{2+} (especially if on diuretics) • Biochemical markers of myocardial injury
Where appropriate	• Blood cultures, CRP, ESR • Thyroid function tests • Drug levels/toxicology screen • Arterial blood gases
Chest X-ray	• Heart size • Evidence of pulmonary edema • Other pathology (e.g., COPD, cancer, AF, pericardial effusion, sinus tachycardia, hypotension ± AF)

Box 9.6 Narrow vs. wide complex tachyarrhythmia

• Narrow complex tachycardias originate in the atria or AV node (i.e., supraventricular tachycardias [SVT]).
• Irregular, narrow complex tachycardia is most commonly AF or atrial flutter with varying AV block.
• Wide complex tachyarrhythmias may originate from either the ventricles (VT) or from the atria or AV node (SVT) with aberrant conduction to the ventricles (RBBB or LBBB configuration or preexcictation).
• If the patient has previous documented arrhythmias, compare the morphology of the current arrhythmia to old ECGs. The diagnosis of VT vs. SVT and thus the appropriate therapy may be evident from review of the prior ECG or history.

Tachyarrhythmias: classification

Tachyarrhythmias are generally classified via an anatomical approach that can then be subdivided on the basis of arrhythmia mechanism (see also Box 9.7). This provides a simple foundation for understanding the ECG morphology and the tachycardia mechanism.

Atrial tachyarrhythmias originate in the atria (or SAN).
- Sinus tachycardia
- Sinus node reentrant tachycardia
- Atrial fibrillation
- Atrial tachycardia
  - Focal atrial tachycardia
  - Macro-reentrant atrial tachycardia (aka atrial flutter)

Atrioventricular tachyarrhythmias are dependent on activation in or conduction via the AV node for maintenance of the arrhythmia.
- Atrioventricular reentry tachycardia (AVRT)
- Atrioventricular nodal reentry tachycardia (AVNRT)
- Junctional tachycardia

Ventricular tachyarrhythmias originate in the ventricle(s).
- Ventricular tachycardia (VT)
  - Monomorphic VT
  - Polymorphic VT (e.g., torsades de pointes)
- Ventricular fibrillation

Features of wide complex tachycardia suggesting a ventricular origin
- AV dissociation or lack of 1:1 AV relationship (although, VA conduction may be present during VT)
  - P waves with no clear association to the QRS
  - Capture and fusion beats
- QRS width >140 ms (if RBBB appearance) or >160 ms (if LBBB appearance)
- QRS axis < −30 or > +90
- Concordance of QRS complexes in precordial leads (all positive or all negative)
- Delayed/slurred initial forces (>100 ms)

Supraventricular causes of a wide complex tachycardia
- SVT with aberrancy (bundle branch block)
- SVT with pre-excitation (activation of the ventricle via antegrade conduction over an accessory pathway other than the AV node) e.g., antidromic AVRT
- SVT + class Ic drug (flecainide)

Box 9.7 Supraventricular tachycardias

Regular tachycardia
- Sinus tachycardia
- Sinus node reentrant tachycardia (SNRT)
- Atrial tachycardia
  - Focal atrial tachycardia
  - Macro-reentrant atrial tachycardia (atrial flutter)
- Atrioventricular reentry tachycardia (AVRT) (i.e., with accessory path, e.g., WPW)
- AV nodal reentry tachycardia (AVNRT)

Irregular tachycardia
- Atrial fibrillation (AF)
- Atrial flutter with variable block
- Multifocal atrial tachycardia

ECG diagnosis of tachyarrhythmias

By following simple rules when interpreting the ECG, any tachycardia can be classified into the categories described earlier; however, the ECG should always be considered in the clinical context. A wide complex tachycardia (WCT) should *always* be diagnosed as VT in the acute setting, as treating such patients incorrectly may be fatal. Review the ECG in both tachycardia and the patient's usual rhythm to aid in diagnosis (e.g., may see features of Wolff Parkinson–White [WPW]) (see also Fig. 9.5).

For narrow complex tachycardias (NCTs) use carotid sinus massage, vagal maneuvers or IV adenosine to facilitate identification of the underlying atrial rhythm.

A simple approach follows.

1. Is the tachycardia regular?
Grossly irregular RR intervals generally indicate AF or flutter with variable block (or VF, but expect the patient to be unconscious!). A slight variability in rate can occur in other tachycardias, particularly at their onset. Alternatively, multiple atrial and/or ventricular ectopic beats or atrial tachycardia with variable AV block can give irregularity.

2. Is the QRS complex wide (>120 ms)?
Yes—ventricular or SVT with aberrancy; no—supraventricular.

SVT should only be considered for a wide complex tachycardia in the appropriate clinical setting (e.g., young patient, no previous cardiac history, normal RV and LV function, no accompanying cardiovascular compromise) and after review with senior colleagues.

Note: Look at the baseline, sinus ECG (if available) for pre-existing bundle branch block or pre-excitation (suggesting an accessory pathway).

3. Identify P waves, their morphology, and P:QRS ratio
- *1:1 P:QRS, normal P-wave morphology:* sinus tachycardia, focal atrial tachycardia originating from close to the SA node (high crista terminalis or right superior pulmonary vein), or, rarely, sinus node reentry tachycardia.
- *1:1 P:QRS, abnormal P-wave morphology:* focal atrial tachycardia. AVRT or AVNRT (if slow ventricular to atrial conduction = long RP tachycardia).
- *P waves not visible:* AVRT or AVNRT (with rapid ventricular to atrial conduction). Compare QRS morphology in tachycardia with that in NSR, as a slight deflection in the tachycardia QRS complex not seen in NSR may represent a retrograde P wave.
- *P:QRS 2:1, 3:1, or greater:* focal or macro-reentrant atrial tachycardia with AV nodal block and varying AV conduction.
- *P wave rate >250 bpm:* atrial flutter (macro-reentrant atrial tachycardia). Usually there will be a 2 or 3:1 P:QRS ratio. In typical atrial flutter, a characteristic saw tooth baseline is seen in the inferior leads with upright P waves (dart-and-dome) in leads V1 and V2.

4. Response to AV block (adenosine or carotid massage)

If a rapid P-wave rate persists despite induced AV nodal block, then the tachycardia is independent of the AV node, i.e., macro-reentrant or focal atrial tachycardia or SNRT.

If tachycardia is terminated by AV nodal block, it is dependent on the AVN (either AVRT or AVNRT, rarely junctional tachycardia). Focal atrial tachycardia and sinus node reentry may also be terminated by adenosine, not through AV nodal block but because they are adenosine sensitive.

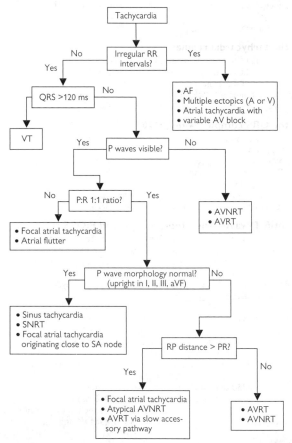

Figure 9.3 ECG diagnosis of tachycardia.

Tachycardia: emergency management

History

This includes previous cardiac disease, palpitations, dizziness, chest pain, symptoms of heart failure, and medication. Ask specifically about conditions known to be associated with certain cardiac arrhythmias (e.g., AF—alcohol, thyrotoxicosis, mitral valve disease, CAD, pericarditis; VT—previous MI, LV aneurysm, cardiomyopathy).

Examination

Check BP and assess for heart sounds and murmurs that are signs of heart failure and carotid bruits.

Management (see Fig. 9.4)

Hemodynamically unstable patients

Tachyarrhythmias causing severe hemodynamic compromise (cardiac arrest, systolic BP <90 mmHg, severe pulmonary edema, evidence of cerebral hypoperfusion) require urgent treatment, usually with external defibrillation/cardioversion. Drug therapy needs time to take effect and hemodynamic stability but may be considered for some awake patients.

- Sedate awake patients with midazolam (2.5–10 mg IV) ± fentanyl (25–50 µg/IV) for analgesia. Monitor for respiratory depression and have flumazenil and naloxone readily available.
- General anesthesia with propofol is preferred, but remember the patient may not have an empty stomach and precautions should be taken to prevent aspiration (e.g., cricoid pressure, ET intubation).
- For a monophasic defibrillator use 360 J synchronized shock and for biphasic defibrillators use 200 J or the maximum available. synchronized shock.
- If tachyarrhythmia recurs or is unresponsive, try to correct $\downarrow P_aO_2$, $\uparrow P_aCO_2$, acidosis or $\downarrow K^+$. Give Mg^{2+} (2 g IV) and shock again. Amiodarone 150–300 mg bolus IV may also be used, but be aware that it may increase defibrillation thresholds.
- Give specific antiarrhythmic therapy (see p. 614).
- If there is ongoing VT in the context of cardiac arrest or recurrent VT episodes, causing hemodynamic compromise and requiring repeated DC cardioversions, then give IV amiodarone (150 mg IV over 10 minutes bolus x 1 with a repeat x 1, followed by 1 mg/min IV x 6 hour followed by 0.5 mg/min IV x 18 hour). Alternately, IV lidocaine may be administered (1 to 1.5 mg/kg bolus over 3–5 minutes with repeat dose in 2 minutes) (max dose 300 mg in 1 hour) followed by 2–4 mg/min. Follow ACLS guidelines for treatment of unstable tachyarrhythmias.

Hemodynamically stable patients

- Admit patient to telemetry and obtain a 12 lead ECG.
- Try vagal maneuvers (e.g., Valsalva/carotid sinus massage) after ensuring that the patient has no carotid bruits.
- If type of arrhythmia is apparent, then initiate appropriate treatment.
- If there is a question regarding the diagnosis, give adenosine 6 mg rapid IVP followed immediately by 5 mL saline flush. If there is no response, try 6 and then 12 mg in succession with continuous ECG rhythm strip.

- Definitive treatment should start as soon as the diagnosis is known. First episodes of AVNRT, AVRT, and focal atrial tachycardia may need no further treatment. Patients with all other diagnoses and WPW should undergo further investigation and management in conjunction with a cardiologist or electrophysiologist as necessary.

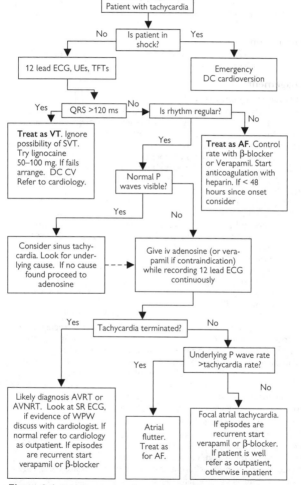

Figure 9.4 Guidelines to the safe management of arrhythmias in the emergency department. Adapted from Barts and the London A+E guidelines.

Drug treatment of tachyarrhythmias

Table 9.1 Drug treatment of tachyarrhythmias

Sinus tachycardia	Identify and treat underlying cause		
Atrial fibrillation **Atrial flutter** **SVT**	*Rate control* *(AV node)* • β-Blockade • Calcium blocker (e.g., diltiazem) • Digoxin	*Conversion to SR* • Amiodarone • Ibutilide • Dofetilide • Sotalol • Flecainide • Disopyramide • Synchronized DC shock • Propafenone • Dronedarone	*Prevention* • Amiodarone • Sotalol • Flecainide • Dofetilide • Quinidine • Disopyramide • Propafenone • Dronedarone
AV nodal reentrant tachycardia (AVNRT)	• Adenosine • β-Blockade • Verapamil • Vagal stimulation • Flecainide • Dronedarone • Propafenone	• Amiodarone • Digoxin • Flecainide • Synchronized DC shock • Dronedarone • Propafenone	
Accessory pathway tachycardias (i.e., AVRT)	*At AV node* • Adenosine • β-Blockade	*At accessory pathway* • Ibutilide • Sotalol • Flecainide • Disopyramide • Quinidine • Amiodarone • Propafenone • Dronedarone	*Termination only* • Synchronized shock
Ventricular tachycardia	*Termination and prevention* • Lidocaine • Amiodarone • Magnesium if Torsades (TdP) • DC shock	• Flecainide • Disopyramide • Propafenone • β-Blockade • Procainamide • Dronedarone • Mexiletine • Amiodarone	

Supraventricular tachycardia

This section deals with the diagnosis and pharmacological management of individual supraventricular tachycardias (SVTs) (see Fig. 9.5). Their mechanisms and ablation are discussed in detail in Chapter 13.

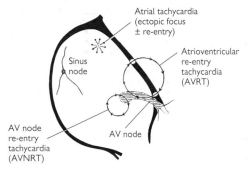

Figure 9.5 Types of supraventricular tachycardia. Reproduced with permission from Ramrakha P, Moore K (2004). *Oxford Handbook of Acute Medicine*, 2nd ed. Oxford, UK: Oxford University Press.

Sinus tachycardia

Defined as a sinus rate >100 for an adult, this may be physiological (e.g., exercise or emotion) or pathological. Look for and treat underlying causes—anemia, drugs (e.g., caffeine, cocaine, etc.), hyperthyroidism, pain, hypoxia, fever and infection, hypovolemia, and cardiac tamponade.

If no underlying cause is found and the rate is stable without normal variation, consider sinus node reentrant tachycardia (SNRT) or focal atrial tachycardia as alternative diagnoses. These will be paroxysmal in nature, have sudden onset or offset, and are often terminated by IV adenosine. If, after a thorough search, no underlying cause is found it may be termed *inappropriate sinus tachycardia.*

β-Blockers are useful for symptomatic persistent inappropriate sinus tachycardia and are vital in controlling the sinus rate in hyperthyroidism and post-MI in the absence of overt heart failure.

Sinus nodal reentrant tachycardia

This is a rare cause of narrow complex tachycardia due to a micro-reentrant circuit within the SAN. The P wave on the ECG is identical to sinus tachycardia, making diagnosis difficult.

β-Blockers or calcium channel blockers are the first-line treatment. Modification of the SA node by radiofrequency ablation (RFA) is reserved for drug-refractory cases or those not wishing to take drugs.

Atrial tachycardia

The term *atrial tachycardia* (AT) describes all regular atrial rhythms with a P rate >100 regardless of the mechanism, and this should be prefixed by either *focal* or *macro-reentrant* unless the mechanism is unknown.

Focal atrial tachycardias

These are due to an automatic focus of atrial cells firing faster than the SA node. The P wave morphology and axis during tachycardia can be used to predict the location of the source. They are characteristically paroxysmal with short bursts at a rate of 150–200 bpm, but they may be incessant, increasing the risk of tachycardia-induced cardiomyopathy.

They occur in normal hearts but are also associated with many forms of cardiac disease as well as metabolic disarray, digitalis toxicity, and pulmonary disease. They are generally long-RP/short-PR tachycardias.

Treatment is needed only for symptomatic patients or incessant tachycardia. β-Blockers and calcium channel blockers can be used to slow the atrial rate and the ventricular response by AV nodal blockade. Class 1c (flecainide and propafenone) or class III drugs (amiodarone and sotalol) may suppress the tachycardia. RFA can be curative. Some ATs may be terminated with IV adenosine.

Macro-reentrant atrial tachycardia (atrial flutter)

Atrial flutter (AFL) is an ECG definition of a P wave rate >240 bpm and an absence of an isoelectric baseline between deflections. It is caused by a reentry circuit over large areas of the right or left atrium. The circuit is not influenced by adenosine, and block of the AVN reveals the underlying rhythm seen as a "saw-tooth" pattern to the P waves on ECG.

It may be associated with underlying heart disease or seen in patients with structurally normal hearts. AFL with rapid ventricular rates can exacerbate heart failure symptoms and, if incessant, worsen LV function.

Synchronized DC cardioversion effectively restores sinus rhythm (SR), but AFL often recurs. Drug therapy is not very effective. AVN blockade is difficult to achieve and the high doses of β-blockers, calcium channel blockers, and digoxin required may have unwanted side effects. Class Ic and III drugs as well as amiodarone can be used to maintain SR; however, propafenone and flecainide can paradoxically accelerate the ventricular rate in AFL by slowing the tachycardia rate sufficiently to allow the AVN to conduct 1:1. They should always be used in combination with an AVN blocking agent. Amiodarone is an alternative agent, particularly if LV function is impaired.

RFA is the most effective way of maintaining SR and is frequently curative. If curative ablation is not possible and effective rate control is not achieved with drugs, then ablation of the AV node and implantation of a permanent pacemaker is a palliative solution. Anticoagulation recommendations for patients with AFL are identical to those with AF.[1]

---

1 Blomstrom-Lundqvist C, Scheinman MM, Aliot EM, et al. (2003). ACC/AHA/ESC guidelines for the management of patients with supraventricular arrhythmias *J Am Coll Cardiol* **42**:1493–1531.

Atrioventricular nodal reentrant tachycardia (AVNRT)

This is the most common cause of a narrow complex tachycardia in patients with normal hearts, typically in young adults, occurring more often in women than men. AVNRT characteristically causes paroxysms of severe palpitations, with a pounding in the neck (due to reflux of blood into the jugular veins caused by simultaneous atrial and ventricular contraction). It has a benign prognosis and may require no treatment. The ECG in SR is usually normal (see Fig. 9.6).

The tachycardia is terminated by IV adenosine or vagal maneuvers. The underlying reentrant circuit is entirely within the AV node and therefore can be controlled long term with β-blockers, verapamil, or diltiazem. Alternative second-line agents are flecainide, propafenone, or sotalol. The first-line treatment for recurrent symptomatic episodes, however, is RFA, which can be curative.

When symptoms are very infrequent a "pill in the pocket" approach is sometimes helpful, i.e., a large oral dose of, e.g., verapamil is taken to terminate the event.

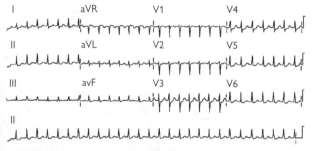

Figure 9.6 Typical presenting ECG of AVNRT or AVRT, showing a narrow complex tachycardia without visible P waves.

Atrioventricular reentrant tachycardia (AVRT)

This is due to an AV reentrant circuit involving a connection between the atria and the ventricles other than the AV node (Fig. 9.7). As these accessory pathways (AP) are present at birth, arrhythmias usually present much younger than AVNRT (infancy or childhood).

Rapid paroxysmal palpitations are the usual symptom. It is usually narrow complex as the ventricle is activated by antegrade conduction via the AVN (orthodromic). However a WCT is also possible if the antegrade conduction to the ventricle is via the accessory pathway (antidromic). The presence of symptomatic AP-mediated SVT is associated with an increased risk of sudden death and referral to a specialist is mandatory.

RFA of the AP is the treatment of choice. The most useful drugs are flecainide and propafenone, which slow conduction in the accessory pathway and the AV node. Verapamil, diltiazem, and β-blockers should be used only when there is no history of atrial fibrillation, there is no antegrade conduction during tachycardia, or the AP is known to have a long antegrade refractory period.

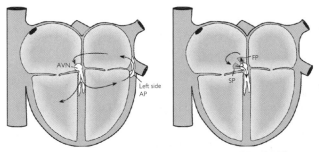

Figure 9.7 Mechanism of AVNRT and AVRT. Both AVNRT and AVRT have reentrant mechanisms. Orthodromic AVRT via a left-sided accessory pathway (AP) (above). Activation from A to V is down the atrioventricular node (AVN), then across the ventricular myocardium and back from V to A up the AP, thus completing the circuit. The ventricle therefore is an essential part of the circuit. Antidromic AVRT (not shown) would activate in the opposite direction. Typical AVNRT (below) activates from the atrium to the AVN via the slow pathway (SP) and from the AVN to the atrium via the fast pathway (FP) thus completing the circuit. The ventricle is activated as a bystander via the bundle of His and is not an essential part of the circuit. Atypical AVNRT (not shown) activates in the opposite direction.

Junctional tachycardia

This term should only be used for focal tachycardias that originate from the AV nodal tissue directly. They are rare in adult cardiology. Distinction from other forms of narrow complex tachycardia is only possible at the EP study.

RFA is high risk as the AV node may be damaged. β-Blockers and flecainide, and propafenone are effective.

Atrial fibrillation

Atrial fibrillation (AF) is the most common sustained cardiac arrhythmia with a prevalence of 0.5%–1% in the general population but 10-fold greater in those aged over 65. It is an atrial arrhythmia where uniform activation is replaced by chaos, such that coordinated contractile function is lost and the atria dilate. It is characterized by an ECG lacking consistent P waves and a rapid, often irregular ventricular rate.

Classification

Previously, many terms were used to classify AF. However, now an international consensus on nomenclature has been reached,[1] allowing the correct selection of management options for patients. All episodes of AF lasting >30 seconds should be described as follows:

• *First detected* or a *recurrent episode*
• *Self terminating* or *not self terminating*
• *Symptomatic* or *asymptomatic*
• *Paroxysmal* (if self-terminating within 7 days)
• *Persistent* (if cardioverted to SR by any means or lasts >7 days regardless of how it terminates)
• *Permanent* (if it does not terminate or relapses within 24 hours of cardioversion)
• *Lone* (in the absence of underlying structural heart disease) or *idiopathic* (in the absence of any disease)

Causes (see Table 9.2)

AF is a common end point for many forms of cardiac disease where atrial myocytes are damaged or subject to adverse stress generated by ischemia, cyanosis, elevated intracavity, or pericardial pressures. These changes are hypothesized to alter the conduction properties of the myocardium facilitating fibrillation.

---

1 Levy S, Camm AJ, Saksena S, et al. (2003). International consensus on nomenclature and classification of atrial fibrillation. *J Cardiovasc Electrophysiol* 14:443–445.

Table 9.2 Causes of atrial fibrillation

Common	Potentially reversible	Rare
• Hypertension	• Alcohol binge	• Congenital heart
• Left ventricular	• Hyperthyroidism	disease
failure (any cause)	• Acute MI	• Autonomic "vagal"
• Coronary artery	• Acute pericarditis	overactivity
disease	• Myocarditis	• Pericardial effusion
• Mitral or tricuspid	• Exacerbation of	• Cardiac metastases
valve disease	pulmonary disease	• Myocardial
• HCM	• Pulmonary embolism	infiltrative diseases
• COPD	• Cardiac surgery	(e.g., amyloid)
		• Atrial myxoma

Symptoms and signs

Palpitations, dyspnea, fatigue, presyncope, syncope, and chest pains are common. However, 30% of patients present with AF as an incidental finding only. Ambulatory monitoring reveals that even patients with symptomatic paroxysmal AF have many asymptomatic episodes.

Physical findings are an irregular pulse (which, if rapid, will be faster at the apex than wrist), variable intensity of the first heart sound, and absent a-waves in the JVP.

Atrial fibrillation: evaluation

A reversible cause should be sought early to allow appropriate treatment. The most important investigations are the following:

- *ECG:* irregular ventricular rate and absence of P waves. V rate depends on intact AV nodal function. In the presence of complete AV nodal block a slow regular junctional or ventricular escape rhythm is present. The QRS will be broad if there is aberrant conduction; ST-T wave changes may be due to rapid rate, digoxin, or underlying cardiac disease.
- *CXR:* cardiomegaly, pulmonary edema, intrathoracic precipitant, valve calcification (MS)
- *Chemistries:* hypokalemia, renal impairment; check Mg^{2+}, Ca^{2+}
- *Cardiac enzymes:* ?MI. Small rise after DC shock
- *Thyroid function:* thyrotoxicosis may present as AF only.
- *Liver function tests*
- *Drug levels:* especially if patient is taking digoxin
- *Arterial blood gas (ABG):* if hypoxic, in shock or ?acidotic
- *Echocardiogram (TTE ± TEE):* for LV function, valve lesions, and pericardial effusion, and to exclude intracardiac thrombus prior to conversion to SR. LA size is an important predictor of likely future maintenance of SR.
- *Other investigations* depend on suspected precipitant.

Other investigations when patient is stable

Use a 24-hour ambulatory monitor to assess heart rate control and look for intermittent AF or bradycardia. CXR, exercise testing (or other ischemia stress test), and coronary angiography can also be used.

Management

There is some controversy regarding the ideal strategy for management of atrial fibrillation. However, depending on the clinical situation and the patient's level of symptoms, a rate or rhythm control strategy may be preferable.

Currently available antiarrhythmic drugs (AADs) are limited by their toxicity, including proarrhythmia, and if a rhythm control strategy is chosen, AAD administration should be undertaken in concert with a specialist. Patients should remain on anticoagulation with warfarin to decrease the incidence of thromboembolic complications regardless of whether a rate or rhythm control strategy is chosen.

Emergency management

If the patient is hemodynamically compromised, then urgent external synchronized DC cardioversion under general anesthesia or sedation is needed. This is rarely necessary; usually rate control is sufficient to acutely control symptoms.

If symptoms persist despite rate control, cardioversion can be attempted pharmacologically with ibutilide 1 mg over 10 minutes repeated ×1, flecainide (2 mg/kg, max 150 mg, infused via a peripheral line over 30 minutes) or if LV dysfunction is suspected, amiodarone (5 mg/kg, max 300 mg; generally, 150 mg IV over 10 minutes repeated × 1).

Patients must be monitored throughout for possible ventricular arrhythmia, bradycardia, and hypotension. If AF has been present for >48 hours, cardioversion should be preceded by a TEE to exclude atrial thrombus.

All patients should be anticoagulated with Coumadin for at least 4 weeks post-cardioversion. Decisions regarding long-term anticoagulation should be made on the basis of the patient's risk profile.

Atrial fibrillation: management

Rate control
Drugs
The first-line agents are β-blockers or nondihydropyridine calcium-channel antagonists (verapamil or diltiazem), which are effective during both exercise and rest. Digoxin is effective only at rest and should be considered a second-line agent.

Rhythm control
If symptoms are not improved by rate control alone, the restoration and maintenance of SR should be attempted. The trials of rate vs. rhythm control underrepresent younger patients (<65 years old), so in this group an aggressive strategy of rhythm control may be warranted regardless of symptoms.

Drugs
Flecainide, sotalol, dofetililide, propafenone, disopyramide, and quinidine are more effective than placebo in maintaining SR. They may contribute to QT prolongation or prolongation of the action potential duration and can be associated with the development of VT/VF. They should initially be administered while under the supervision of a specialist and are relatively contraindicated in patients with impaired LV function and/or underlying coronary artery disease.

Amiodarone is the most effective antiarrhythmic drug and is not associated with VT/VF, as seen in the other AADs. However its use is limited by noncardiac toxicities and is not tolerated in up to 25% of patients.

Pacemakers
While various pacemaker strategies are hypothesized to be useful in maintaining SR, the data are limited. Atrial pacing modes (AAI or DDD) are preferable to reduce the AF burden.
- "Vagal AF" is prevented by pacing.
- SA node disease symptoms are improved by a "block and pace" regimen: rate-controlling drugs for AF and pacing for bradycardic episodes.
- Trigger suppression. Atrial ectopy that initiates AF may be prevented by use of pacemakers with specific algorithms to pace the atrium just faster than the native rhythm or briefly pace rapidly following detection of an atrial ectopic. This is currently a class III indication for implantation of a permanent pacemaker in the absence of another indication for pacemaker therapy.
- Multisite pacing. By reducing the intra- and interatrial activation time, the tendency to AF may be reduced.

Atrial defibrillators
With limited data and not commonly used, they are thought to work by promptly cardioverting each episode of AF, preventing remodeling of the atria. AF episodes may be reduced and quality of life may improve. However, even though shocks are low energy (1–2 J) they are painful. Careful patient selection is required, and current clinical use is limited.

Catheter and surgical ablation
Pace and ablate When adequate rate or symptom control is not possible with drugs or their side effects are not tolerated, a permanent pacemaker may be implanted followed by radiofrequency ablation of the AVN. This achieves rate control and therefore symptom improvement but renders the patient pacer dependent and should only be chosen as a last resort.

Anticoagulation
Both aspirin (325 mg daily) and warfarin (INR 2–3) reduce strokes in AF. Decisions regarding anticoagulation strategy depend on the patient's overall stroke risk, and no distinction should be made between paroxysmal, persistent or permanent AF.

The CHADs score is a clinical prediction tool used to estimate the risk of stroke in nonvalvular atrial fibrillation.[1] Patients receive a risk score based on the presence of congestive heart failure, hypertension, age >75, diabetes, and prior stroke or TIA. The risk increases with the number of features present. Those patients having two or more features are categorized as having moderate to high risk of stroke per year (≥4%/year), and it is suggested that they be maintained on warfarin therapy. Those with one risk factor are at moderate risk (2.8%/year), and 0 are low risk.

The ACC/AHA/ESC guidelines (Table 9.3) for anticoagulation in atrial fibrillation take into account the risk factors included in the CHADs model as well as additional factors.

1 Gage BF, van Walraven C, Pearce L, et al. (2004). Selecting patients with atrial fibrillation for anticoagulation: stroke risk stratification in patients taking aspirin. *Circulation* 110(16):2287–2292.

Table 9.3 Guidelines for anticoagulation in atrial fibrillation (modified from ACC/AHA/ESC guidelines for AF 2006[†])

Condition	Recommendation
<60 years old Normal heart (lone AF)	Aspirin 81–325 mg/day or no therapy
<60 years with heart disease but no other risk factors	Aspirin 81–325 mg/day
Age 60–74 with no risk factors	Aspirin 81–325 mg/day
Age 65–74 with diabetes mellitus or CAD	Warfarin (INR 2–3)
>75 years old	Warfarin (INR 2–3)
Age 65 or older, heart failure	Warfarin (INR 2–3)
LV ejection fraction <35%	Warfarin (INR 2–3)
Rheumatic heart disease	Warfarin (INR 2–3 or higher)
Prosthetic heart valves	Warfarin (INR 2–3 or higher)
Persistent atrial thrombus on TEE	Warfarin (INR 2–3 or higher)
Prior thromboembolism[*]	Warfarin (INR 2–3 or higher)

[*]Risk factors for thromboembolism: heart failure, LV ejection fraction <35%, hypertension, previous thromboembolic event.

[†]Fuster V, Ryden LE, Cannom DS, et al. (2006). ACC/AHA/ESC Guidelines for the Management of Patients with atrial fibrillation. *Circulation* 114:e257–e354.

Ventricular tachycardia

This section deals with diagnosis and pharmacological management. Mechanisms and ablation are discussed in detail in Chapter 13. The most important distinction is the presence of structural heart disease. Impaired LV function is the strongest predictor of a poor prognosis.

VT in the normal heart ("benign") VT)

Right ventricular outflow tract (RVOT) tachycardia

This is due to the automatic firing of cells in the RVOT, giving a characteristic ECG pattern of LBBB with a strongly inferior axis (see Fig. 9.8). Paroxysms of palpitation may be related to exercise. The tachycardia is often adenosine sensitive.

Usually symptoms are well controlled by verapamil or a β-blocker, but RFA is a potentially curative option.

Care must be taken to exclude arrhythmogenic right ventricular cardiomyopathy (ARVC), particularly if the ECG or echocardiogram is not typical. LVOT tachycardia (RBBB + inferior axis) is also recognized.

Fascicular tachycardia

This is a reentrant tachycardia emerging most commonly from the left posterior fascicle. ECG typically shows RBBB with superior axis (see Fig. 9.9). It is often sensitive to IV verapamil (which normally slows then terminates it) but not adenosine. Symptoms are well controlled with oral verapamil or class Ic AADs, but RFA offers a cure.

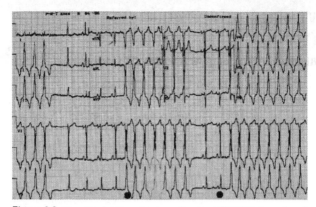

Figure 9.8 Intermittent right ventricular outflow tract (RVOT) tachycardia and sinus rhythm. During the tachycardia beats, notice the left bundle branch block appearance and the positivity in leads II, III, and aVF, indicating an inferior axis.

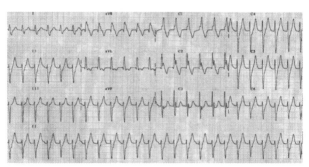

Figure 9.9 12 lead ECG of fascicular tachycardia suggested by broad complex tachycardia with right bundle branch block appearance and superior axis.

VT with impaired LV function

Symptoms
Palpitations, chest pain, presyncope, syncope, dyspnea, pulmonary edema, and sudden death can all occur. How well patients tolerate the arrhythmia depends mainly on their LV function and the tachycardia rate.

Etiology
Any cause of impaired LV function can predispose to VT. Common causes are coronary artery disease, dilated cardiomyopathy, and HCM. VT is often due to reentry around areas of scarred or diseased myocardium. VT may rapidly deteriorate to VF, and these patients may present with sudden death.

General management
It is essential to treat the underlying heart failure and cause (ACE inhibitors, β-blockers, diuretics, nitrates, statins). This reduces not only the symptoms but also the incidence of arrhythmia.

Preventing SCD
Implantable cardiac defibrillators (ICDs) have dramatically improved survival for these patients and are indicated for both primary and secondary prevention.

Long-term antiarrhythmic treatment
β-Blockers may reduce arrhythmia and SCD, but the impact of other drugs is minimal and may be harmful. Flecainide, propafenone, and sotalol have been associated with *increased* mortality and should be avoided, except in patients with ICDs under supervision of an electrophysiologist.

Amiodarone and mexilitine have a neutral impact on prognosis but may reduce the number of VT episodes and thus ICD therapy.

RFA is possible in certain situations when the VT is slow and relatively well tolerated.

Arrhythmogenic right ventricular cardiomyopathy (ARVC)

This is an uncommon genetic disorder resulting in fatty fibroinfiltration of the RV myocardium. The scarring predisposes to VT of RV origin.

The ECG in tachycardia has an LBBB appearance but in SR it may be normal or have a terminal notch in the QRS (epsilon wave) or T-wave inversion in V1–V3.

It is a progressive disease, associated with worsening RV function (leading to symptoms of heart failure), arrhythmia, and sudden death.

The diagnosis is indicated by a typical ECG VT appearance and evidence on echocardiogram (late) or MRI (early) of RV impairment, dilatation, and fatty infiltration. RV biopsy is not necessary. Signal-averaged ECG is often abnormal and may be used to differentiate ARVC from RVOT VT.

An ICD is warranted to decrease the risk of sudden cardiac death (SCD). Drug management includes flecainide, sotalol, amiodarone, and β-blockers. However, they have limited potential in preventing SCD.

Disarticulation of the RV from the LV (thus electrically isolating RV arrhythmias) has been used in difficult cases.

Brugada syndrome

This is an important form of idiopathic VT and VF. It is an autosomal domi-nant condition with variable penetrance and is characterized by a defect in the *SCN5A* gene, causing loss of function in the sodium channel. Patients are mainly found in Southeast Asia and are mostly men (M:F 8:1).

The heart is otherwise normal and the first manifestation may be VF or a very rapid, unstable VT. The hallmark feature is an RBBB appearance with ST elevation in leads V1–V3. A flecainide challenge will reveal the ECG abnormality if not already present (see Fig. 9.10).

Perform serial ECGs after administration of flecainide 2 mg/kg body weight IV in 10 minutes, or procainamide 10 mg/kg IV in 10 minutes. The test is positive if an additional 1 mm ST elevation appears in leads V1, V2, and V3. All positive individuals should undergo EP studies and further specialist evaluation.

The primary therapy is ICD to prevent SCD, although there is a sugges-tion that quinidine may be helpful.

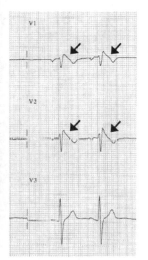

Figure 9.10 Brugada ECG with flecainide challenge. A typical Brugada ECG with arrows marking the characteristic prominent coved ST-segment elevation in the right precordial leads, ≥2 mm at its peak, followed by a negative T wave with little or no isoelectric separation. Intravenous flecainide (2 mg/kg, max. 150 mg; in 10 minutes) exaggerate the ST changes or reveals them if initially absent.[1]

1 Wilde AA, Antzelevitch C, Borggrefe M, et al. (2002). Proposed diagnostic criteria for the Brugada syndrome. Consensus report. *Circulation* 106:2514–2519.

Bundle branch tachycardia

This is a reentry circuit when activation circuits up one bundle branch and down the other (in either direction). It only occurs in diseased ventricles with delayed conduction in the bundles. It is confirmed only during EP study and is treated with RFA.

Torsades de pointes (TdP)

See Long QT Syndrome (p. 391).

Long QT syndrome

Long QT syndrome (LQTS) is a fascinating condition of which our understanding of the genes, molecular function of the myocyte, and clinical expression of the disease has evolved rapidly over recent years. The identification of genetic mutations that code for protein elements of specific ion channels has taught us more about the link between genotype and phenotype than any other cardiologic disorder.

Pathology

LQTS is due to prolonged repolarization of the ventricular myocyte, which is manifest as a lengthened QT interval on the ECG and predisposes to ventricular tachycardia in the form of torsades de pointes (TdP), VF, and sudden cardiac death.

The cardiac action potential is generated by at least 10 distinct but finely balanced ionic currents (principally gating the flow of Na^+, K^+, and Ca^{2+} ions across the cell membrane). A functional abnormality in any of these, whether acquired or genetic, that accentuates depolarizing currents or attenuates repolarizing currents, can potentially lead to LQTS.

Congenital LQTS

Two inherited forms of LQTS are well known. The more common Romano–Ward syndrome (autosomal dominant with variable penetrance) has no other phenotypic features, and the much rarer Jervell Lange–Nielson syndrome (autosomal recessive) is associated with deafness. A modern gene-based classification, however, has now replaced these eponymous syndromes, and 10 chromosome loci (LQTS1–10) coding for 10 genes have been identified (see Table 9.4). Each genetic syndrome can also be characterized by distinct clinical features.

There is an interaction between congenital and acquired forms. Carriers of genetic abnormalities may not manifest the overt ECG changes. However, if challenged by a QT-prolonging drug such as erythromycin, they are at risk of developing torsades and sudden death.

Acquired LQTS (see Table 9.5)

Clinical features

The unmistakable hallmark of LQTS is recurrent syncopal episodes precipitated by emotion or physical stress or at rest. The arrhythmia is torsades de pointes, often preceded by a short–long–short cardiac cycle (Fig. 9.11). This bradycardia-related phenomenon is more common in the acquired form. The clinical features of the congenital form are related to the specific genetic mutation (see Table 9.4). Unfortunately, the first clinical event can be sudden cardiac death.

ECG. QTc values are typically >460 ms but may be as long as 600 ms. The T-wave pattern may give a clue to the gene involved. In affected families a normal QT interval does not rule out genetic carrier status. The degree of QT prolongation varies across the ventricle, so QT dispersion, if measured, is also greater.

$$\text{Normal QTc} = \frac{QT}{\sqrt{(RR\ interval)}} = \frac{0.38\text{–}0.46\ sec}{(9\text{–}11\ small\ squares)}$$

Table 9.4 Characteristics of currently identified congenital LQTS

LQTS subtype	Gene	Frequency	Effect	Clinical features ECG finding
1	KVLQT1	30%–35%	↓K$^+$ efflux	Syncope with exercise or acute emotional reactions Broad, late-onset T wave
2	HERG	25%–30%	↓K$^+$ efflux	Syncope with exercise, emotions, or awakening to an alarm Widely split, low-amplitude T wave
3	SCN5A	5%–10%	Prolonged Na$^+$ influx	Symptoms at rest rather than when excited. Young age and usually presents as sudden death Biphasic or peaked, late-onset T wave
4	Ankyrin-B	1%–2%	Increased Na+ within the cell and Ca^{2+} outside the cell	Variable QT prolongation
5	Mink	1%	↓K$^+$ efflux	Not defined
6	MiRP1	Rare	↓K$^+$ efflux	Not defined
7	KCNJ2	Rare	↓K$^+$ efflux	Modest QT prolongation
8	CACNA1C	Rare	Prolonged Ca^{2+} influx	Exaggerated QT prolongation
9	CAV3	rare	Prolonged Na$^+$ influx	Not defined
10	SCN4β	Extremely rare—1 family	Prolonged Na$^+$ influx	Not defined

* Potassium currents (I$_k$) are repolarizing and the sodium currents (I$_{Na}$) are depolarizing. The ankyrin-B gene codes not for an ion channel but for a cellular structural protein that binds sodium ion channels.[1]

1 Splawski I, Shen J, Timothy KW, et al. (2000). Spectrum of mutations in long-QT syndrome genes. *Circulation* 102:1178–1185.

Table 9.5 Common causes of acquired LQTS

Drugs*	
Antiarrhythmics	Quinidine, procainamide, disopyramide, flecainide, propafenone, sotalol, ibutilide, dofetilide, amiodarone (rare)
Antimicrobials	Erythromycin, clarithromycin, trimethprim, ketoconazole, itraconazole, chloroquine
Antihistamines	Terfenadine
Other drugs	Amitriptyline, fluvoxamine, chlorpromazine, domperidone, cisapride, glibenclamide
Other causes	
Electrolyte imbalance	Hypokalemia, hypomagnesemia, hypocalcemia
Severe bradycardia	Complete heart block, sinoatrial node disease, hypothyroidism, hypothermia

*Note: This is not a comprehensive list, and LQTS is the most common single reason for new drugs being withdrawn.

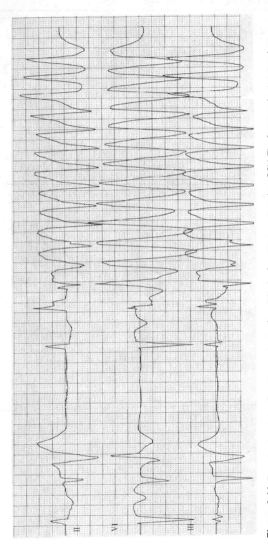

Figure 9.11 Torsades de pointes. A continuous tracing from 3 leads of a patient monitored on CCU. The first complex is a sinus beat followed by 2 ectopics. There is then a long pause (2s) followed by another sinus beat.

Long QT syndrome: management

Usually episodes of torsades de pointes (TdP) are short-lived and terminate spontaneously. However, a prolonged episode causing cardiovascular compromise needs immediate treatment with DC cardioversion.

For recurrent bursts or following a cardiac arrest, give IV magnesium bolus and infusion, followed by urgent temporary pacing (at rate 90–110) if necessary. An isoproterenol infusion may be used to increase the ventricular rate and shorten the QTc while pacing is being arranged.

Acquired

The underlying cause should be identified and reversed. Stop the offending drugs. Give Mg^{2+} before getting blood results. K^+ can be checked rapidly with a blood gas analyzer; replace if <4 mmol/L and aim to achieve high normal levels.

Long-term treatment is not usually necessary. However, a permanent pacemaker is required if nonreversible heart block was the cause or if there is significant underlying bradycardia predisposing to TdP.

Congenital

As most events are triggered by sudden increases of sympathetic activity, treatment is aimed at preventing this. The first choice is β-blockade. Propanolol reduces events in symptomatic patients. If full β-blockade cannot be achieved or is not tolerated, surgical left cardiac denervation is an alternative.

Cardiac pacing is useful to alleviate the β-blocker-induced bradycardia and where pauses have been identified to precipitate symptoms (LQT3). Pacing is never the sole treatment in congenital LQTS.

ICDs should only be used with careful consideration, i.e., for patients at high risk of SCD or when a resuscitated cardiac arrest was the first event. ICDs prevent SCD but not TdP, and recurrent distressing shocks for non-sustained episodes can ruin a patient's life.

Careful patient selection, concomitant use of β-blockers, and shrewd device programming minimize inappropriate therapies.

Asymptomatic patient

Screening of affected families reveals patients with LQTS who have never had symptoms. Most patients do not die from LQTS but all are at risk (13% incidence of fatal events over a lifetime if untreated). A balance must be struck between lifelong treatment with associated side effects and the risk of sudden death.

Predicting risk is extremely difficult but is helped by knowledge of the baseline QTc and of the genetic abnormality. A recent study suggested treatment in LQT1 if QTc >500 ms (men + women); in LQT2 for all men if QTc >500 ms and all women; and in LQT3 for all patients. All patients need individual counseling.[1]

---

1 Priori SG, Schwartz PJ, Napolitano C, et al. (2003). Risk stratification in the long-QT syndrome. *N Engl J Med* 348:1866–1874.

Arrhythmia in special situations

Pediatrics

Arrhythmia may occur at any stage in the pediatric population, from fetal life to adolescence.

Fetus and neonate

AVRT and atrial flutter are the usual cause of tachycardia. If persistent, hydrops fetalis may result. The majority of AVRT cases resolve spontaneously in utero or by 1 year of age, although recurrences later in life may occur. Ablation may be necessary.

Congenital heart block occurs mediated by maternal anti-Ro/SSA antibodies and if severe may also cause hydrops fetalis. This always persists after birth and usually requires permanent pacing, although timing depends on the stability of the subsidiary pacemaker.

Infancy and childhood

AVRT is the usual (80%) cause of tachycardia. AVNRT is rare in infancy, but becomes increasingly common in teenage years. Focal atrial tachycardias and a specific form of AVRT mediated by a slow atrial septal accessory pathway (persistent junctional reciprocating tachycardia) both lead to incessant tachycardia and profound ventricular dysfunction (tachycardia-induced cardiomyopathy).

This usually completely resolves with successful therapy. Radiofrequency ablation is now commonly performed in older children and may also be used in refractory arrhythmias in neonates and young infants when necessary.

Congenital heart disease

Arrhythmias in association with congenital cardiac lesions are poorly tolerated, and if uncontrolled may lead to a rapid decline in ventricular function and cardiac output.

Supraventricular tachycardia

These are a major cause of both morbidity and mortality in congenital heart disease. Accessory pathways are associated with Ebstein's anomaly and congenitally corrected transposition of the great arteries and this results in AVRT. Macro-reentrant–atrial tachycardia is common late following the Mustard, Senning, or Fontan procedures.

This condition is notoriously difficult to control with medication, and although ablation (either percutaneous or surgical) is commonly successful acutely, arrhythmia recurrence is a problem. Pacing has also been used.

Ventricular tachycardia

VT is seen in Ebstein's anomaly and following repair of tetralogy of Fallot. Treatment may involve radiofrequency ablation, antiarrhythmic drugs, or an ICD.

Pregnancy

The hemodynamic and hormonal changes associated with pregnancy may unmask arrhythmic substrates for the first time or exacerbate pre-existing arrhythmic conditions. Gestational palpitations are common, and most frequently there is an increased awareness of physiological tachycardia.

If new ventricular arrhythmias occur, peripartum cardiomyopathy should be actively excluded. Attention should be given to the safety of medications and diagnostic procedures considered during pregnancy.

Permanent pacemakers

Introduction

Permanent pacemakers can pace and sense in one, two, and/or even three chambers of the heart. There are two types of lead: unipolar, which has one electrode in the heart, the other being the casing of the pulse generator ("active can"), and bipolar, where there are two closely spaced electrodes in the heart.

International code

This three-letter identification code describes the basic function of the pacing system. The first letter is the chamber(s) paced and the second letter is the chamber(s) sensed: V = ventricle, A = atrium, D = dual (i.e., A+V). The third letter indicates how the device responds to a sensed event: I = inhibits, T = triggers, D = dual (i.e., I+T), and O = nothing. Often a fourth letter is used to describe added features of the device, e.g., R = rate responsiveness.

Implantation

Most pacemakers are implanted transvenously using the cephalic or subclavian vein. An incision is made about 2 cm below the clavicle across the deltopectoral groove. The cephalic vein is isolated and is often of sufficient caliber to accept two pacing wires.

Alternatively, a guide wire can be introduced followed by introducer sheaths to provide access. Sometimes the cephalic vein is not suitable and the leads have to be introduced via puncture of the subclavian vein using the Seldinger technique. The ventricular lead is most commonly placed in the RV apex. RV outflow tract or on the septum, an active fixation lead is required.

The atrial lead is placed in the right atrial appendage ideally, but anywhere in the RA with adequate pacing parameters is acceptable although likely to require an active fixation lead (Table 9.6).

After both leads are placed in acceptable positions, they are then secured and attached to the pulse generator, which is placed either subcutaneously or beneath the pectoral muscles.

Indications for permanent pacing are listed in Box 9.8.

Table 9.6 Acceptable pacing parameters for new leads

	Atrium	Ventricle
Threshold*	<1.5 V	<1.0 V
Sensitivity	>1.5 mV	>4.0 mV
Slew rate	>0.2 V/sec	>0.5 V/sec
Impedance	400–1000 ohms	400–1000 ohms

*Using a pulse width of 0.5 ms.

Box 9.8 Indications for permanent pacing

Definite indications
- Symptomatic third-degree heart block
  - Bradycardia with symptoms
  - Pauses ≥3 seconds
  - Awake ventricular rates <40 bpm
- Symptomatic advanced second-degree heart block
- Third-degree or advanced second-degree heart block in patients with atrial fibrillation and bradycardia with pauses of >5 seconds
- Advanced second-degree heart block with pauses ≥3 seconds
- Bifasicular block with intermittent third-degree, second-degree block or alternating bundle branch block
- Trifasicular block with intermittent third-degree or second-degree block
- After STEMI in the presence of persistent high-grade AV block
- Symptomatic sinus node dysfunction
- Symptomatic chronotropic incompetence
- Carotid sinus hypersentivity with recurrent syncope
- Sustained VT caused by pauses
- Conditions requiring drugs that result in symptomatic bradycardia

Relative indications
- Asymptomatic third degree block with V rate <40 or second degree (type II) with distal heart block
- Sinus node dysfunction (SND) with HR <40 and where symptom–ECG correlation is not available
- Syncope and SND evident on EPS
- High-risk patients with long QT syndrome
- Chronic chronotropic incompetence (HR <40)
- Neurocardiogenic syncope with significant bradycardia on tilt testing
- Symptomatic HCM with outflow gradient

Adapted from ACC/AHA/'NASPE 2008 Guidelines. *J Am Coll Cardiol* 2008; 51(21):2085–2105.

Which pacing modality?

The vast majority of patients should have atrial-based pacing (i.e., either AAI or DDD) (see Fig. 9.12). Ventricular-only pacing leads to a greater incidence of AF and potential pacemaker syndrome.

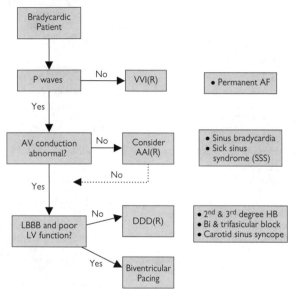

Figure 9.12 Algorithm to select the optimal pacing mode.

Complications of pacing

Pacemaker syndrome

This occurs in patients with intact VA conduction during VVI pacing. Symptoms include presyncope, syncope, lightheadedness, fatigue, exercise intolerance, malaise, lethargy, dyspnea, headache, chest pain, and nonspecific symptoms.

Loss of AV synchrony can decrease cardiac output by 20% at rest. There is atrial contraction against a closed mitral and tricuspid valve, leading to cannon waves. There is also activation of atrial stretch receptors with release of atrial natriuretic peptide (ANP).

The treatment is to restore AV synchrony by either reducing the pacing rate or inserting an atrial lead.

Endless loop tachycardia (pacemaker-mediated tachycardia [PMT])

This occurs in dual-chamber pacing (VDD, DDD, or DDDR) and is caused by inappropriate sensing of retrograde P waves, which trigger a ventricular response. The treatment is to increase the postventricular atrial refractory period (PVARP) to prevent sensing of the retrograde P wave or activate a variety of anti-PMT algorithms.

Other tachycardias

Atrial flutter or fibrillation can cause rapid ventricular pacing in dual-chamber systems by sensing and tracking the atrial rate. To overcome this, the pacemaker can either mode-switch to VVI or be reprogrammed to DDI so that the atrial rate cannot be tracked.

Interference

MRI is generally contraindicated in a patient with a pacemaker, as it can cause serious malfunction. However, recommendations are changing and MRI-compatible systems are being developed.

Radiation therapy can damage pacemaker electronics or result in erosion of the generator. The radiation dose is cumulative. Shielding is mandatory. The pulse generator should be interrogated after therapy and may need to be replaced.

Cautery pacemaker needs to be checked before and after surgery as the electronics of the generator can be damaged. It should be reprogrammed to a non-sensing mode (VOO) prior to surgery or have a magnet applied during cautery to force the device to pace (see below).

Magnet response

When the pacemaker is within a sufficiently strong magnetic field, it reverts to its magnet mode. This is non-sensing fixed pacing at the device's "magnet rate" usually 70–80 /min, i.e., DOO (dual chamber) or VOO/AOO (single chamber).

Additional potential complications of pacing include lead malfunction, device recalls, and device infection. Evaluation and management of these problems should be done in consultation with a cardiovascular specialist.

Pacemaker follow-up

The device is interrogated every 6–12 months. The battery voltage is measured, and below a critical level the elective replacement indicator (ERI) activates. There are approximately 6 months between ERI and the dangerous EOL (end of life).

The lead(s) function is assessed by checking pacing threshold, sensitivity (the size of sensed electrogram detected), and pacing impedance. Any change in these parameters could indicate a problem, e.g., low impedance suggests an internal insulation break, while high impedance might suggest a conductor problem.

Modern devices store the time and duration of many changes of pacemaker function, which is helpful for arrhythmia detection. Most can also store electrograms that help in the diagnosis of arrhythmias and pacemaker malfunction.

Remote or transtelephonic monitoring may also aid in careful patient follow-up.

Pacemakers for chronic heart failure

Cardiac resynchronization therapy (CRT)

CRT is a novel treatment for symptomatic heart failure (NYHA Class III–IV). In patients with a ventricular conduction delay, coordination of wall motion in the left ventricle can be improved by pacing the lateral LV (via the coronary sinus) and septum (via the RV) simultaneously. This improves cardiac output and symptoms. Ventricular filling may be improved by optimizing the AV delay.

Current indications

- NYHA Class III–IV heart failure
- On optimal medical therapy
- Sinus rhythm
- QRS duration >120 ms
- LVEF ≤35%
- LVEDD >55 mm

Electrical vs. mechanical dyssynchrony

Looking at QRS width on a 12 lead ECG is simple and widely available but is a very crude tool for assessing mechanical dyssynchrony and may explain why as many as 30% of patients in clinical trials have not responded to CRT. However, LBBB is more prevalent in CHF and associated with increased mortality.

Mechanical dyssynchrony consists of the following:

- Atrioventricular dyssynchrony
- Interventricular dyssynchrony (delay between RV and LV contraction)
- Intraventricular dyssynchrony (differences in regional wall motion)

There are various ways to assess mechanical dyssynchrony, including the 12 lead ECG, cardiac MRI, radionuclide ventriculography, and echocardiography, which is probably the most useful because of its availability and simplicity. Interventricular dyssynchrony can be measured by the difference in the aortic and pulmonary pre-ejection times (measured from the beginning of the QRS to aortic or pulmonary valve opening). A significant difference is 40 ms.

Intraventricular dyssynchrony can be assessed using tissue Doppler imaging (TDI), looking at the time to peak systolic contraction in different segments of the LV, in particular the difference between the septum and the lateral wall. Strain rate in different segments and color TDI can reveal significant intraventricular dyssynchrony.

Implantation

The RA and RV leads are inserted by conventional techniques as described earlier. The coronary sinus (CS) is the preferred route for pacing the left ventricle (see Fig. 9.13). Normally, a venogram of the CS is performed using an occlusive balloon and a suitable lateral or posterolateral vein identified. The unipolar or bipolar LV lead is then inserted either with a stylet or using an over-the-wire (OTW) technique into a stable position with acceptable pacing parameters and no diaphragmatic stimulation.

With increasing evidence for the prevention of sudden cardiac death in patients with heart failure, most biventricular pacemakers will include a defibrillator. A thorascopic approach to LV lead placement has also been used.

Future directions

There is evidence of mechanical dyssynchrony in some patients with heart failure and a narrow QRS who may benefit from CRT.

Patients who have had AV nodal ablation for symptomatic AF have better exercise tolerance with biventricular pacing than with RV pacing alone. Pacing the apex of the RV is not the optimal site for ventricular function, and high septal or His pacing may improve hemodynamics.

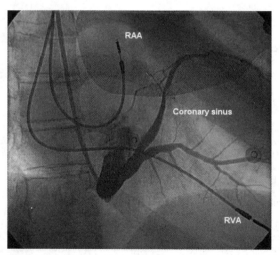

Figure 9.13 Location of the coronary sinus (CS) prior to placing a left ventricular lead. Shown is a fluoroscopic image of the heart from the RAO projection. There is an active fixation lead in the conventional right atrial appendage (RAA) and a lead in the right ventricular apex. Dye has been injected from below retrogradely up the CS to demonstrate the lateral left ventricular branches, from where pacing stimuli can capture the ventricle.

Chapter 10

Heart disease in pregnancy

Basic principles

Cardiac disease in pregnancy is rare in the United States, Europe, and the developed world, but it is common in developing countries. In the United States, rheumatic heart disease is now extremely rare in women of childbearing age.

Women with congenital heart disease who have undergone corrective or palliative surgery in childhood and survive into adulthood are encountered more frequently. These women may have complicated pregnancies. Women with mechanical prosthetic valves face difficult decisions regarding anticoagulation during pregnancy.

Ischemic heart disease is becoming more common in pregnancy as the mean age of pregnancy increases and the smoking epidemic continues. Dissection of the aorta and its branches occurs more commonly in pregnancy and postpartum. Pregnancy may cause a specific dilated cardiomyopathy—peripartum cardiomyopathy.

Because of significant physiological changes in pregnancy, symptoms such as palpitations and signs such as an ejection systolic murmur are very common and innocent findings.

The care of the pregnant and parturient woman with heart disease requires a multidisciplinary approach and formulation of an agreed-on and documented management plan encompassing management of both planned and emergency delivery.

This chapter covers the most important cardiac conditions relevant to pregnancy.

Physiological changes in pregnancy

Cardiac output increases early in pregnancy, reaching a maximum by the mid second trimester and plateaus at 30%–50% above pre-pregnancy levels. This is achieved by an increase in both stoke volume, as a result of increased blood volume, and heart rate (Table 10.1).

There is peripheral vasodilation and a fall in systemic and pulmonary vascular resistance (Fig. 10.1). The pregnant uterus can require up to 18% of cardiac output. Oxygen consumption increases throughout pregnancy and reaches 30% above pre-pregnancy levels by the time of delivery.

Although there is no increase in pulmonary capillary wedge pressure (PCWP), serum colloid oncotic pressure is reduced. The colloid oncotic pressure–pulmonary capillary wedge pressure gradient is reduced by 28%, making pregnant women particularly susceptible to pulmonary edema. Pulmonary edema will be precipitated if there is either an increase in cardiac preload (such as infusion of fluids) or increased pulmonary capillary permeability (such as in pre-eclampsia), or both.

In late pregnancy in the supine position, pressure of the gravid uterus on the inferior vena cava causes a reduction in venous return to the heart and a consequent fall in stroke volume and cardiac output. Turning from the lateral to the supine position may result in a 25% reduction in cardiac output. Pregnant women should therefore be nursed in the left or right lateral position whenever possible. If the mother has to be kept on her back, the pelvis should be rotated so that the uterus drops forward, and cardiac output and uteroplacental blood flow are optimized. Reduced cardiac output is associated with reduction in uterine blood flow and thus in placental perfusion; this can compromise the fetus.

Labor is associated with further increases in cardiac output (15% in the first stage and 50% in the second stage). Uterine contractions lead to autotransfusion of 300–500 mL of blood back into the circulation. The sympathetic response to pain and anxiety further elevate heart rate and blood pressure. Cardiac output is increased more during contractions than between contractions.

Following delivery, there is an immediate rise in cardiac output due to the relief of inferior vena cava obstruction and contraction of the uterus that empties blood into the systemic circulation. Cardiac output increases by 60%–80% followed by a rapid decline to pre labor values within about 1 hour of delivery. Peripheral vascular resistance also rises.

Transfer of fluid from the extravascular space increases venous return and stroke volume further. Those women with cardiovascular compromise are therefore most at risk for pulmonary edema during the second stage of labor and the immediate postpartum period.

Table 10.1 Physiological changes in cardiovascular system in pregnancy

Cardiac output	↑	40%
Stroke volume	↑	
Heart rate	↑	10–20 beats/min
Blood pressure	↓	First and second trimester
	→	Third trimester
Central venous pressure	→	
Pulmonary capillary wedge pressure (PCWP)	→	
Systemic vascular resistance (SVR) and pulmonary vascular resistance (PVR)	↓	25%–30%
Serum colloid osmotic pressure	↓	10%–15%

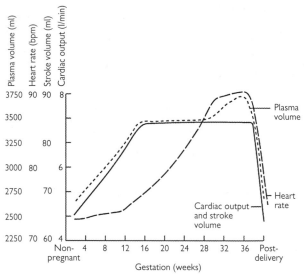

Figure 10.1 Physiological changes in pregnancy. Systemic and pulmonary vascular resistance fall during pregnancy. Blood pressure may fall in the second trimester, rising slightly in late pregnancy. Note that the cardiac output and stroke volume peak by 16 weeks gestation. Reprinted with permission from Throne SA (2004). *Heart* 90(4):450–456.

Normal findings in pregnancy

On examination

Findings may include the following:
- Bounding/collapsing pulse. Prominent a- and v-waves
- Ejection systolic murmur (present in over 90% pregnant women. May be quite loud, and audible all over the precordium)
- Third heart sound
- Relative sinus tachycardia
- Atrial and ventricular ectopy
- Peripheral edema
- Bibasilar rales

On ECG

These findings are partly related to changes in the position of the heart:
- Atrial and ventricular ectopy
- Q wave (small) and inverted T wave in lead III
- ST-segment depression and T-wave inversion inferior and lateral leads.
- QRS-axis leftward shift

Investigations

- The amount of radiation received by the fetus during a maternal CXR is negligible and CXRs should never be withheld if clinically indicated in pregnancy. The fetus should be shielded.
- Transthoracic (TTE) and transesophageal (TEE) echocardiograms are also safe with the usual precautions to avoid aspiration.
- MRIs are safe in pregnancy.
- Routine investigation with electrophysiological studies and angiography are normally postponed until after pregnancy but should not be withheld in, e.g., acute coronary syndromes.

General considerations in pregnancy

The heart has relatively less reserve than that of the respiratory system. Women with heart disease may not be able to increase their cardiac output adequately to cope with pregnancy and delivery.

The outcome and safety of pregnancy are related to the following:
- Presence and severity of pulmonary hypertension
- Presence of cyanosis
- Hemodynamic significance of the lesion (MR and AI are well tolerated whereas AS and MS are more likely to cause problems)
- Functional class as determined by the level of activity that leads to dyspnea (New York Heart Association [NYHA])[1]

Cardiac events such as stroke, arrhythmia, pulmonary edema, and death complicating pregnancies are predicted by the following[2]:
- A prior cardiac event or arrhythmia
- NYHA classification >II
- Cyanosis
- Left ventricular ejection fraction <40%
- Left heart obstruction (mitral valve area <2 cm^2, aortic valve area <1.5 cm^2, aortic valve gradient >30 mmHg)

Women with congenital heart disease are at increased risk of having a baby with congenital heart disease and should therefore be offered detailed scanning for fetal cardiac anomalies.

Women with cyanosis (oxygen saturation <80%–85%) have an increased risk of intrauterine growth restriction, fetal loss, and thromboembolism secondary to the reactive polycythemia. Their chance of a livebirth in one study was <20%.[3,4] In addition, there is a significant mortality risk to the mother.

Women with the above risk factors for adverse cardiac or obstetric events should be managed and counseled by a multidisciplinary team including cardiologists with expertise in pregnancy, obstetricians, fetal medicine specialists, and pediatricians.

Regular antenatal visits and judicious monitoring to avoid or treat expediently any anemia or infection or cardiac decompensation are essential. There should be early involvement of obstetric anesthesiologists and a carefully documented plan for delivery.

1 McCaffrey FM, Sherman FS (1995). Pregnancy and congenital heart disease: the Magee Women's Hospital. *J Matern Fetal Med* 4:152–159.

2 Siu SC, Sermer M, Colman, et al. (2001). Prospective multicenter study of pregnancy outcomes in women with heart disease. *Circulation* 104:515–521.

3 Presbitero P, Somerville J, Stone S, et al. (1994). Pregnancy in cyanotic congenital heart disease. Outcome of mother and fetus. *Circulation* 89:2673–2676.

4 Weiss, BM, Zemp L, Seifert B, Hess OM (1998). Outcome of pulmonary vascular disease in pregnancy. *J Am Coll Cardiol* 31:1650–1657.

Pulmonary hypertension and pregnancy

Pulmonary vascular disease, whether secondary to a reversed large left-to-right shunt such as a VSD (Eisenmenger's syndrome) or lung or connective tissue disease (e.g., scleroderma) or due to primary pulmonary hypertension, is extremely dangerous in pregnancy.

Women known to have pulmonary vascular disease should be advised from an early age to avoid pregnancy and be given appropriate contraceptive advice. Maternal mortality is 40%.[1] The danger relates to fixed pulmonary vascular resistance (PVR) and an inability to increase pulmonary blood flow with refractory hypoxemia. Most deaths can be attributed to thromboembolism, hypovolemia, or pre-eclampsia.

Pulmonary hypertension is defined as a nonpregnant elevation of mean (not systolic) pulmonary artery pressure ≥25 mmHg at rest or 30 mmHg on exercise in the absence of a left-to-right shunt. Pulmonary artery systolic (not mean) pressure is usually estimated by using Doppler ultrasound to measure the regurgitant jet velocity across the tricuspid valve. This should be considered a screening test.

There is no agreed-upon relation between the mean pulmonary pressure and the estimated systolic pulmonary pressure. If the systolic pulmonary pressure estimated by Doppler is thought to indicate pulmonary hypertension, a specialist cardiac opinion is recommended. If there is pulmonary hypertension in the presence of a left-to-right shunt, the diagnosis of pulmonary vascular disease is particularly difficult and further investigation including cardiac catheterization to calculate pulmonary vascular resistance is likely to be necessary.

Pulmonary hypertension as defined by Doppler studies may also occur in mitral stenosis and with large left-to-right shunts that have not reversed. Although such women may not have pulmonary vascular disease and a fixed PVR (or this may not have been established prior to pregnancy), they have the potential to develop it and require very careful monitoring with serial echocardiograms.

Management

- In the event of unplanned pregnancy, a therapeutic termination should be offered.[1] Elective termination carries a 7% risk of mortality, hence the importance of avoiding pregnancy if possible.
- If such advice is declined, multidisciplinary care, elective admission for bed rest, oxygen, and thromboprophylaxis are recommended.[2]
- There is no evidence that monitoring the pulmonary artery pressure pre- or intrapartum improves outcome. Indeed, insertion of a pulmonary artery catheter increases the risk of thrombosis, which may be fatal in such women.[3]

1 Yentis SM, Steer PJ, Plaat F (1998). Eisenmenger's syndrome in pregnancy: maternal and fetal mortality in the 1990s. *Br J Obstet Gynaecol* 105:921–922.

2 Avila WS, Grinberg M, Snitcowsky, et al. (1995). R. Maternal and fetal outcome in pregnant women with Eisenmenger's syndrome. *Eur Heart J* 16:460–464.

3 Rosenthal E, Nelson-Piercy C (2000). Value of inhaled nitric oxide in Eisenmenger syndrome during pregnancy (letter). *Am J Obstet Gynecol* 183:781–782.

- Vasodilators given to reduce the pulmonary artery pressure will (with the exception of inhaled nitric oxide and prostacyclin), inevitably result in a concomitant lowering of the systemic pressure, exacerbating hypoxemia and affecting fetal perfusion.
- There is no evidence that abdominal or vaginal delivery or regional vs. general anesthesia improves outcome in pregnant women with pulmonary hypertension.
- Maternal mortality is extremely high whatever measures are taken. Most fatalities occur during delivery or the first week postpartum.

Marfan's syndrome and pregnancy

Eighty percent of Marfan patients have some cardiac involvement, most commonly mitral valve prolapse and regurgitation. Pregnancy increases the risk of aortic rupture or dissection, usually in the third trimester or early postpartum.

The adverse affects of hormonal and physiologic changes on the abnormal aorta result in an unpredictable maternal risk of aortic dissection or rupture. Progressive aortic root dilation and an aortic root dimension >4 cm are associated with increased risk (10%). Those with aortic roots >4.6 cm should be advised to delay pregnancy until after aortic root repair.[1]

Conversely, in women with minimal cardiac involvement and an aortic root <4 cm, pregnancy outcome is usually good,[2] although those with a family history of aortic dissection or sudden death are also at increased risk. Genetic counseling is vital prior to pregnancy.

Management
- Monthly echocardiograms if documented aortopathy
- β-Blockers for those with hypertension or aortic root dilation
- Vaginal delivery for those with stable aortic root measurements but elective cesarean section with regional anesthesia if there is an enlarged or dilating aortic root*

---

*Associated with neonatal complications (prematurity, respiratory distress, IUGR, intraventricular haemorrhage, death).

1 Lipscomb KJ, Clayton Smith J, Clarke B, et al. (1997). Outcome of pregnancy in women with Marfan's syndrome. *Br J Obstet Gynaecol* 104:201–206.

2 Rossiter JP, Repke JT, Morales AJ, et al. (1995). A prospective longitudinal evaluation of pregnancy in the Marfan syndrome. *Am J Obstet Gynecol* 173(5):1599–1606.

Valvular heart disease in pregnancy

Valvular heart disease affects ~1% of pregnancies and may be associated with an increased risk of adverse maternal, fetal, and neonatal outcomes. High-risk features include the following:
- Impaired LV function (EF <40%)
- Left-sided valve stenoses* (atrial stenosis [AS] with valve area <1.5 cm^2 or mitral stenosis [MS] with valve area <2.0 cm^2)
- Previous maternal cardiovascular event (CCF, TIA, CVA), or
- Symptoms* (NYHA class II or higher)
  Risk increases with each additive factor; see Box 10.1.

Box 10.1 Classification of valvular heart disease risk in pregnancy

Low maternal and fetal risk
- Asymptomatic AS with mean gradient <50 mmHg and normal LV function
- AR, NYHA Class I/II and normal LV function
- MR, NYHA Class I/II and normal LV function
- MV prolapse with no MR or with mild–moderate MR and normal LV.
- Mild–moderate MS (MV area >1.5 cm^2, gradient <5 mmHg), no severe pulmonary hypertension
- Mild–moderate PS

High maternal and fetal risk
- Severe AS with or without symptoms
- AR and NYHA Class III or IV symptoms
- MS with NYHA Class II or higher
- MR with NYHA Class III or IV symptoms
- AV disease, MV disease, or both, resulting in severe pulmonary hypertension (PA pressure >75% systemic pressure)
- AV disease, MV disease, or both, with LV dysfunction (LVEF <40%)
- Maternal cyanosis
- Reduced functional status (NYHA Class III or IV)

High maternal risk
- Impaired LV systolic function (LVEF <40%)
- Previous heart failure
- Previous CVA or TIA

High neonatal risk
- Maternal age <20 or >35 years
- Use of anticoagulant therapy throughout pregnancy
- Smoking during pregnancy
- Multiple gestations

Adapted from Reimold SC, Rutherford JD (2003). Valvular heart disease in pregnancy. *N Engl J Med* 349(1):52–59.

Mitral stenosis and pregnancy

Mitral stenosis (MS) is important in pregnancy; although it is asymptomatic at pregnancy onset, women may deteriorate secondary to tachycardia, arrhythmias, or the increased cardiac output. The most common complication is pulmonary edema secondary to increased left atrial pressure, and precipitated by increased heart rate or increased volume (such as occurs early in the third trimester or during the third stage of labor or following injudicious intravenous fluid therapy).[1]

The risk is increased with severe MS (mitral valve area <1 cm^2), moderate or severe symptoms prior to pregnancy, and in those diagnosed late in pregnancy.[1]

Management

Women with severe mitral stenosis should be advised to delay pregnancy until after valvotomy or, if the valve is not amenable to valvotomy, until after mitral valve replacement.

β-Blockers decrease heart rate, increase diastolic filling time,[2] and decrease the risk of pulmonary edema.

Diuretics should be continued in pregnancy. If medical therapy fails, or for those with severe mitral stenosis, balloon mitral valvotomy may be safely and successfully used in pregnancy if the valve is suitable. Percutaneous balloon valvotomy carries a risk of major complications of about 1%, whereas for surgical valvotomy the figures are closed valvotomy, fetal mortality 5%–15%, maternal 3%; open valvotomy, fetal mortality 15%–33%, maternal 5%.

Women with mitral stenosis should avoid the supine and lithotomy positions as much as possible for labor and delivery. Fluid overload must be avoided, and even in the presence of oliguria, without significant blood loss, the temptation to give intravenous colloid must be resisted.

If pulmonary edema occurs it should be treated in the usual way with oxygen and diuretics. Introduction or reintroduction of a β-blocker may be useful to slow the heart rate.

1 Desai DK, Adanlawo M, Naidoo DP, et al. (2000). Mitral stenosis in pregnancy: a four-year experience at King Edward VIII Hospital. *Br J Obstet Gynaecol* 107:953–958.

2 al Kasab SM, Sabag T, al Zaibag M, et al. (1990). Beta-adrenergic receptor blockade in the management of pregnant women with mitral stenosis. *Am J Obstet Gynecol* 163:37–40.

Other valve lesions

Mitral regurgitation

MR is usually due to mitral valve (MV) prolapse. It is well tolerated as systemic vascular resistance is low in pregnancy. LV function is important in assessing risk (normal function carries a good prognosis).

The most likely time for problems is immediately after delivery, because of autotransfusion, increased venous return, and increased peripheral vascular resistance.

Aortic stenosis

AS is usually congenital. If it is severe or symptomatic, advise the patient to defer pregnancy until this is surgically corrected.

If the patient is already pregnant and symptomatic early on, consider termination of the pregnancy. Surgical replacement and balloon valvuloplasty are both associated with significant risks.

Aortic regurgitation

AR is usually well tolerated as reduced systemic vascular resistance in pregnancy reduces the regurgitant volume. Vasodilators and diuretics are usually sufficient treatment (stop ACE inhibitors and replace with nifedipine, hydralazine, etc.).

Risks are the same as those for MR.

Mechanical heart valves in pregnancy

The optimal management of women with prosthetic mechanical heart valve replacements in pregnancy is controversial since the interests of the mother and the fetus are in conflict. These women require lifelong anticoagulation (see Box 10.2), and this must be continued in pregnancy because of the increased risk of thrombosis.

Warfarin is associated with warfarin embryopathy if given between 6 and 12 weeks gestation[1] and with increased risks of miscarriage, stillbirth, and fetal intracerebral hemorrhage.[2] There is some evidence that the adverse effects of warfarin are related to the dose required to maintain the INR >2, with doses in excess of 5 mg being associated with higher risks of teratogenesis, miscarriage, and stillbirth.[3]

Heparin and low-molecular-weight heparin, even in full anticoagulant doses, are associated with increased risks of valve thrombosis and embolic events[1-4] but are not associated with fetal malformations and offer greater flexibility as delivery nears.

Management

There are three basic options:
- Continue warfarin throughout pregnancy, stopping only for delivery. This is the safest option for the mother.[1,2]
- Replace the warfarin with high-dose unfractionated or low-molecular-weight heparin from 6 to 12 weeks gestation to avoid warfarin embryopathy and then resume warfarin and switch back to heparin as delivery nears.
- Use high-dose unfractionated or low-molecular-weight heparin throughout pregnancy.

The option is chosen will depend on several factors:
- The type of mechanical valve. The risk of thrombosis is less with the newer bileaflet valves (e.g., CarboMedics) than with the first-generation ball and cage (e.g., Starr–Edwards) or second-generation single tilting disc (e.g., Bjork–Shiley) valves.
- The position of the valve replacement. Valves in the aortic rather than the mitral position are associated with a lower risk of thrombosis.[4,5]
- The number of mechanical valves
- The dose of warfarin required to maintain a therapeutic INR
- Any previous history of embolic events

Whichever management option is chosen, warfarin should be discontinued and substituted with heparin for 10 days prior to delivery to allow

1 Chan WS, Anand S, Ginsberg JS (2000). Anticoagulation of pregnant women with mechanical heart valves. *Arch Intern Med* 160:191–196.

2 Sadler L, McCowan L, White H, et al. (2000). Pregnancy outcomes and cardiac complications in women with mechanical, bioprosthetic and homograft valves. *Br J Obstet Gynaecol* 107:245–253.

3 Cotrufo M, De Feo M, De Santo L, et al. (2002). Risk of warfarin during pregnancy with mechanical valve prostheses. *Obstet Gynecol* 99:35–40.

4 Meschengieser SS, Fondevilla CG, Santarelli MT, et al. (1999). Anticoagulation in pregnant women with mechanical heart valve prostheses. *Heart* 82:23–26.

5 Elkayam U (1999). Pregnancy through a prosthetic heart valve. *J Am Coll Cardiol* 33:1642–1645.

clearance of warfarin from the fetal circulation. For delivery itself, heparin therapy is interrupted.

Warfarin is recommended postpartum. In the event of bleeding or the need for urgent delivery in a fully anticoagulated patient, warfarin may be reversed with fresh frozen plasma (FFP) and vitamin K, and heparin with protamine sulfate. Vitamin K should be avoided if possible since it renders the woman practically unable to anticoagulate with warfarin after delivery.

Women with prosthetic valve replacements all require antibiotic endo-carditis prophylaxis for delivery regardless of the mode of delivery.[6,7]

Urgent vaginal delivery should be avoided in a woman anticoagulated with Coumadin because of risk of fetal intracerebral hemorrhage.

Box 10.2 Anticoagulation in pregnancy

Unfractionated heparin
- Often given in early and late pregnancy in patients with mechanical heart valves and valvular heart disease with AF. Used early in pregnancy, as it is not teratogenic. In peripartum period it is used for rapid control (and reversal) of anticoagulation in case emergency delivery undertaken. Not as effective as other forms of anticoagulation
  - *Side effects:* hemorrhage (fetal and maternal), thrombocytopenia (monitor FBC), osteoporosis, alopecia

Low-molecular-weight heparin
- Effective anticoagulant. Easier to monitor dosage schedule. Less likely to cause thrombocytopenia (but does still occur)
  - *Side effects:* maternal and fetal hemorrhage

Warfarin
- Effective oral anticoagulant. Studies show it to be more effective than unfractionated heparin at preventing valve thrombosis.
  - *Side effects:* hemorrhage, teratogenic in first trimester, therefore avoid during this period if at all possible (use heparin).

Aspirin
- Occasionally used in high-risk patients (AF, LV dysfunction, previous emboli) or those with previous prosthetic valve thrombosis
  - *Side effects:* hemorrhage, prolonged labor, low birth weight (in high doses), constriction of ductus, fetal renal dysfunction, and hemostatis abnormalities

---

6 Endocarditis Working Party of the British Society for Antimicrobial Chemotherapy (1982). *Lancet* 2:1323–1326.

7 Dajani AS, Taubert KA, Wilson W, et al. (1997). Prevention of bacterial endocarditis. Recommendations by the American Heart Association. *JAMA* 277:1794–1801.

Ischemic heart disease

The risk factors for myocardial infarction (MI) in pregnancy are the same as for the nonpregnant woman. The risk is increased in multigravid women and in those who smoke, and in women with diabetes, obesity, hypertension, and hypercholesterolemia.

Infarction most commonly occurs in the third trimester and affects the anterior wall of the heart.[1] Maternal death rate is 20%. In pregnancy the underlying etiology is more likely to be due to nonatherosclerotic conditions (such as coronary artery thrombosis or dissection) than in the nonpregnant woman.[2]

Management

- Management of acute MI is as for the nonpregnant woman.
- Angiography should not be withheld if clinically indicated. The fetus should be shielded.
- Intravenous and intracoronary thrombolysis and percutaneous transluminal coronary angioplasty and stenting have all been successfully performed in pregnancy.
- Both aspirin and β-blockers are safe in pregnancy.
- There are less data for clopidogrel and glycoprotein IIb/IIIa inhibitors, although there are case reports of their successful use.
- Statins should be discontinued for the duration of pregnancy as they are associated with an increased risk of malformations.[2]
- ACE inhibitors and ARBs are similarly contraindicated during pregnancy.

1 Roth A, Elkayam U (1996). Acute myocardial infarction associated with pregnancy. *Ann Intern Med* 125:751–757.

2 Edison RJ, Muenke M (2004). Central nervous system and limb anomalies in case reports of first trimester statin exposure. *N Engl J Med* 350:1579–1582.

Hypertrophic obstructive cardiomyopathy (HOCM)

The danger in pregnancy relates to left ventricular outflow tract obstruction that may be precipitated by hypotension or hypovolemia. Provided these are avoided, pregnancy is usually well tolerated.

Management

β-Blockers should be continued in pregnancy or initiated for symptomatic women.[1]

Epidural anesthesia/analgesia carries the risk of vasodilation and hypotension with consequent increased left ventricular outflow tract obstruction. Any hypovolemia will have the same effect and should be rapidly and adequately corrected.

1 Oakley GD, McGarry K, Limb DG (1979). Management of pregnancy in patients with hypertrophic cardiomyopathy. *BMJ* 1:1749–1750.

Peripartum cardiomyopathy

This pregnancy-specific condition is defined as the development of cardiac failure between the last month of pregnancy and 5 months postpartum, in the absence of an other identifiable cause or recognizable heart disease prior to the last month of pregnancy, and left ventricular systolic dysfunction.

The diagnosis should be suspected in the puerperal patient with shortness of breath, tachycardia, or signs of heart failure. It is confirmed with echocardiography.

Echocardiographic criteria for peripartum LV dysfunction[1]

- Left ventricular ejection fraction <45%
- Fractional shortening <30%
- LVEDP (left ventricular end diastolic pressure) >2.7 cm/m^2
- Often, echocardiography shows that the heart is enlarged with global dilation of all four chambers and markedly reduced left ventricular function

Risk factors

- Multiple pregnancy
- Hypertension (be it pre-existing or related to pregnancy or pre-eclampsia)
- Multiparity
- Increased age
- African American race

Management

Treatment is as for other causes of heart failure:

- Oxygen
- Diuretics
- Vasodilators
- ACE inhibitors if postpartum
- Inotropes if required
- Heart transplantation

About 50% of women make a spontaneous and full recovery. Most case fatalities occur close to presentation. Recent data show a 5-year survival of 94%.[2] Prognosis and recurrence depend on the normalization of left ventricular size and function within 6 months of delivery.[3] Those women with severe myocardial dysfunction, defined as LV end diastolic dimension ≥6 cm and fractional shortening ≤21%, are unlikely to regain normal cardiac function on follow-up.[4] Those whose LV function and size do not return to normal within 6 months and prior to a subsequent pregnancy are at significant risk of worsening heart failure (50%) and death (25%) or recurrent peripartum cardiomyopathy with a future pregnancy. They should therefore be advised against pregnancy.[5]

1 Pearson GD, Veille JC, Rahimtoola S, et al. (2000). Peripartum cardiomyopathy. National Heart, Lung and Blood Institute and Office of Rare Diseases (NIH). Workshop recommendations and review. *JAMA* 283:1183–1188.

2 Felker GM, Thompson RE, Hare JM, et al. (2000). Underlying causes and long-term survival in patients with initially unexplained cardiomyopathy. *N Engl J Med* 342:1077–1084.

3 Elkayam U, Tummala PP, Rao K, et al. (2001). Maternal and fetal outcomes of subsequent pregnancies in women with peripartum cardiomyopathy. *N Engl J Med* 344:1567–1571.

4 Witlin AG, Mabie WC, Sibai BM (1997). Peripartum cardiomyopathy: a longitudinal echocardiographic study. *Am J Obstet Gynecol* 177:1129–1132.

5 Shotan A, Ostrezega E, Mehra A, et al. (1997). Incidence of arrhythmias in normal pregnancy and relation to palpitations, dizziness and syncope. *Am J Cardiol* 79:1061–1064.

Arrhythmias in pregnancy

Atrial and ventricular premature complexes (APC, VPC) are common in pregnancy. Many pregnant women are symptomatic from forceful heart beats that occur following a compensatory pause after a VPC or from physiological sinus tachycardia. Most women with symptomatic episodes of dizziness, syncope, and palpitations do not have arrhythmias.[1]

An unusually fast sinus tachycardia requires investigation for possible underlying pathology, such as

- Blood loss
- Infection
- Heart failure
- Thyrotoxicosis
- Pulmonary embolus

The most common arrhythmia encountered in pregnancy is supraventricular tachycardia (SVT). First onset of SVT (both accessory pathway-mediated and AV nodal reentrant) is rare in pregnancy, but 22% of 63 women with SVT had exacerbation of symptoms in pregnancy.[2] Half of SVTs do not respond to vagal maneuvers.

Management

- Propranolol, verapamil, and adenosine have FDA approval for acute termination of SVT. Adenosine has advantages over verapamil, including probable lack of placental transfer, and may be safely used in pregnancy for SVTs that do not respond to vagal stimulation.[3,4]
- Flecainide is safe and is also used in the treatment of fetal tachycardias.
- Propafenone and amiodarone should be avoided,[5] the latter because of interference with fetal thyroid function.
- Temporary and permanent pacing, cardioversion, and implantable defibrillators are also safe in pregnancy.[3]

1 Lee SH, Chen SA, Wu TJ, et al. (1995). Effects of pregnancy on first onset and symptoms of paroxysmal supraventricular tachycardia. *Am J Cardiol* 76:675–678.

2 Page RL (1995). Treatment of arrhythmias during pregnancy *Am Heart* 130:871–876.

3 Mason BA, Ricci-Goodman J, Koos BJ. (1992). Adenosine in the treatment of maternal paroxysmal supraventricular tachycardia. *Obstet Gynecol* 80:478–480.

4 James PR (2001). Cardiovascular disease. In Nelson-Piercy C (Ed.), Prescribing in Pregnancy. *Bailliere's Best Practice and Research in Clinical Obstetrics and Gynaecology* 15:903–911.

5 Magee LA, Downar E, Sermer M, et al. (1995). Pregnancy outcome after gestational exposure to amiodarone. *Am J Obstet Gynecol* 172:1307–1311.

Cardiac arrest in pregnancy

This should be managed according to the same protocols used in the nonpregnant woman, with two very important additions.

Pregnant women (especially those in advanced pregnancy) should be "wedged" to relieve any obstruction to venous return from pressure of the gravid uterus on the inferior vena cava. This can be most rapidly achieved by turning the patient into the left lateral position. If CPR is required, then the pelvis can be tilted while keeping the torso flat to allow external chest compressions.

The obstetric team should be present. This is to ensure that obstetric causes of the collapse are considered (e.g., amniotic fluid embolism, massive postpartum hemorrhage) and appropriately treated. In addition, emergency caesarean section may be required to aid maternal resuscitation and rescue the fetus if of viable age.

Endocarditis prophylaxis

Antibiotic prophylaxis is mandatory for those with prosthetic valves, complex congenital heart disease, or heart transplant and for those with a previous episode of endocarditis.[1]

Many cardiologists recommend that women with structural heart defects (e.g., VSD) also receive prophylaxis.

Recommendations of the American Heart Association stratify cardiac conditions into high, moderate, and negligible (not requiring antibiotic prophylaxis) risk (see Table 10.2).[1]

Fatal cases of endocarditis in pregnancy have occurred antenatally, rather than as a consequence of infection acquired at the time of delivery.

The current U.S. recommendations[1] are as follows:

- **Amoxycillin 2 g po or ampicillin 2 g IV or cefazolin 1 g IV** at the onset of labor or ruptured membranes or prior to caesarean section, followed by amoxycillin 500 mg po (or IM/IV depending on patient's condition) 8 hours later.
- For women who are allergic to penicillin, give cephalexin 2 g po or clindamycin 600 mg po or azithromycin 500 mg po, for IV cefazolin or ceftriaxone 1g IV or clindamycin 600 mg IV.

Table 10.2 Stratification of cardiac conditions according to risk of bacterial endocarditis

High risk Endocarditis prophylaxis recommended	• Prosthetic valves (metal, bioprosthetic and homografts) • Previous bacterial endocarditis • Complex cyanotic congenital heart disease (Fallot's, transposition of great arteries) • Surgical systemic/pulmonary shunts
Moderate risk Endocarditis prophylaxis not recommended	• Other congenital cardiac malformations • Acquired valvular disease • Hypertrophic cardiomyopathy • Mitral valve prolapse with mitral regurgitation
Negligible risk Endocarditis prophylaxis not recommended	• Isolated secundum atrial septal defects • Surgically repaired ASD, VSD, PDA • Mitral valve prolapse without regurgitation • Physiological heart murmurs • Cardiac pacemakers

1 Nishimura RA, Carabello BA, Faxon DP, et al. (2008). ACC/AHA 2008 guideline update on valvular heart disease: focused updated on infective endocarditis. *Circulation* 118:887–896.

2 Endocarditis Working Party of the British Society for Antimicrobial Chemotherapy (1982). *Lancet* 2:1323–1326.

Multisystem disorders

Libman–Sacks endocarditis

Associations
- Systemic lupus erythematosus (SLE)
- Primary and secondary anti-phospholipid antibody syndrome

Epidemiology
- Present in at least 50% of fatal SLE patients who undergo postmortem examination. Up to 43% of cases with echocardiography
- 6%–10% of primary anti-phospholipid antibody syndrome cases with echocardiography
- Young, African/Caribbean women typically

Pathology
- Classically sterile, verrucous vegetations on the ventricular aspect. Diffuse leaflet thickening is thought to be the chronic, healed stage.
- Commonly mitral and aortic valves. Other valves and endocardial surfaces are also affected.
- Usually valve regurgitation; stenosis is rare.
- It is uncertain whether the association with anti-phospholipid antibodies is causal. Antigens are negatively charged phospholipids in endothelial cell membranes. Prevalence and severity of valve disease are similar, whether antibodies are present or not.
- Sites of endothelial damage due to turbulence and jet impaction may act as foci for thromboses and further damage.
- Valve thickening and regurgitation are more common after chronic steroid therapy and in older patients.

Clinical features
- Usually asymptomatic with a normal cardiovascular examination
- General lupus features, such as a malar rash, arthritis, sweats, and alopecia
- Recurrent miscarriage, arterial and venous thromboses, and thrombocytopenia suggest anti-phospholipid antibody syndrome.
- Symptoms and signs due to heart failure and valve disease could be present.

Imaging findings in lupus
- Valve abnormalities in 28%–74% of cases. Vegetations occur in 4%–43% of cases, particularly those with anti-phospholipid antibodies. Thickening occurs in 19%–52% of cases, with associated regurgitation in 73%.
- Pericardial effusion or thickening, left ventricular hypertrophy (due to hypertension), left ventricular dilatation, left ventricular segmental dysfunction, left ventricular global dysfunction, and pulmonary hypertension.

Imaging findings in primary anti-phospholipid antibody syndrome

- Valve abnormalities in 30%–32% of cases, particularly those with peripheral arterial thromboses. Vegetations are found in 6%–10% and thickening in 10%–24%.
- Regurgitation occurs in 10%–24% of cases.

Blood tests

- Blood cultures to exclude infective endocarditis
- Full blood count, clotting profile, autoantibody screen

Treatment

- No specific therapy is recommended.
- Treat underlying conditions and complications.

Prognosis in lupus

- Cardiovascular death is ranked third in lupus patients.
- Combined incidence of heart failure, valve replacement, thromboembolism, and infective endocarditis is 22%.

Marfan's syndrome

Epidemiology
- Incidence is 1 in 5,000 to 1 in 10,000 persons.
- There are no known geographical, racial, or gender predilections.
- It is diagnosed prenatally through to adulthood.

Pathology
- Autosomal dominant point mutations occur in fibrillin-1 gene on chromosome 15. Over 200 mutations are described.
- Fibrillin-1 glycoprotein is an integral component of microfibrils in connective tissues.
- Structural integrity of ocular, skeletal, cardiovascular, and other tissues is compromised.
- Phenotype is highly variable because of varying genotype expression.

Ghent criteria for diagnosis
- The index case has no contributory family or genetic history, with major criteria in at least two different organ systems plus involvement of a third organ system. Alternatively, there is contributory family or genetic history, one major organ system criterion, plus involvement of second organ system.
- Relative of the index case has a major criterion in family history, major criterion in organ system, plus involvement of a second organ system.

Imaging
- Radiographs, CT, and MRI scans are used to assess axial skeleton, hip joints, hands, and feet.
- Echocardiography and MRI are used to assess the mitral and aortic valves, aortic root, and ascending aorta.
- Slit-lamp examination is used to look for retinal detachment, supero-lateral lens dislocation, cataracts, severe myopia, and open-angle glaucoma. Globe ultrasound and keratometry help in assessing the cornea.

Genetic testing
This has a limited role in diagnosis and is used primarily to diagnose family members if a mutation is known. Linkage analysis can be applied in families with several affected relatives.

Treatment
- β-Blockers (possibly calcium channel blockers) delay and attenuate aortic root dilation
- Antibiotic chemoprophylaxis for bacteremia-prone procedures
- Surgery for aortic root and valve disease, skeletal and ocular complications
- Gentle exercise
- Some preliminary studies suggest that ACE inhibitors are useful and may improve outcomes

Prognosis
- Life expectancy is about two-thirds of normal.
- Cardiovascular death occurs in over 90% of cases from aortic dissection or heart failure.

Ghent criteria for Marfan's syndrome

Table 11.1 Skeletal system involvement (2 major *or* 1 major and 2 minor criteria)

Major criteria	Minor criteria
1. Pectus carinatum	1. Moderately severe pectus excavatum
2. Pectus excavatum requiring surgery	2. Joint hypermobility
3. Reduced upper to lower segment ratio or arm span to height ratio >1.05	3. High arched palate with teeth crowding
4. Wrist and thumb signs	4. Facial appearance (dolichocephaly, malar hypoplasia, down-slanting palpabral fissures, retrognathia)
5. Scoliosis exceeding 20° *or* spondylolisthesis	5. Enophthalmos
6. Elbow extension <170°	
7. Medial displacement of medial malleolus causing pes planus	
8. Protrusio acetabulae	

Ocular system involvement (1 major *or* 2 minor criteria)

Major criteria	Minor criteria
1. Ectopia lentis	1. Abnormally flat cornea
	2. Axial globe lengthening
	3. Iris or ciliary muscle hypoplasia

Cardiovascular system involvement (1 major *or* 1 minor criterion only)

Major criteria	Minor criteria
1. Ascending aortic dilation involving at least the sinuses of Valsalva with or without aortic regurgitation *and*	1. Mitral valve prolapse with or without mitral regurgitation
2. Ascending aortic dissection	2. Main pulmonary artery dilation
	3. Mitral annulus calcification
	4. Descending thoracic or abdominal aortic dilation or dissection

Pulmonary system involvement (requires 1 minor criterion)

1. Spontaneous pneumothorax or apical blebs

Skin and integument involvement (requires one of the following):

1. Striae atrophicae without marked weight change, pregnancy, or repetitive stress
2. Recurrent or incisional herniae

Dural involvement (1 major criterion)

1. Lumbosacral dural ectasia

A contributory family or genetic history (1 major criterion)

1. Parent, child, or sibling meeting diagnostic criteria independently
2. Known fibrillin-1 mutation
3. Presence of haplotype around fibrillin-1 inherited by descendent known to be associated with unequivocally diagnosed Marfan's syndrome in the family

Ehlers–Danlos syndrome

Epidemiology
- 1 in 5,000 live births. Incidence is about 1 in 400,000.
- It typically presents between childhood and early adulthood.
- No racial or gender bias is known.

Pathology
- Inherited (autosomal dominant or recessive and X-linked recessive) defects in synthesis and metabolism of different types of collagen produce connective tissue defects.
- A new form recently described shows deficiency of tenascin-X (extracellular matrix protein) with normal collagen.
- Six different subtypes are described: classic, hypermobile, vascular, kyphoscoliosis, arthrochalasia, and dermatosparaxis. There is much overlap between types in up to 50% cases.
- Increased tissue elasticity with decreased strength and poor healing.

Clinical features
- Typically there is joint hypermobility, skin hyperextensibility, tissue fragility, and poor wound healing. Classically, patients get "cigarette paper" scarring over their knees.
- Mitral valve prolapse is typically seen in classic, hypermobile, and vascular forms. A minority of patients progress to severe mitral regurgitation requiring surgery. Recent echocardiographic studies suggest that cardiac defects may be less frequent than previously thought, although coronary artery aneurysm can be devastating.
- Aortic root ectasia with dilated sinuses of Valsalva is found. This is rarely severe or progressive, and aortic root replacement is exceptional.
- The vascular form also exhibits prominent veins, low weight, short stature, spontaneous pneumothorax and rupture of medium-sized and large arteries, and bowel perforation. Joints are affected less frequently. The skin is fragile but not hyperextensible.
- Differential diagnoses include Marfan's syndrome, Menkes kinky hair disease, Williams syndrome, Stickler syndrome, cutis laxa, and pseudoxanthoma elasticum.

Treatment
- No specific medical therapy is indicated. High-dose vitamin C may provide some benefit but there are no controlled studies.
- Provide patient education and preventive strategies. Patients should avoid excess and repetitive lifting and contact sports.
- Avoid suturing wounds, if possible.
- Regular eye and dental assessments are required.
- Genetic counseling is recommended. There is a limited role for genetic testing.

Prognosis

- Increased mortality occurs in the vascular form. Median age is 50 years, with death from spontaneous arterial and gastrointestinal rupture.
- Patients with other forms usually have normal life expectancy with increased morbidity from recurrent dislocations, poor wound healing, and scarring.

Kawasaki disease

Epidemiology

More than 90% of cases are in children under 10 years of age. Peak incidence is at age 18–24 months in the United States and 6–12 months in Japan. It is more common in males and in children of Japanese descent.

Pathology

- Etiology is unknown but likely to be infectious. Possible agents include Parvovirus B19, meningococcus, *Coxiella burnetii*, bacterial toxin-mediated superantigens, HIV, *Mycoplasma pneumoniae*, adenovirus, *Klebsiella pneumoniae*, *Parainfluenza* type 3 virus, rotavirus, measles, and human lymphotropic virus.
- Other determinants may be genetic and immunological factors, vectors, and passive maternal immunity.
- Generalized vasculitis is most severe in medium-sized arteries affecting all layers of the wall. There is smooth muscle necrosis with splitting of internal and external elastic laminae and aneurysm formation.
- Subsequent vessel fibrosis, stenosis, thrombosis, and aneurysm rupture occur.

Clinical features

- *Acute stage* (days 1–11) is characterized by high fever, irritability, non-exudative bilateral conjunctivitis (90%), iritis (70%), perianal erythema (70%), acral erythema and edema that impede ambulation, strawberry tongue, lip fissures, hepatic, renal, and gastrointestinal dysfunction, myocarditis, pericarditis, and cervical lymphadenopathy (75%).
- *Subacute stage* (days 11–30) is characterized by persistent irritability, anorexia, conjunctival injection, decreased temperature, thrombocytosis, acral desquamation, and aneurysm formation.
- *Convalescent/chronic phase* (after 30 days) is characterized by aneurysm expansion, possible myocardial infarction, and resolution of smaller aneurysms (60% of cases).

Diagnosis requires exclusion of other illnesses with similar clinical signs, fever lasting more than 5 days, and four out of the following: polymorphous rash, bilateral conjunctival injection, mucous membrane changes (diffuse injection of oral and pharyngeal mucosa, erythema or fissuring of the lips, and strawberry tongue), acute, nonpurulent cervical lymphadenopathy (one lymph node must be >1.5 cm), and extremity changes (erythema of palms or soles, indurative edema of hands or feet, and membranous desquamation of the fingertips).

Other features include heart failure, mitral regurgitation, aseptic meningitis, facial palsy, stroke, arthralgias or arthritis, pleural effusion, pulmonary infiltrates, vulvitis, urethritis, extremity gangrene, pustules, and erythema multiforme–like lesions.

Imaging
- Echocardiogram at baseline, 3 weeks, and 1 month after blood work have normalized. Look for coronary artery aneurysms and evidence of valvulitis, myocarditis, and pericarditis.
- Diffuse coronary dilation is seen in 50% of cases by day 10.
- An alternative is magnetic resonance angiography.

Blood work
- Normocytic anemia, granulocytosis, thrombocytosis (weeks 2–3), and thrombocytopenia (with severe coronary disease)
- Elevated ESR, CRP, α_1-antitrypsin and serum complement (may be normal)
- Mild transaminitis (40%) and raised bilirubin (10%)

Treatment
- Intravenous gammaglobulin
- Aspirin (small aneurysms). Dipyridamole (large aneurysms). Consider anticoagulation.
- Hospitalization until patient is afebrile and inflammatory markers have normalized
- Influenza vaccine if patient is on long-term aspirin therapy.

Prognosis
- Mortality is 0.1%–2%. Cardiac complications occur in 25% of patients if untreated.
- Recurrence rate is 1%–3%.

Takayasu arteritis

Epidemiology
- Global incidence of 2.6 cases per million population annually
- Typically affects women (80%–90% of cases) in their second and third decade

Pathology
- Idiopathic, segmental, granulomatous vasculitis of large and medium-sized arteries occurs, particularly involving the aorta and its branches, the pulmonary arteries, and, consequently, all major organs.
- Subsequent arterial stenosis (90% of cases), occlusion, thrombosis, and aneurysm formation (27% of cases) produce end-organ ischemia. Heart failure due to hypertension, myocarditis, and aortic regurgitation is common.
- It is associated with HLA-A10, B5, Bw52, DR2, and DR4 in Japan and Korea, but with HLA-B22 in the United States.

Clinical features
- *Systemic:* fever, night sweats, fatigue, weight loss, myalgia, arthralgia or arthritis, rash (erythema nodosum, pyoderma gangrenosum or lupoid), headaches, dizziness, and syncope
- *Local:* heart failure, angina, hypertension (may be paroxysmal), stroke, transient ischemic attack, visual disturbances, carotidynia, abdominal pain, limb claudication, asymmetric pulses (common), absent pulses (rare), post-stenotic dilations producing bounding pulses (common), and bruits (over subclavian arteries and aorta).
- *Pregnancy* does not affect the vasculitis. Patients may have problems with hemodynamic monitoring, malignant hypertension, pre-eclampsia and fetal complications.

Imaging
Angiography shows stenosis, occlusions, or aneurysms of the aorta and its primary branches or large arteries in the proximal upper or lower extremities. Changes are focal or segmental and not due to atherosclerosis, fibromuscular dysplasia, or similar causes.

Magnetic resonance imaging, magnetic resonance angiography, and computed tomography are useful for serial examinations and diagnosis in the early stages. They show mural thickening and thrombi of aorta and stenosis. Distal vessels are not imaged as well. Contrast may reveal pre-stenotic inflammatory lesions that may be missed on angiography.

Echocardiography is used to assess ventricles, aortic root, and valve.

Blood work
- No specific markers
- Normochromic normocytic anemia (50% of cases), mild leucocytosis, thrombocytosis, and elevated ESR (more than 50 mm initially)
- Transaminitis, hypoalbuminemia, negative ANA, and positive rheumatoid factor (15% of cases)

Treatment

- Give high-dose steroids for 4–6 weeks until ESR is normalized.
- If patient is steroid-resistant or relapses, consider weekly intravenous methylprednisolone or methotrexate, daily or monthly intravenous cyclophosphamide, cyclosporine (renal toxicity and hypertension), azathioprine, or mycophenolate mofetil.
- Antihypertensives, antiplatelet drugs, and anticoagulants.
- Balloon angioplasty and stenting, bypass surgery, and replacement with synthetic grafts.

Prognosis

- This is determined by the severity of vascular and end-organ damage.
- 60% of patients respond to steroids but 40% relapse. Survival can be up to 95% at 15 years.

Polyarteritis nodosa and other systemic vasculitides

Epidemiology
- 4–9 cases per million-population per year
- Typically affects men between the ages of 40–70 years

Pathology
- Usually involves small and medium-sized muscular arteries
- Fibrinoid necrotizing vasculitis beginning in the tunica media and spreading to the intima and adventitia. Immune complex mediated
- Sequelae: aneurysm formation, hemorrhage, and thrombosis
- Macroscopic ("classic") form affects kidneys (80%–90%), heart (<70% and excluding pulmonary arteries), gastrointestinal tract (50%–70%), liver (50%–60%), spleen (45%), and pancreas (25%–35%). Microvasculature is typically spared.
- Microscopic ("microscopic polyangiitis") form also involves the microvasculature, typically glomeruli and pulmonary capillaries.

Clinical features
- Fever, malaise, weight loss (>50% cases)
- Arthralgia, arthritis, tender subcutaneous nodules (15% cases), abdominal pain, nausea and vomiting (>60% cases), retinopathy, gastrointestinal hemorrhage (6% cases), bowel perforation (5% cases), and infarction (1.4% cases)
- Renal failure, hypertension, myocardial infarction, heart failure, and pericarditis
- Unique features of Churg–Strauss syndrome include allergic rhinitis, polyposis, recurrent bronchitis, and asthma. The heart is involved in 85% cases, causing pericardial effusion, myocarditis, and restrictive cardiomyopathy with systolic and diastolic dysfunction.
- Wegener's granulomatosis rarely causes pericarditis and coronary arteritis (10%–20% cases antemortem). It can cause myocardial infarction and sudden death.

Imaging
- Selective angiography remains the gold standard.
- Saccular microaneurysms (2–5 mm diameter) are seen in 60%–80% of cases, with usually at least 10 per single visceral circulation. They are typically at branching points and bifurcations.
- Vessel ectasia and irregularity, segmental stenosis, occlusions, and hypervascularity are also found.
- Similar appearances are found in vasculitis associated with rheumatoid disease, SLE, and Churg–Strauss syndrome.

Blood work

- Elevated ESR, positive anti-neutrophilic cytoplasmic antibodies (ANCA), hypergammaglobulinemia, and hepatitis B surface antigenemia (30% cases)
- Churg–Strauss syndrome is characterized by peripheral blood eosinophilia (90% untreated cases), high serum IgE levels, and positive rheumatoid factor (70% cases). Hepatitis B surface antigen testing is usually negative.

Treatment and prognosis

- High-dose steroids and cyclophosphamide produce remission in 90% of cases.
- The relapse rate is up to 40%.
- Five-year survival if untreated is 15%, with death from progressive renal failure or gastrointestinal complications.
- Morbidity and mortality in Churg–Strauss syndrome are mainly due to severe asthma, heart failure, and gastrointestinal complications. Prognosis is similar to that of polyarteritis nodosa.

Ankylosing spondylitis

Epidemiology

- Incidence is 0.1%–1% in the general population and 1%–2% among HLA-B27-positive individuals.
- It is usually seen in northern Europeans, with onset during late adolescence and early adulthood. Juvenile onset (before 16 years) occurs especially among Native Americans, Mexicans, and in developing countries.
- It is three times more frequent in males.

Pathology

- Chronic multisystem inflammatory disease. Other seronegative spondyloarthropathies include reactive arthritis (Reiter's syndrome), juvenile chronic arthritis, and those in association with psoriasis and inflammatory bowel disease.
- There is a strong association with HLA-B27 and genetic predisposition.
- 10%–20% of first-degree relatives positive for HLA-B27 develop the disease.
- Typically it affects ligament and capsule attachments to bone in sacroiliac joints and axial skeleton-enthesitis. It culminates in joint erosion, fibrosis, and ossification producing vertebral fusion.
- Cardiac involvement usually manifests late but occasionally precedes overt joint disease.
- Aortic regurgitation (1%–10% cases) causes 1) ascending aortitis (1%–10% cases), resulting in thickening, stiffness, and dilation of aorta; 2) aortic valve fibrosis, causing cusp thickening, nodularity, and shortening.
- Pericarditis (<1% of cases)
- Myocardial fibrosis causing systolic and diastolic dysfunction appears on echocardiography. It may progress to dilated cardiomyopathy. Myocardial function may be further compromised by secondary amyloidosis.
- Atrioventricular node conduction problems with complete heart block.

Clinical features

- Fever and weight loss
- Insidious low back pain progressing proximally in a relapsing–remitting pattern
- Chronic pain and morning stiffness (>70% cases); fatigue (65% cases); reduced mobility (47% cases)
- Depression (20% cases, especially females) and neurological deficits
- Acute unilateral iritis (25%–30% cases)
- Chest tightness and breathlessness from restricted chest movements

Imaging

- Erosions and sclerosis of sacroiliac joints
- Squared-off vertebral bodies and syndesmophytes culminating in the bamboo spine

Bloods

- No diagnostic tests are needed.
- Elevated ESR and CRP (75% cases) are found.

Treatment

- Nonsteroidal anti-inflammatory drugs and sulfasalazine
- Specialist treatment for complications. Patients may require spinal or cardiac surgery.
- Genetic counseling

Prognosis

- Disease of the aorta and valves is more frequent with increasing disease duration. It may be progressive or resolve.
- Death can be due to cardiac complications such as complete heart block.

Polymyositis and dermatomyositis

Cardiac involvement is frequent but usually subclinical. Fifteen percent of cases are symptomatic and 55% are noted on echocardiography.

T cell–mediated cytotoxicity against muscle fibers is found in polymyositis. Complement-mediated lysis of cell membranes with vascular smooth muscle hyperplasia, coagulation, and infarction occurs in dermatomyositis. This produces a small vessel and capillary vasculopathy that does not cause significant deterioration in ventricular function.

One-quarter of cases have myocarditis at postmortem with microscopic interstitial fibrosis, nonspecific inflammatory infiltrates, and necrosis. Ventricular function is usually preserved.

Conducting tissues are particularly affected, producing nonspecific ST- and T-wave changes, atrial arrhythmias, and atrioventricular and bundle branch block. These problems are more commonly seen in children.

Pericarditis is rare and seen in 25% of cases on echocardiography.

Coronary vasospasm may occur, and provocation testing has demonstrated endothelial dysfunction with vasoconstriction in response to intracoronary acetylcholine.

Cor pulmonale may occur secondary to primary lung disease and pulmonary hypertension.

Overt cardiac complications should be treated using steroids, immunosuppressive drugs, and calcium channel blockers. Cardiac complications are an important cause of death, together with malignancy and lung problems.

Rheumatoid disease

This multisystem disease is characterized by a symmetrical, deforming, peripheral arthropathy.

Prevalence is 1%. Typically it affects females, with peak onset in the fifth decade.

Cardiac involvement is seen in 60% of cases echocardiographically with 10%–15% being symptomatic. It is directly related to the severity of joint disease and the presence of nodules.

Half of cases have a subclinical fibrinous pericarditis with effusions seen in 40% of cases on echocardiography. From 1% to 2% of cases are symptomatic. This is usually independent of disease duration and may precede it. Cardiac tamponade and constrictive pericarditis are rare and usually respond to treatment with steroids and disease-modifying drugs.

More than 50% of patients with subcutaneous nodules have myocardial and endocardial nodular granulomas. They rarely compromise cardiac function through mitral valve deformity and regurgitation or conduction problems such as first-degree (most common), left bundle branch, and complete heart block.

Of patients with severe disease, 20% have a diffuse myocarditis with nonspecific inflammatory infiltrates, myocyte necrosis, and fibrosis that may cause biventricular failure, arrhythmias, and conduction problems. Ventricular function may also be compromised by secondary amyloidosis.

Coronary arteritis is noted in 20% of cases postmortem. It is now appreciated that many autoimmune and systemic inflammatory diseases contribute to the progression, sometimes in accelerated fashion, of clinically significant coronary artery disease. Rheumatoid patients have an increased incidence of clinical coronary artery disease, compared with age-matched controls.

Nonspecific valvulitis produces fibrotic, hyalinized valves with occasional incompetence. The aortic valve is affected more commonly than the mitral valve.

Stress testing and cardiac imaging

Exercise ECG

This is a commonly used test involving a treadmill, BP measurement, and continuous electrocardiogram (ECG) monitoring. Overall sensitivity for coronary heart disease is around 68% and specificity is 77%. This increases when considering prognostically significant disease, for which the test has a sensitivity of 86%.

In intermediate- to high-risk patients (e.g., men with ischemic symptoms), the test has a predictive accuracy of >90%. The test is of least value in populations who are least likely to be suffering from ischemic heart disease, e.g., asymptomatic middle-aged women, for whom the test has a positive predictive value of <50%.

Indications

- Diagnosis of coronary artery disease in select patients (those with higher pretest probability of disease [see above].
- Post-MI in patients treated with thrombolytics: pre-discharge (submaximal test in days 4–7 to assess prognosis, decide on exercise rehabilitation program, and evaluate adequacy of treatment and need for invasive evaluation/revascularization) or late post-discharge (symptom limited 3–6 weeks) testing may be used.
- Pre- and post-revascularization, especially if symptomatic, to determine the degree of exercise limitation.
- Evaluation of arrhythmias: optimizing rate-responsive pacemaker function, evaluation of known or suspected exercise-induced arrhythmias, and evaluation of treatment of these disorders.
- Preoperative evaluation in select patients.
- Cardiopulmonary stress testing to evaluate congestive heart failure (CHF) patients for heart transplant.
- Evaluating the physiological significance of valvular lesions in asymptomatic patients, usually done with echocardiography (i.e., assessing for exercised-induced pulmonary hypertension in patients with mitral stenosis).

Contraindications

- Fever or acute viral illness
- Myo- or pericarditis
- Symptomatic severe aortic stenosis
- Aortic dissection
- Severe uncontrolled hypertension
- Decompensated heart failure
- Unstable angina or acute-phase of myocardial infarction (MI)
- Significant resting arrhythmia (e.g., uncontrolled atrial fibrillation or complete heart block)
- Known severe left main disease
- Physical disability impairing ability to exercise
- ECG abnormality rendering interpretation of ST segment difficult (e.g., LBBB, LVH with strain or digoxin effect, WPW/pre-excitation). In such patients, addition of exercise imaging is generally necessary to assess inducible ischemia.

When to stop

- Target heart rate achieved (>85% age-predicted maximal heart rate [= 220 minus age in years])
- Exercise-limiting angina or dyspnea
- Dizziness
- Fatigue or patient requests to stop
- Atrial arrhythmia other than ectopic beats
- Frequent ventricular ectopic beats or VT
- ST-segment elevation in leads without Q waves or ST depression more than 5 mm
- Hypotension (implies global LV ischemia and decreased cardiac output with exercise)
- Exaggerated hypertensive response to exercise (SBP >220 mmHg or DBP > 120 mmHg)
- New high-grade AV block or bundle branch block

Criteria for a positive test (see Fig. 12.1)

- **Flat or down-sloping ST depression** of at least 1 mm 80 ms after the J point (junction between the QRS and ST segment). Up-sloping ST depression at least 1.5 mm (less specific).
- ST elevation*
- Increase in QRS voltage (ischemic LV dilatation)
- Failure of BP to rise or hypotension during exercise (ischemic LV dysfunction)*
- Ventricular arrhythmias*
- Typical ischemic symptoms during exercise
- Inability to increase heart rate
- Also ST depression at low workload (<<6 min Bruce) in multiple lead groups, persisting into recovery, >2 mm, down-sloping pattern

* These features are indications for **urgent angiography**.

Causes of false-positive ECG exercise tests are listed in Box 12.1.

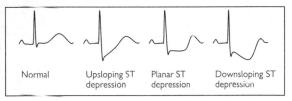

| Normal | Upsloping ST depression | Planar ST depression | Downsloping ST depression |

Figure 12.1 Criteria for a positive test.

Box 12.1 Causes of false-positive tests

- Cardiomyopathies
- Hypertension
- LVOT obstruction
- Mitral valve prolapse
- Hyperventilation
- Resting ECG abnormality (LBBB, LVH with strain, pre-excitation, digoxin)
- Electrolyte abnormalities (hypokalemia)
- Tricyclic antidepressants
- Syndrome X
- Coronary artery spasm
- Sympathetic overactivity

Transthoracic echocardiography (TTE)

Introduction

Despite dramatic advances in new cardiac imaging technologies, echocardiography remains the most widely used diagnostic imaging tool in clinical practice. Since its development by Edler and Herz almost five decades ago and routine clinical implementation a decade later, echocardiography has developed into a comprehensive and practical method to rapidly and repeatedly evaluate cardiac morphology and function.

There are now published guidelines regarding the appropriate use of echocardiography in clinical practice. Correct interpretation of an echocardiogram first requires an understanding of the physical principles underlying the available modalities.

Ultrasound physics

All forms of ultrasonic imaging are based on generation of high-frequency (>1 mHz) acoustic pressure waves from a transducer comprised of one or more piezoelectric crystals. Current is passed across the crystal leading to material deformation and wave transmission. The piezoelectric element also serves as a receiver, and waves returning from insonified objects (e.g., walls, valves) deform the crystal(s), which in turn generate a current that can be sampled over time.

Because the velocity of sound is constant, object location (spatial resolution) can be determined through timing of the returning signal. The amplitude of the returning signal is based on the angle of incidence (surfaces perpendicular to the ultrasound beam are stronger reflectors) and the interface of acoustic impedances (greater differences, as occurs in the left ventricle at the tissue–blood interface, lead to greater reflectivity).

Returning ultrasound information is processed for maximum image integrity and then mapped to pixels for display and storage. Although images may be stored on videotape, current methods of digital storage and retrieval enable optimal image integrity, easy access to archived studies for comparison and research purposes, and offline processing.

M-mode

This was the first clinically available form of echocardiography and, while still available on modern machines, has been virtually replaced in current practice by newer two-dimensional (2-D) imaging techniques. M-, or "motion-", mode images depict a single line of ultrasound data over time (Fig. 12.2).

Its advantage lies in its high sampling rate (>1 kHz) and superb temporal resolution, resulting in the ability to depict rapidly moving structures. It is especially useful for measuring chamber dimensions and the timing of various events during the cardiac cycle.

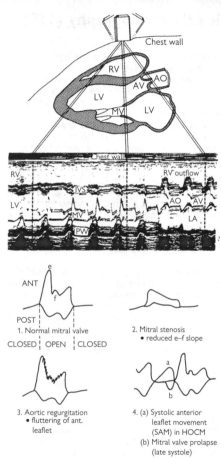

Figure 12.2 Normal M-mode echocardiogram. AO, aortic valve; IVS, interventricular septum; LA, left atrium; LV, left ventricle; MV, mitral valve; PW, posterior wall of LV; RV, right ventricle. Adapted from R Hall, *Med International* 17: 774. Reprinted with permission from Longmore M, Wilkinson I, Rajagopalan S (2004). *Oxford Handbook of Clinical Medicine*, 6th ed. Oxford University Press.

Two-dimensional or sector scanning

When an ultrasound beam is swept across a chosen cardiac window, rapid sequential sampling can be performed, leading to a display of multiple "scan lines" of information and a sector image created nearly instantaneously. Since a finite number of scan lines is possible, interpolation of data between lines is performed and an image slice or sector (hence, the term *sector scanning*) is stored in digital form.

Through reiterative acquisition over a cardiac cycle, a movie composed of sequentially acquired sectors is created demonstrating structural motion, which can then be displayed on a monitor. Beam sweeping can be performed by mechanical rotation of one or more crystals or through the use of programmed firing of a bank of crystals (phased array).

Sampling rates were previously dictated and limited by videotape standards but, with digital capabilities appearing in some form on virtually all machines and replacing outdated tape technology, higher frame rates are possible.

The availability of harmonic tissue imaging has substantially improved image resolution by eliminating artifact and improving the signal-to-noise ratio. Low-level signals emanating from tissue and comprising the first harmonic of the transmitted ultrasound are selectively sampled. In this way, extraneous reflections such as reverberations are filtered out, leaving a cleaner image.

Three-dimensional imaging

While 2-D echocardiography presents user-selected sector or tomographic information, 3-D echocardiography has the potential to provide a comprehensive evaluation of cardiac anatomy similar to that of more quantitatively mature technologies such as magnetic resonance imaging (MRI) or computerized tomography (CT) (see Figs. 12.3 and 12.4).

Three-dimensional echocardiography can be performed using the "free-hand" approach in which multiple 2-D sectors are acquired from a probe positionally mapped using a "spark gap" or magnetic tracking system.

Both image and position data are stored for post-hoc 3-D reconstruction. The development of the matrix array transducer and improved computational capabilities has made post-hoc, 3-D chamber reconstruction a reality, with accurate volumetric assessment comparable to that of MRI. More recently, real-time acquisition of spatially limited cardiac segments has been made available.

Although there are still some limitations with the currently available technology, it is likely that this modality will gain wider application in future clinical practice.

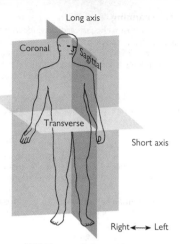

Figure 12.3 The so-called anatomical position. The subject is upright and facing the observer. Any structure within the body can be described within the references of the three orthogonal planes—two in the long axis and the third in the short axis. Reprinted with permission from Anderson RH, Ho SY, Brecker SJ (2001). Anatomic basis of cross-sectional echocardiography. *Heart* 85(6):716–720.

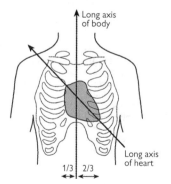

Figure 12.4 The heart lies in the mediastinum with its own long axis tilted relative to the long axis of the body. Appreciation of this discrepancy is important in the setting of cross-sectional echocardiography. Reprinted with permission from Anderson RH, Ho SY, Brecker SJ (2001). Anatomic basis of cross-sectional echocardiography. *Heart* 85(6):716–720.

Transthoracic Doppler imaging

- Analysis and quantification of object motion within the heart is performed using Doppler-based technologies. In brief, the same equipment described earlier propagates ultrasound aimed at moving red blood cells or tissue.
- Frequencies of returning ultrasound are shifted upward and downward by cells traveling toward and away from the transducer, respectively.
- The frequency shift is proportional to an object's velocity as described by the Doppler equation.
- The signal intensity is dependent on the number of cells moving at a particular velocity.
- Velocity information is depicted graphically as a spectral pattern over time (similar to the M-mode display) or mapped to pixels as color overlaying the 2-D or 3-D image (color Doppler).
- The ultrasound beam must be as parallel as possible to the target, as off-axis angulation by >20° causes significant underestimation of velocities.

Doppler is restricted in its ability to sample high velocities by the *Nyquist limit*, which is dependent on the sampling rate (the lower the frequency, the higher the evaluable velocity) and object depth (the deeper the object, the lower the sampling rate). When the frequency shift of moving objects (i.e., velocity) exceeds the Nyquist limit, *aliasing* occurs, precluding velocity assessment.

Pulsed Doppler

Pulsed Doppler imaging allows accurate sampling of blood velocities averaged within a limited region of interest or "sample volume." Transducer elements serve both as transmitters and receivers, which allows for the selective sampling of reflected ultrasound with accurate range and spatial information.

Pulsed Doppler spectral displays portray velocity vectors over time (see Box 12.2).

Laminar flow is found within normal vessels and chambers and characterized by a gradual increase in flow velocities from the vessel wall to the center of the lumen. It is characterized by a narrow spectral trace representing a relatively discrete population of blood velocities.

Box 12.2 Flow quantification from pulsed Doppler

Quantification

Pulsed Doppler spectral traces can provide important information regarding flow quantification and timing. By assuming that sampling occurs at an orifice with a relatively fixed area over the cardiac cycle (e.g., the left ventricular outflow tract) and integrating the time velocity spectral curve (*time–velocity integral* [TVI]), the area under this curve can be multiplied by the area of the orifice (determined from 2-D or M-mode Echo), resulting in the stroke volume.

Turbulent flow occurs across stenotic or regurgitant orifices (valves, shunts, etc.) where high pressure gradients lead to high red cell kinetic energy and disordered, high-velocity motion. It is graphically portrayed as spectral broadening. Aliasing often occurs with high-velocity jets, leading to "wraparound."

Continuous wave (CW) Doppler permits beam steering. Transducer elements are shared for purposes of CW and intermittent 2-D imaging. A virtual cursor positioned over the 2-D image can be moved to guide and minimize off-axis sampling angulation.

CW Doppler velocities are depicted as a filled-in spectral tracing as all of the velocities along the sampling cursor (or ultrasound beam) are measured. Blood cells traveling at the fastest velocities are represented at the outer edge of the spectral trace (peak) or darkest line of the trace (modal) velocities.

Color Doppler flow imaging employs multigate pulsed Doppler to portray blood flow overlying the 2-D image. Information is used to detect regurgitant or stenotic lesions and shunts. Qualitative assessment of velocity amplitude and direction is possible using color maps.

- Pixels are assigned a color based on user-configurable mapping parameters. Pixel color is based on average velocity in the pixel region of interest.
- By convention, a color map system is used in all machines, with **blue** representing flow away from the transducer and **red** depicting flow toward the transducer (see Fig. 12.5).
- The lighter the color, the higher the velocity.
- Turbulent velocities can be displayed as a green hue with variance mapping.
- Aliasing is depicted as a mix of colors, or a "mosaic" pattern.

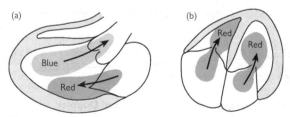

Figure 12.5 Color Doppler (red: flow toward transducer; blue: flow away from transducer). (a) Top: systolic blue flow of left ventricular ejection; bottom: red flow of diastolic mitral inflow, shown from parasternal long-axis window. (b) Left: red flow of diastolic tricuspid inflow; right: red flow of diastolic mitral inflow shown from apical four-chamber window.

Tissue Doppler imaging (TDI) is used to assess low-velocity displacement of myocardium. A high pass filter excludes higher frequency blood flow signals, leaving only low-velocity shifts attributable to tissue motion.
- Mitral or tricuspid annular motion can be tracked and correlates with systolic and diastolic performance of the associated ventricles.
- Regional wall motion can be assessed for displacement that may be affected by overall cardiac motion or local tethering.

Strain rate imaging can measure regional thickening and thinning independent of the external influences on wall motion that can affect tissue Doppler measurements. With strain rate imaging, two sampling sites are simultaneously acquired and intersample displacement (strain) over time (strain rate) can be determined. Strain and strain rate can be determined in the radial, longitudinal, and circumferential directions.

For calculations from Doppler measurements, see Box 12.3.

Box 12.3 Calculations from Doppler measurements

Valve gradients

The velocity of blood cells traveling through a narrow orifice is directly proportional to the pressure gradient at that point in time. This relationship is approximated by the simplified Bernoulli formula:

Gradient (mmHg) = $4 V^2$ (where V = peak Doppler velocity in m/sec)

In situations where there are high flow velocities (e.g., aortic stenosis with high LVOT velocities), the flow before the stenosis must be accounted for.

Gradient (mmHg) = $4(V_2^2 - V_1^2)$ (where V_2 = velocity across the lesion and V_1 = velocity proximal to the lesion)

Both peak and mean gradients can be determined by measuring the maximal velocity and velocity–time integral (VTI).

Valve area (continuity equation)

This is based on the principle that flow proximal to the valve = flow across the valve. The most common application is the calculation of aortic valve area in patients with aortic stenosis, as shown below.

LVOT flow = LVOT area × LVOT (VTI) by pulsed Doppler

LVOT area = ϖ (LVOT diameter in PLAX/2)^2

Aortic valve flow = Aortic valve area × Aortic valve VTI
                                     by CW Doppler

Aortic valve flow = LVOT flow,

Aortic valve area = (LVOT VTI/Aortic valve VTI) × LVOT area

The standard TTE

Most laboratories employ imaging protocols incorporating acquisition of images from standard views in a specific sequence. Image quality is maximized by avoiding overlying lung artifacts and rib reflections. Pulsed and color flow Doppler is performed following 2-D imaging in each view.

Standard echo windows (and views) and the main cardiovascular structures visualized are as follows:

Left parasternal window

- Long axis (PLAX): left atrium and ventricle, aortic root, mitral and aortic valves, and right ventricle (see Figs. 12.6 and 12.7)
- Short axis (PSAX): 4 levels
  - Aortic valve/left atrial level: includes tricuspid valve (TV), right ventricular outflow tract (RVOT), pulmonic valve (PV), and pulmonary artery (Pa) (see Fig. 12.6)
  - Left ventricular base/mitral valve
  - Mid-left ventricle/papillary muscle
  - Left ventricular apex
- Right ventricular inflow

Apical window

- 4 chamber (A4C): both atria, ventricles and AV valves, inferior septal and anterolateral LV walls (Fig. 12.7). Pulmonary veins may also be seen.
- 5 chamber (A5C): A4C angled anteriorly to LV outflow tract (the "fifth chamber" in this view is the aortic root)
- 2 chamber (A2C): left atrium, anterior and inferior LV walls
- 3 chamber/apical long axis (A3C): apical version of PLAX view with anteroseptal, posterior or inferolateral walls and LV outflow tract

Suprasternal window (SS)

- Aortic arch and head vessels
- Proximal descending thoracic aorta

Subcostal window (SC)

- 4 chamber and short axis views are often imaged
- The inferior vena cava (IVC) and descending aorta can also be seen

Right parasternal window (optional)

- Ascending aorta and CW Doppler of aortic valve

Chamber evaluation

Chambers are routinely measured from M-mode tracings or, more commonly, using digital calipers to perform assessment from 2-D images. The PLAX view is the standard for most chamber measurements.

Area tracings provide enhanced accuracy but require adequate endocardial visualization for optimal accuracy.

Chamber volumes are derived from 2-D measurements using geometric modeling. The most common volumetric approaches include the modified Simpson's biplane method of disks and the area–length formula.

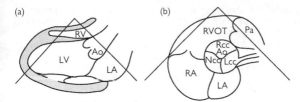

Figure 12.6 (a) Parasternal long axis view; (b) parasternal short axis view (aortic level). Ao, aorta; LA, left atrium; Lcc: left coronary cusp; LV, left ventricle; Ncc: noncoronary cusp; Pa, pulmonary artery; RA, right atrium; Rcc Ao: right coronary cusp of aortic valve, RVOT, right ventricular outflow tract.

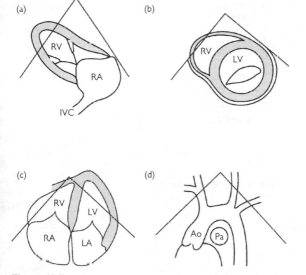

Figure 12.7 (a) Parasternal long axis view (RV inflow); (b) parasternal short axis (mitral valve level); (c) apical 4 chamber view; (d) suprasternal long axis view. For abbreviations see Figure 12.6; IVC, inferior vena cava.

3-D echo has also been validated as an accurate and reproducible method of chamber volume quantification and is superior to standard 2-D imaging if done properly.

Most clinical labs perform measurements in real time during image acquisition, though modern workstations allow for comprehensive off-line analysis. End-diastole is usually defined as the beginning of the QRS complex and end-systolic measurements are performed at maximum LV contraction. The American Society of Echocardiography has published guidelines for standard chamber quantification and it is recommended that these can be applied in routine clinical practice.

Left atrium
- Measure at ventricular end-systole.
- Linear (anteroposterior [AP]) measurement is made from PLAX view at aortic cusp level.
- Area (A4C) and volume (modified Simpson's formula or area–length method using the A4C and A2C views) are also often quantified.

Left ventricle
- Measure chamber diameter from PLAX at mitral leaflet tips at end-diastole and end-systole.
- Septal and posterior wall thickness should be measured from PLAX at mitral leaflet tips in end-diastole.
- Volumes (modified Simpson's biplane method of disks)
- Derived variables
  - *Fractional shortening:*

    $FS = ([LVIDd - LVIDs]/LVIDs) \times 100$

    where $LVID = LV$ internal diameter in diastole (d) and systole (s).

  - *Ejection fraction* (from 2-D- or 3-D-generated volumes or derived from M-mode [e.g., Teicholz formula])
  - *Mass* can be derived from M-mode measures (ASE-modified Penn formula), 2-D volumetric models, or 3-D reconstruction. M-mode mass calculations tend to overquantify LV mass.

Aortic root and ascending aorta
- Linear measurements from 2-D PLAX view or M-mode at end-diastole.

The root is measured at cusp level, and aorta is measured at sinotubular junction and 2 cm above this.

Right atrium
- Area, inferior/superior and lateral/medial diameter measurements from A4C view

Right ventricle

- Irregular shape makes standardized quantification and geometric modeling difficult.
- Diameter typically is measured in A4C view at base or mid-ventricle.
- Qualitative comparison of size relative to left ventricle (if normal in size).

Pulmonary artery

- Diameter measurement in PSAX at aortic valve level.

Assessment of wall motion

Overall assessment is based on review of wall segments from multiple standard views. In general, abnormalities of LV regional function should be apparent in more than one view.

Regional wall motion is best described using the standard 16-segment model recommended by the American Society of Echocardiography:

- **Basal (6):** anteroseptal, anterior, anterolateral, inferolateral (or posterior), inferior, inferoseptal
- **Mid LV (6):** same as above
- **Apical (4):** anterior, lateral, inferior, and septal. (In some systems the tip of the apex is included as a 17th segment.)

Regional functional assessment

Systolic function should be classified as *normal*, *globally hypokinetic*, or demonstrating the presence of *regional wall motion abnormalities*.

Global hypokinesis is consistent with cardiomyopathy, either ischemic or nonischemic. Some degree of regional wall motion abnormality may be present in nonischemic cardiomyopathy.

The presence of distinct regional wall motion abnormalities with large areas of normal regional function is suggestive of underlying coronary artery disease, either areas of infarct or stunned/hibernating myocardium.

Evaluation of regional wall thickening is preferable to endocardial motion, which may be influenced by tethering of adjacent segments. Unfortunately, this is not always possible when endocardial or epicardial border definition is suboptimal.

Each regional segment is classified as follows:
1. Normal or hyperkinetic
2. Hypokinetic
3. Akinetic
4. Dyskinetic
5. Aneurysmal

A **wall motion score index** can be calculated on the basis of analysis of each segment using the 16-segment model (see Fig. 12.8) and assigning a score based on the categories above:

- Sum of individual wall motion scores/number wall segments visualized.
- A normal score is 1 (i.e., 16/16).
- A higher score indicates more severe coronary disease and is predictive of future cardiac events.
- This index may be especially useful in stress echocardiography.

Identification of hyperechogenic, thinned areas suggests the presence of scarring.

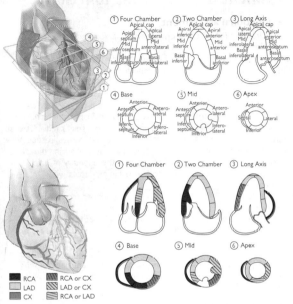

Figure 12.8 A 17-segment wall segment model (top). Coronary perfusion territories (bottom). Reprinted with permission from Lang et al. (2005). *J Am Soc Echo* 18:1440–1463.

Assessment of LV systolic function

Global functional assessment

- *Ejection fraction (EF) estimation* is usually performed qualitatively (see Table 12.1).
- *2-D echo ejection fractions* can be quantified most efficiently on or offline by means of the following methods:
  - *Simpson's modified biplane method of disks:* A4C and A2C LV traces are obtained and the apex–annulus length is divided into a standard number of equal segments, the length of which serves as disc height. Cross-sectional disc area is calculated from the elliptical formula (ϖ $r_1 r_2$), where r_1 and r_2 are the endocardial medial–lateral dimension of each segment in the A4C and A2C views, respectively.
  - *Area Length method:* Volume is determined by measuring the LV endocardial area (A) on the PSA view at the papillary muscle level and the longest apex–annulus length (L) in any apical view. Volume = 5/6 AL.
- *LV stroke volume:* LVOT VTI × LVOT area (derived from diameter in PLAX view).
- *Systemic cardiac output:* LV stroke volume × heart rate.
- *Pulmonary stroke volume:* RVOT VTI × RVOT area (derived from systolic medial–lateral dimension at level of Doppler sampling).
- *RV output:* Pulmonary stroke volume × heart rate.
- *Pulmonic/systemic shunt ratio (Qp/Qs):* pulmonary cardiac output/ systemic cardiac output, aids in describing the degree of intracardiac shunting, e.g., in atrial septal defects.

Stress echocardiography

This is performed in conjunction with exercise (usually treadmill) or after administration of a pharmacological stress agent (i.e., dobutamine). Standard views are PLAX, PSAX mid-ventricle, A4C, and A2C.

Images are acquired at rest and immediately post-stress following exercise or at rest, low-dose, peak-dose, and post-dobutamine infusion. Images are displayed in quad screen format for direct comparison of rest and stress images.

Sensitivity and specificity are 75%–85% and 80%–90%, respectively, and are comparable to SPECT perfusion imaging. In patients with coronary

Table 12.1 Assessment of LV ejection fraction

LV ejection fraction	Qualitative assessment
>75%	Hyperdynamic
55%–75%	Normal
40%–54%	Mildly reduced
30%–39%	Moderately reduced
<30%	Severely reduced

artery disease, sensitivity for detection of flow-limiting stenosis increases with the number of coronary arteries involved.

A **wall motion score index (WMSI)**, as described previously, can be calculated at rest and following stress to determine the extent of scarring and/or ischemia. An exercise WMSI above 2 predicts a high risk (>5%/year) of future cardiac events (see Table 12.2).

A normal exercise echocardiogram is associated with a very low rate of future cardiac events (<1%/year).

Contrast can be administered to improve endocardial border definition.

Common applications

- Diagnosis of coronary disease in patients with chest pain or angina (or equivalent)
- Determine physiological significance of a coronary stenosis prior to revascularization
- Risk stratification following myocardial infarction (MI)
- Viability testing using dobutamine stress
  - Biphasic response to dobutamine suggests hibernating myocardium and predicts functional recovery and improved outcome following revascularization.
- Preoperative risk stratification in selected patients at increased risk for postoperative cardiac complications following noncardiac surgery, especially those with intermediate or major clinical predictors of increased risk and poor baseline functional status
- Follow-up of patients after coronary revascularization, especially if symptomatic
- Assess physiological significance of valvular lesions, particularly mitral stenosis and mitral regurgitation
- Differentiate true aortic stenosis from "pseudo-"aortic stenosis in patients with low transvalvular gradient due to low cardiac output

Findings of high risk

- Decreased LVEF or increase LV end-systolic volume during stress
- Extensive ischemia (multiple dysfunctional segments with stress) suggesting multivessel disease
- Ischemia at low workload
- Resting LVEF <40%
- Resting wall motion abnormalities with remote ischemia

Table 12.2 Interpretation of stress echocardiogram

Resting wall motion	Stress wall motion	Interpretation
Normal	Hyperdynamic	Normal
Normal	Abnormal	Ischemia
Abnormal	Unchanged	Scar
Abnormal	Improved	Nontransmural scar without ischemia
Abnormal	Worse	Ischemia

Assessment of LV diastolic function

Evaluation of LV diastolic function includes measurement of the various phases of diastole, including isovolumic relaxation, early filling, diastasis (atrioventricular [AV] pressure equilibration without LV filling), and atrial systole. The characteristics of these filling phases are generally age and heart-rate dependent and affected by LV loading conditions to variable degrees (see Fig. 12.9).

Pulsed Doppler mitral inflow: E wave (peak early diastolic velocity), A wave (peak atrial systolic velocity), E/A ratio, and transmitral deceleration time (DT, time interval from peak E wave to its return to baseline).

The following should be taken into account when assessing these parameters:
- The E/A ratio is particularly dependent on sample-volume placement (annulus, mitral tips, etc.) and loading conditions.
- E/A ratio decreases with age and assessment must be age-normalized. An E/A ratio <1.0 is common among the elderly (age >65 years) and often represents normal aging.
- Increasing LV filling pressures (e.g., in heart failure) lead to pseudonormalization of the E/A ratio, which often reverts to an abnormal pattern following maneuvers to reduce LV preload (e.g., diuresis, nitroglycerin, or Valsalva maneuver).
- The DT correlates with invasive measures of LV stiffness, whereas other measures largely reflect LV relaxation.

Pulsed Doppler of pulmonary veins: Assessment of LA filling, which is affected by the diastolic properties of the LV. Usually the right upper pulmonary vein is sampled in the A4C view and guided by color flow Doppler, though optimal visualization is often difficult. S, D, and A waves represent systolic and diastolic atrial filling. The A wave is generated by reverse flow into the pulmonary veins during atrial contraction.
- The S/D ratio increases with age as LV diastolic relaxation declines.
- A pulmonary vein A wave duration >30 ms greater than transmitral A wave durations suggests elevated LV filling pressure.

CW Doppler of LV outflow/mitral inflow: Isovolumic relaxation time (IVRT) is the interval between aortic valve closure and mitral valve opening. Changes in IVRT tend to parallel those seen in DT with increasing diastolic dysfunction.

Tissue Doppler of septal and lateral mitral annuli (E', A')
- This is less dependent on loading conditions.
- The septal mitral annular velocity is the preferred measurement.
- The E/E' ratio correlates with LV end-diastolic pressure and a ratio >15 is strongly suggestive of elevated filling pressure, with a ratio <8 strongly suggestive of normal filling pressure.

Color Doppler M-mode: Rate of blood flow into the LV from annulus to apex is determined by measuring the slope of the line along the edge of the color Doppler M-mode tracing. Normal propagation velocity (Vp) is >45–50 cm/sec. Ratio of E/Vp >2 correlates with elevated LA pressure.

These parameters are used to determine the severity of diastolic dysfunction (see Fig.12.9). In general:

- Markers of impaired relaxation (e.g., decreased E and E' are accompanied by compensatory enhancement of A and A'), reduced pulmonary venous D, and reduced Vp.
- Increases in LV filling pressure lead to pseudonormalization of the transmitral Doppler E/A ratio, reversal of the pulmonary vein S/D ratio, and increased E/E' ratio.
- As compliance decreases, the transmitral DT drops below 130 ms, early Doppler filling velocity is increased and, because of elevated late diastolic LV pressures, atrial contraction and associated velocities are reduced.
- If E/E' ratio <8 and LA is of normal size, symptoms are unlikely to be due to diastolic heart failure.

Do not miss **constriction**. Look for the following:

- Septal "bounce" and dyssynchrony
- IVC dilatation
- Hepatic vein expiratory reversal
- Excessive mitral inflow respiratory variation
- Restrictive filling pattern on mitral inflow Doppler with normal tissue Doppler mitral annular velocities

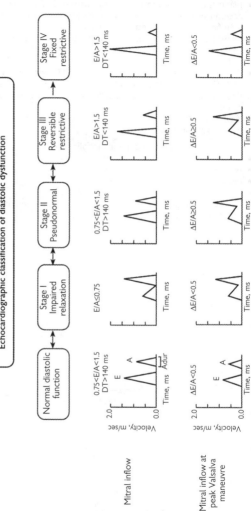

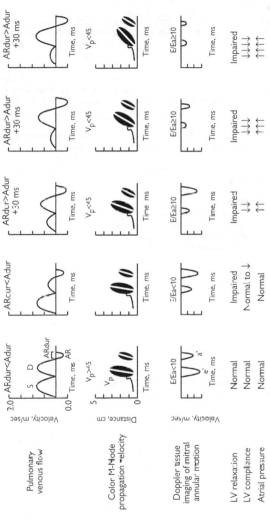

Figure 12.9 Echocardiographic classification of diastolic dysfunction.

Echocardiography in aortic stenosis

Etiology

Aortic stenosis (AS) can be congenital (i.e., unicuspid or bicuspid valve) or, more commonly, degenerative. In late stages, severe fibrocalcification precludes etiologic identification even on direct intraoperative visualization. Chronic severe AS is usually accompanied by concentric LV hypertrophy due to pressure overload.

Bicuspid aortic valve is diagnosed best on short axis view and can display various configurations. Often a "raphe" is observed representing the undeveloped commissure where persistent cuspal fusion is present. Systolic cuspal "doming" is consistent with congenital AS, as is best seen in the PLAX view.

Degenerative AS typically starts in the annulus fibrosis (most commonly in the noncoronary cusp area) and gradually proceeds to invade the cusp bases, body, and, in later stages, the tips. Valve thickening without hemodynamic stenosis is termed *sclerosis*, and is a common cause of murmur in asymptomatic adults.

Hemodynamics

Stenosis is defined as a hemodynamically significant reduction in valve area as indicated by a rise in transvalvular pressure gradient.

Pressure gradient is dependent on flow and, in the setting of low cardiac output, may be minimally elevated despite significant stenosis (i.e., low-gradient aortic stenosis).

Aortic stenosis severity is categorized according to the valve area, transvalvular velocity, and mean pressure gradient (see Table 12.3).

ECHO diagnosis

- Assess cusp separation or presence of doming. A trileaflet valve with one cusp opening fully (approaching edge of the root) is probably not significantly stenotic.
- CW Doppler-derived gradients are reported as instantaneous peak and/or mean. The mean gradient is more reliable in determining stenosis severity.
- Cath lab gradients are "peak to peak" with pressure measurements that are usually not acquired simultaneously and often do not correlate with the peak gradient by Doppler, which reflects the maximal instantaneous pressure. The mean gradients obtained by ECHO and catheterization are comparable.

Table 12.3 2006 ACC/AHA classification of AS severity

Measurement	Normal	Mild	Moderate	Severe
Jet velocity (m/sec)	<2.0	2.0–3.0	3.0–4.0	>4.0
Mean gradient (mmHg)	<10	10–25	25–40	>40
Valve area (cm²)	3–4	1.5–2.0	1.0–1.5	<1.0

- CW Doppler can underestimate the transvalvular gradient if the ultrasound beam is not parallel to the direction of flow.
- Peak transvalvular velocity >2.5 m/sec (instantaneous gradient of 25 mmHg) suggests some degree of stenosis.
- Elevated cardiac output or significant aortic regurgitation will increase transvalvular flow and gradient but should not affect calculations of valve area.
- **The dimensionless index (DI)** is the ratio of LVOT velocity or VTI (pulsed Doppler)/transvalvular velocity or VTI (CW Doppler) and essentially corrects for abnormal cardiac output. General guidelines are as follows:
  - DI <0.5: significant stenosis
  - DI 0.25–0.5: moderate stenosis
  - DI <0.25: severe stenosis

Aortic valve area is calculated using the following *continuity equation*:

Aortic valve area = (LVOT VTI/Aortic valve VTI) × LVOT area

Measuring wall thickness for LVH, assessing LV systolic function, and looking for coexistent mitral regurgitation are other essential aspects to the echocardiographic evaluation of aortic stenosis.

Transesophageal echocardiography (TEE)

TEE is a minimally invasive test that has advantages over TTE due to the higher ultrasonic frequency (5–7 MHz) and improved spatial resolution, particularly for structures located in proximity to the esophagus (i.e., atria, valves; see Fig. 12.10) (see Box 12.4 for common indications).

The transesophageal approach also allows for an unobstructed echocardiographic window in those patients with poor transthoracic acoustic windows. It is also valuable in the intraoperative setting without interfering with the operative field. Virtually all TEE probes have multiplane scanning capability.

Patient preparation

The procedure is performed using topical anesthesia and IV conscious sedation.

Prior to procedure

• The patient is NPO for 4–6 hours prior to the procedure.
• Obtain patient history to determine if there are contraindications or risk factors for complications from the procedure and/or sedation (i.e., known esophageal pathology or dysphagia, pulmonary disease such as COPD or sleep apnea).
• Perform physical exam with particular attention to oropharynx/airway.
• Any dentures are removed and the back of the throat may be sprayed with lidocaine (Xylocaine®) or benzocaine (note that these agents can have adverse side effects that are dose-dependent). Viscous lidocaine can also be gargled and swallowed for local anesthesia.
• Short-acting IV benzodiazepenes (i.e., midazolam) and opiate analgesics (i.e., fentanyl) may be administered for sedation. Continuous pulse-oximetry, BP, and HR monitoring is required.
• Reversal agents (i.e., Narcan, flumazenil) should be readily available.
• Perform under general anesthesia if conscious sedation is not possible or if deemed unsafe.

Procedure

• Oxygen and wall suction should be available. A nurse should assist in monitoring during and after the procedure. A bite guard is used.
• The patient is placed in the supine or left lateral position with the neck flexed.
• The TEE probe is lubricated with gel and introduced gently to the pharynx. Once the patient swallows, the probe is advanced into the esophagus. Excessive force should be avoided, especially if resistance is felt during intubation.

Post-procedure

The patient should be NPO for 1–2 hours post-procedure to allow recovery of the gag reflex.

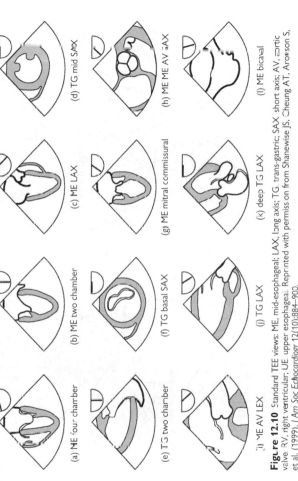

(a) ME four chamber

(b) ME two chamber

(c) ME LAX

(d) TG mid SAX

(e) TG two chamber

(f) TG basal SAX

(g) ME mitral commissural

(h) ME ME AV SAX

(i) ME AV LAX

(j) TG LAX

(k) deep TG LAX

(l) ME bicaval

(continued)

Figure 12.10 Standard TEE views: ME, mid-esophageal; LAX, long axis; TG, trans-gastric; SAX, short axis; AV, aortic valve; RV, right ventricular; UE, upper esophageal. Reprinted with permission from Shanewise JS, Cheung AT, Aronson S, et al. (1999). *J Am Soc Echocardiogr* 12(10):884–900.

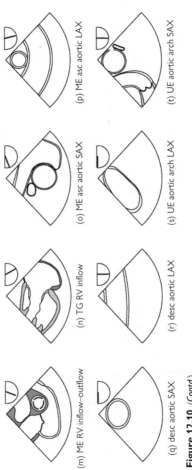

(m) ME RV inflow–outflow

(n) TG RV inflow

(o) ME asc aortic SAX

(p) ME asc aortic LAX

(q) desc aortic SAX

(r) desc aortic LAX

(s) UE aortic arch LAX

(t) UE aortic arch SAX

Figure 12.10 (Contd.)

Box 12.4 Common indications for TEE

- Valvular disease, especially prior to surgery (i.e., MVP with severe MR) and prosthetic valve dysfunction
- Infective endocarditis
- Cardiac source of embolism, including patent foramen ovale (PFO)
- Aortic pathology (aortic, rupture, aneurysm, atheroma)
- Atrial fibrillation prior to DC cardioversion
- Cardiac masses
- Pericardial disease
- Congenital heart defects
- Intraoperative monitoring during cardiac surgery
- Guiding interventional procedures—ASD/PFO closure, mitral valvuloplasty
- Poor transthoracic windows

Pitfalls

Serious complications are rare (0.2%) and include esophageal perforation, bronchospasm/laryngospasm, arrhythmias, and severe hypoxia due to aspiration or respiratory depression from sedation. Mild pharyngeal discomfort is common and self-limited. Mortality rate is <0.01%.

The proximal aortic arch and the upper portion of the ascending aorta is a blind spot because of the interposition of the trachea and right bronchus between the heart and esophagus, and dissection limited to this area could be missed (though this is rare). Given the resolution of TEE, certain normal structures (e.g., Chiari network, aortic valve strands, prosthetic valve sutures) might be inadvertently mistaken as pathological.

TEE for a cardiac source of embolism

Patients who have suffered a cerebral embolic event, especially at a young age (<50 years), may have a cardiac source of emboli that is not evident on transthoracic echocardiogram (TTE). Once a TTE has excluded major causes such as mitral valve disease, a TEE should be performed to examine the following areas.

Key views

- Left atrial thrombus or spontaneous contrast (0° mid-esophageal [ME] four chamber, 90° ME bicaval, two chamber and long axis [LAX])
- Left atrial appendage for thrombus (90° ME two chamber)
- Patent foramen ovale (PFO) (90° ME bicaval)
- Atrial septal aneurysm (90° ME bicaval)
- Atrial myxoma (0° ME four chamber, 90° ME two chamber, 90° ME bicaval)
- LV cavity for left ventricular thrombus, including apex (120° TG LAX)
- Aortic atheroma (>4 mm, mobile and ulcerated aortic plaques have the highest risk of embolization) in ascending arch and descending aorta
- Aortic and mitral valves for vegetations and fibroelastomas

Diagnosis of patent foramen ovale

- Color Doppler imaging to detect right-to-left shunt.

Bubble study

- 10 mL of saline is agitated by injecting between 2 syringes connected by a three-way stop-cock.
- Position the TEE probe at either 0 or 180° at ME level to visualize the right atrium.
- Inject agitated saline.
- Repeat with Valsalva maneuver, if necessary.
- The presence of bubbles in the left heart chambers three cardiac cycles after opacification of the right atrium is consistent with the diagnosis of PFO.
- Sensitivity of detection of R–L shunt can be improved by injecting into the femoral vein rather than an antecubital vein, but this is not routinely done.

Diagnosis of atrial septal aneurysm

- The base of the aneurysm should measure at least 1.5 cm.
- The excursion of the membrane should be at least 1.5 cm in the direction of either atria. M-mode can be useful to accurately measure the excursion of the aneurysm.
- The existence of an atrial septal aneurysm in conjunction with PFO (but not in isolation) has been shown to increase stroke risk.

TEE in aortic dissection

TEE can demonstrate the presence of an intimal flap in the aorta with great accuracy (sensitivity of 99%, specificity of 98%).

Key views

- Presence of intimal flap in the following:
  - Ascending aorta (120° ME AV LAX, 30° ME ascending aortic SAX)
  - Descending aorta (0° desc aortic SAX, 90° descending aortic LAX)
  - Aortic arch (0° UE aortic arch LAX, 90° UE aortic arch SAX)
- Coronary artery involvement (30–45° ME AV SAX)
- Aortic valve for regurgitation, annular dilation, cusp involvement (120° ME AV LAX)
- Site of intimal rupture, color Doppler to determine true and false lumen
- Aortic rupture with collection around aorta
- Pericardial effusion
- Thrombus or spontaneous contrast in false lumen

Blood pressure control (i.e., β-blockers) should be initiated prior to TEE and adequate sedation should be given to avoid hypertension during esophageal intubation.

Pitfalls

There are blind spots in the proximal arch.

Aortic artifacts (imaging artifacts that mimic dissection)

- Artifacts have parallel position to the aortic wall and are motion dependent on true structures.
- Blood flow velocities are similar on either side of the artifact.
- Use superpositioning of color Doppler over the artifact without mosaic pattern to indicate turbulence and flow that does not follow an anatomical structure.

An equivocal TEE examination should prompt the use of another imaging modality such as CT or MRI.

Aortic intramural hematoma (AIH)

This appears as an area of wall thickness >7 mm with or without the presence of an echolucent space in the aortic wall. It may be difficult to differentiate from an atherosclerotic plaque or penetrating aortic ulcer, and other imaging modalities such as CT or MRI may be required.

Diagnosis of AIH

- >7 mm crescent or circular thickening of aortic wall
- Extending 1–20 cm longitudinal
- No intimal flap or Doppler flow in thickened aortic wall

TEE in endocarditis

Box 12.5

TEE is more sensitive (**sensitivity >90%**) than TTE for the detection of vegetations (sensitivity <60%) in infective endocarditis (IE), especially if the vegetations are <5 mm in size.

TEE is the preferred diagnostic test

- Patients with poor TTE windows
- Prosthetic valve endocarditis
- Intermediate or high clinical suspicion for IE with negative TTE
- IE with complications (i.e., abscess, hemodynamically significant valvular insufficiency)

Some authorities feel that all patients with clinical IE should have TEE for early detection of complications such as perivalvular abscess formation, and for *Staphyloccocus aureus* IE, where the risk of complications is high. This approach is also cost-effective.

A negative TTE and TEE has a negative predictive value of 95%. If clinical suspicion remains high, however, TEE should be repeated in 7–10 days, as small vegetations (<2 mm) may be missed on the initial study.

Echocardiographic criteria for diagnosis of IE according to Duke classification

- *Vegetations:* irregular mobile echodensities usually seen along lines of valve closures downstream from regurgitant flow. These are typically located on the *atrial side of the mitral valve* (anterior leaflet more common) and the *ventricular side of the aortic valve.*
- *Myocardial abscess* most commonly occurs in the aortic root followed by ventricular septum, mitral valve, and papillary muscle. TEE has a sensitivity of 80%, compared to 30% for TTE.
- Prosthetic valve dehiscence.
- New valvular regurgitation.

Other complications that can be diagnosed by echocardiography include leaflet perforation, fistula, and chordal rupture.

Key views

- Aortic valve, aortic root (30–45° ME AV SAX, 120° ME LAX)
- Mitral valve views (see p. 37)
- Tricuspid valve (0° ME four chamber, 120° TG LAX)
- Pulmonary valve (90° ME RV inflow–outflow)

TEE is useful prior to surgery to exclude involvement of other valves and to look for an abscess or other complication that may require additional surgical procedures (see Box 12.6). Sensitivity of TEE and of TTE are comparable for the detection of right-sided vegetations.

Pitfalls

Valve strands (Lambl's excrescences), chordal structures from myxomatous degeneration, and nonspecific valvular thickening may be mistaken as vegetations, leading to a false-positive result.

Box 12.6 Echocardiographic features requiring surgical referral

- Acute severe aortic or mitral regurgitation causing LV failure or hemodynamic compromise
- Prosthetic valve dehiscence, especially if hemodynamic compromise
- Myocardial abscess
- Vegetations with recurrent embolization despite antibiotics
- Mitral valve vegetation >10 mm due to associated increased risk of embolism
- Increase in vegetation size after 2–4 weeks of antibiotics

TTE/TEE in mitral regurgitation (MR)

Assessment of mitral valve (MV) morphology is required to determine the mechanism of regurgitation and associated structural abnormalities:

- Elongation or rupture of chords
- Papillary muscle rupture
- Retraction of chords
- Prolapse or tethering of leaflets
- Subvalvular apparatus thickening or calcification
- Annular dilation
- Annular calcification
- LV size and function
- LA size
- Regional wall motion abnormalities may suggest ischemic MR.

Key TEE views (see Fig. 12.11)

- Leaflet prolapse or restriction (0° ME four chamber, 45° ME mitral commissural, 90° ME two chamber, 120° ME LAX)
- Annular diameter (120° ME LAX)
- Leaflet prolapse (0° TG basal SAX)
- Subvalvular apparatus (90° TG two chamber)
- Anterior and posterior leaflets are each divided into three segments to describe location of pathology.

Assessment of MR severity (by TEE or TTE)

- Length/area of regurgitant jet
- Density of spectral Doppler tracing
- Timing of MR: early systolic vs. holosystolic by color M-mode
- Direction of jet: eccentric or central
  - *Coanda effect*: size of eccentric wall-hugging regurgitant jet on color Doppler may underestimate severity of regurgitation
- Pulmonary venous systolic flow reversal (see Table 12.4)
- Calculation of regurgitant volume (RV) and effective regurgitant orifice area (EROA) using PISA or volumetric method
- Other features of severe MR:
  - Regurgitant jet width at its origin (vena contracta) >0.7 cm
  - Peak E-wave velocity >1.5 m/sec

Proximal isovelocity surface area (PISA)

- Identify isovelocity hemispheric shells on ventricular aspect of valve in apical view using color Doppler with adjusted aliasing velocity.
- Measure radius of isovelocity shell (r) and aliasing velocity.
- Measure MR peak velocity and VTI from spectral tracing.
  - **EROA** $(cm^2) = 2\pi r^2 \times$ aliasing velocity/MR peak velocity
  - **RV** (mL) = EROA $\times$ MR VTI

Volumetric method

- RV (mL) = Total stroke volume (SV) – Forward stroke volume
  - Total SV = Mitral inflow volume (in absence of significant AR)
  - MV inflow volume = MV VTI (from PW Doppler) $\times$ MV area (πr^2)
  - Forward SV = LVOT VTI $\times$ LVOT area
- **Regurgitant fraction (RF%)** = RV/Total stroke volume $\times$ 100

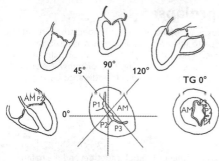

Figure 12.11 Assessment of the mitral valve by TEE. Reprinted with permission from Shanewise JS, Cheung AT, Arouson S, et al. (1999). *J Am Soc Echocardiogr* 12(10):884–900.

Table 12.4 Assessment of MR severity

Parameter	Mild	Moderate	Severe
Jet size	<20% LA area	20%–40% LA area	>40% LA area
LA size	Normal	Normal/mildly dilated	Dilated
Vena contracta	<0.3 cm	0.3–0.7 cm	>0.7 cm
Pulm. vein systolic flow	Normal	Normal/ blunted	Reversal
Regurgitant orifice area	<0.2 cm^2	0.2–0.4 cm^2	>0.4 cm^2
Regurgitant volume	<30 mL	30–60 mL	>60 mL
Regurgitant fraction	<30%	30%–50%	>50%

Mitral valve prolapse

The mitral valve annulus is a nonplanar, saddle-shaped structure. Mitral valve prolapse (MVP) due to myxomatous change is diagnosed when the mitral valve leaflets move beyond the "high points" of the mitral annular plane during systole in the long axis view. The A4C or transverse plane 0° view images the "low points" of the annulus (the distance between low and high points averages 1.4 cm).

Thus, to avoid overdiagnosis of MVP, the criteria for diagnosis are as follows.

Diagnosis

Classical MVP

- Greater than 2 mm displacement of mitral leaflet beyond the mitral annular plane in PLAX view
- Mitral valve thickness >5 mm

Nonclassical MVP

- The prolapsing leaflets are not thickened (<5 mm) and are unaffected by myxomatous degeneration.
- Such patients are not at increased risk of complications such as severe MR, infective endocarditis, and sudden death, compared to those with the classical form of MVP.

MVP causes eccentric mitral regurgitation

- Posterior leaflet prolapse produces an anteriorly directed jet.
- Anterior leaflet prolapse produces a posteriorly directed jet.

Note that when the MR jet hugs the wall of the left atrium (*coanda*), the reported severity should be upgraded. The left and right pulmonary veins should be sampled with pulse wave Doppler imaging to check for systolic flow reversal, suggestive of severe regurgitation.

Perioperative assessment during MV repair

Optimize loading conditions

- Ensure that the patient is fully off bypass with a systolic blood pressure of >120 mmHg before assessing the results of mitral valve repair.
- Give volume or vasoconstrictors as needed to optimize hemodynamics.
- Assess leaflet coaptation and residual regurgitation with color Doppler.
- If there are persistent abnormalities of coaptation with significant MR, surgical revision may be indicated.

Assess left ventricular outflow tract (LVOT)

- LVOT obstruction may occur following mitral valve repair, especially if a rigid annuloplasty ring is used, but is uncommon (1%–2%).
- Obstruction is exacerbated by hypovolemia, and the LVOT gradient should be measured after volume resuscitation.
- If LVOT obstruction persists, the annuloplasty ring may have to be removed.

TEE for MV repair
- Determination of the prolapsing mitral valve segments should be performed to assist in surgical planning.
- Two-thirds of cases of MVP involve the middle scallop (P2 segment) of the posterior leaflet, and most of these cases can be successfully repaired.
- Ruptured chordae and flail mitral valve leaflets should be noted.
- The mitral annulus diameter is also measured (upper limit normal is 35 mm) and presence of annular calcification noted.

Indications for revision surgery after MV repair
- Grade 2+ (moderate) MR
- Persistent LVOT obstruction
- Mitral stenosis (mean gradient ≥ 6 mmHg, MVA <1.5 cm^2)
- Leaflet perforation

TEE in chronic ischemic MR

Mitral valve structure is usually normal and the MR is functional.

Remodeling of the LV causes apical displacement of the papillary muscle and tethering of the mitral valve leaflets, leading to incomplete valve closure. The zone of coaptation is displaced toward the apex and systolic tenting of the mitral valve is seen.

LV remodeling and dilation appears to be necessary for severe MR to develop. Isolated segmental wall motion abnormalities without LV dilation are not generally associated with severe MR. Annular dilatation will exacerbate incomplete leaflet coaptation.

In the presence of an inferior or posterior infarct, the posterobasal wall of the LV may become akinetic or aneurysmal. This can exert asymmetrical traction on the chordae, resulting in tethering of the posterior leaflet and an eccentric anteriorly directed jet of MR.

Key views
- Restriction of leaflet, systolic tenting of MV (0° ME four chamber, 45° ME mitral commissural, 90° ME two chamber, 120° ME LAX)
- Annulus size (120° ME LAX)
- LV assessment especially the posterobasal wall (90° ME two chamber, 0° TG mid SAX)

TTE/TEE for mitral stenosis

Determine the mitral valve area using the *pressure half-time (PHT)* method by measuring the deceleration slope of mitral inflow E-wave velocity (see Assessment of LV Diastolic Function, p. 464, and Fig. 12.8).

PHT is the time interval for the maximal pressure gradient (calculated as $4V_{max}^2$, where V_{max} is the peak E-wave velocity) to decrease to half its level. PHT can also be calculated as $0.29 \times DT$.

Valve area (cm²) = PHT/220

TEE can also be used in the assessment of suitability for percutaneous mitral balloon valvuloplasty (PMBV).

Contraindications to PMBV
- LA or LAA thrombus
- Greater than grade 2 MR

Mitral valve anatomy
1. Loss of mobility
2. Thickening
3. Calcification
4. Subvalvular thickening

Assign a score of 0–4 for each finding and take the sum. A score <8 predicts a favorable outcome following PMBV.

TEE for prosthetic valve dysfunction

TEE is a valuable method for assessing prosthetic valve function and their complications:

- Paravalvular leak
- Intravalvular leak from degeneration of tissue valve
- Prosthetic valve obstruction from pannus or thrombus
- Endocarditis, including valve dehiscence and abscess formation
- Patient–prosthesis mismatch

TEE assessment of mitral valve prosthesis

TEE is especially sensitive in detecting mitral regurgitation in association with prosthetic valves, because the left atrium is imaged in the foreground and is thus devoid of the artifacts generated by mechanical prostheses.

Paravalvular regurgitation

The sewing ring of the mechanical prosthesis appears as a bright ring attached to the mitral annulus. If a significant circumference of the sewing ring separates from the annulus (e.g., from endocarditis), a rocking motion of the valve occurs and is characteristic of valve dehiscence.

Key views

The mitral valve sewing ring should be identified and interrogated with color flow and continuous wave Doppler.
- 0° ME four chamber
- 90° ME two chamber
- 120° ME LAX views of the mitral valve

The motion of the prosthetic valve mechanism (e.g., tilting disc) should be assessed to ensure the discs are moving freely in 120° ME LAX view.

Paravalvular regurgitation is abnormal and may be seen early after valve implantation due to breakdown of the sutures attaching the valve ring to the annulus either from technical failure or infective endocarditis. Paravalvular leaks are more likely in the presence of a calcified mitral annulus.

Intravalvular regurgitation

Mechanical prosthetic valves typically exhibit a small volume of regurgitation during valve closure. These "closing jets" or "closing volumes" are a normal feature inherent in the design of mechanical prostheses and may prevent thrombosis by maintaining continuous blood flow across the valve surface. In general, they can be easily distinguished from pathological regurgitation.

Causes for abnormal intraprosthetic leak include pannus or thrombus preventing the occluder or disks from functioning properly.

Features of normal closing jets
- Short jets <3 cm length
- Narrow base <5 mm
- Early systolic leak

Bioprosthetic mitral prosthesis

The prosthetic valve should be assessed for the following:
- Prolapse or flail leaflets
- Thickened cusps (>3 mm—higher risk of dysfunction)
- Regurgitation (intravalvular and paravalvular)
- Stenosis/obstruction

Prosthetic mitral valve obstruction

This may be due to thrombus or pannus formation. Echocardiographic findings include the following:
- Limited movement of the occluder or disk.
- High peak transvalvular velocity (>2.5 m/sec) or a prolonged pressure half-time (>200 ms) (see Table 12.5).

Table 12.5 Upper limit of pressure half time (ms) for commonly used valves

Valve type	Max t1/2 (ms)
Starr–Edwards	170
St Jude	131
CarboMedics	117
Carpentier Edwards	171
Native valve	60

Echocardiography in aortic regurgitation

Both TTE and TEE are invaluable in determining the etiology of aortic regurgitation:
- Aortic root dilation
- Ascending aortic dissection causing cusp prolapse
- Vegetations causing cusp perforation or flail
- Congenital abnormalities (i.e., bicuspid valve)
- Acquired abnormalities (i.e., rheumatic heart disease)

Color Doppler is used to identify the origin and direction of the regurgitant jet, either central or eccentric. Occasionally, the regurgitant jet may impinge on the anterior mitral leaflet, limiting MV opening in diastole.

M-mode can be used to evaluate timing of valve opening and closure and, with color Doppler, measure the regurgitant jet width.

The severity of aortic regurgitation should be determined in all cases. These findings suggest severe regurgitation:
- Jet diameter/LVOT diameter >65%
- Vena contracta (diameter of the regurgitant jet at its narrowest downstream of the orifice) width >0.6 cm
- Pressure half-time <200 ms
- Systolic flow reversal in the descending aorta
- LV dilation (especially if chronic)
- Early diastolic mitral valve closure (best seen on M-mode)

Key TTE views
- PLAX, PSAX at aortic valve level, A5C

Key TEE views
- 30–45° ME AV SAX
- 120° ME AV LAX
- 0° deep TG LAX
- 120° TG LA

TEE for aortic valve prosthesis

Given the orientation of the aortic valve, the sewing ring will obstruct the view of the valve orifice for mechanical and stented tissue prostheses. Thus assessment of aortic paravalvular leak on 2-D imaging is limited compared to mitral valve assessment.

Continuous wave interrogation is not possible because the LVOT is orientated perpendicular to the ultrasound beam, when the aortic valve is assessed from the standard mid-esophageal views.

A combined TTE and TEE approach is required, because TTE is ideally suited for Doppler interrogation of the aortic valve given the parallel alignment of the ultrasound beam with aortic valve blood flow in the apical 5-chamber view.

Deep transgastric view

This view allows imaging of the aortic valve in the foreground and proper alignment of the Doppler signal from the aortic valve (0° deep TG LAX and 120° TG LAX views). This view is useful to assess the following:

- Movement of the aortic prosthetic valve mechanism
- Color flow Doppler interrogation for aortic regurgitation
- Continuous wave assessment of aortic regurgitation
- Continuous wave measurement aortic valve gradient

The use of the deep transgastric TEE view is especially useful for assessment of aortic prosthetic valve function when a mechanical mitral prosthesis is also present (see Box 12.7). This is because acoustic shadowing from the mitral valve obscures the LVOT in all mid-esophageal TEE views of the aortic valve. However, this view is not obtainable in all patients.

Regurgitation is most commonly intravalvular in bioprosthetic valves. The following may be visible on TEE:

- Cusp thickening (>3 mm predicts risk of valve failure)
- Cusp tear
- Cusp prolapse or flail
- Valve dehiscence

Mechanical aortic valves may normally exhibit a mild degree of early diastolic regurgitation, similar to that described above for mechanical mitral valves. Paravalvular regurgitation is usually abnormal and suggests valve dehiscence or technical failure.

Key views

The aortic valve prosthesis is assessed in the following:

- 30–45° ME AV SAX
- 120° ME AV LAX
- 0° deep TG LAX
- 120° TG LAX

Box 12.7 Echocardiographic assessment of prosthetic aortic valves

Normal mean transvalvular gradient

- St Jude Medical
- Medtronic Hall
- Bioprosthetic valve

- 14 ± 7 mmHg
- 14 ± 3 mmHg
- 13 ± 6 mmHg

Significant stenosis or obstruction likely

- Peak velocity of >4 m/sec or mean velocity of 3 m/sec
- Valve area by continuity equation <1 cm^2
- Mean gradient >26 mmHg
- Dimensionless index <0.25

Stentless aortic valves

- Freestyle or Toronto valve or aortic homografts do not have the disadvantage of a sewing ring casting an acoustic shadow on the aortic valve orifice and TEE gives excellent views of valve cusps. These valves may be indistinguishable from native valves on echocardiogram.

Intraoperative TEE

Indications

AHA Class I indications

- Valve repair, congenital heart surgery, HOCM surgery
- Hemodynamic compromise where LV function is unknown or has not responded to therapy
- Complex endocarditis surgery where perivalvular extension is suspected
- Complex valve replacement, such as homograft valve replacement with coronary reimplantation
- Ascending aortic dissection with aortic valve involvement
- Pericardial window surgery in posterior or loculated effusions
- Intracardiac device placement (i.e., LVAD)

AHA Class II indications

- Surgical procedures in patients at increased risk of myocardial ischemia, myocardial infarction, or hemodynamic disturbances
- Valve replacement
- Cardiac tumor resection, cardiac aneurysm repair, pericardial surgery
- During and after off-pump coronary bypass surgery for the evaluation of regional wall motion (see Box 12.8)
- Evaluation of myocardial perfusion, coronary anatomy, or graft patency
- Ascending aortic dissection without aortic valve involvement
- Cardiac trauma
- Intracardiac thrombectomy or pulmonary embolectomy
- Evaluating anastomotic sites following heart and/or lung transplantation
- Detect air emboli during cardiotomy

Key views to assess LV function (see Fig. 12.12)

- 0° ME four chamber
- 90° ME two chamber
- 120° ME LAX
- 0° TG mid SAX

Box 12.8 TEE in intraoperative and perioperative period (in ICU) to assess hemodynamic instability

- *Coronary artery bypass graft failure:* examine LV in all three coronary distributions to assess for regional wall motion abnormalities. The transgastric view shows all three coronary distributions in one view.
- *Hypovolemia:* reduced LV cavity size and end systolic cavity obliteration
- Pericardial effusion/hemopericardium
- Severe LV or RV failure
- Unsuspected severe mitral regurgitation
- Unsuspected aortic dissection

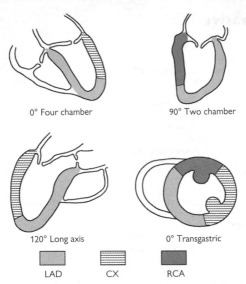

0° Four chamber

90° Two chamber

120° Long axis

0° Transgastric

LAD   CX   RCA

Figure 12.12 Assessment of LV function by TEE. Reprinted with permission from Shanewise JS, Cheung AT, Arouson S, et al. (1999). *J Am Soc Echocardiogr* 12(10):884–900.

Echocardiographic assessment of cardiac masses

Normal anatomy that should not be mistaken for pathology:
- *Chiari network* within the right atrium
- Eustachian valve near the inferior vena cava in the right atrium
- Trabeculations/pectinate muscles in the left atrial appendage
- Ridge separating left pulmonary vein and left atrial appendage
- Highly trabeculated left ventricle as seen in noncompaction
- False cords in left ventricle (anomalous mitral cordal apparatus not connected to valve leaflets)

Myxomas are the most common primary cardiac tumor and specific features can be delineated on echocardiogram:
- They are attached by a stalk to the interatrial septum near the fossa ovalis in 90% cases.
- 75% are in the LA.
- They may have speckled, cystic appearance with frond-like projections.
- They may be multiple. If they occur elsewhere they may be mistaken for thrombus (can be homogeneous in appearance) or other tumors.
- They may cause valve obstruction.

Fibroelastomas are benign tumors attached to cardiac valves. They have a frond-like appearance and may mimic vegetations or myxomas.

Primary malignant cardiac tumors and cardiac metastases can infiltrate the epicardium, myocardium, and endocardium, or they present as an intracavity mass. Pericardial involvement in malignant disease is often associated with a pericardial effusion.

Administration of ultrasound contrast can aid in the identification of intracardiac masses. Vascular masses, such as certain tumors, will take up contrast, whereas nonvascular structures such as thrombus or vegetation are less likely to enhance with contrast.

SPECT perfusion imaging

Single photon emission computed tomography (SPECT) is an important and well-validated tool used to diagnose obstructive epicardial coronary disease and provide important prognostic data in patients with known coronary disease. It is the standard test to evaluate myocardial perfusion in current practice.

SPECT involves the administration of radiolabeled perfusion tracers at rest and during exercise or pharmacological stress. The radionuclides decay and emit gamma photons, which are detected by a gamma camera.

Myocardial tracer uptake is proportional to regional blood blow, hence allowing one to assess for heterogeneity in perfusion as occurs in patients with physiologically significant coronary stenoses. In order for SPECT imaging to accurately diagnose coronary disease, the stressor, either exercise or pharmacologic, must induce a flow disparity between regions supplied by normal and stenotic arteries.

The sensitivity and specificity are 88% and 77%, respectively, for the diagnosis of coronary disease in intermediate-risk patients.

The two most commonly used radioisotopes in nuclear cardiology are thallium-201 and technetium-99m (sestamibi and tetrofosmin) (see Table 12.6). Technetium-99m labeled compounds are preferred because the higher energy gamma photons improve image resolution (less scattering and soft tissue attenuation) and there is little to no redistribution, which makes acquisition more practical and allows for reimaging, if necessary.

The major disadvantage with technetium-99m is hepatic and gastrointestinal uptake.

The primary components of a gamma camera are the following:
- Lead collimator, which allows only photons traveling at 90° to pass
- Sodium iodide crystal, converting energy of incoming photons into light
- Photomultiplier tubes, which amplify and convert the light signal into electrical current

Table 12.6 Radioisotopes used in nuclear cardiology

	Thallium-201	Technetium-99m
Production	Cyclotron	Mo-99m generator
Half-life	73 hr	6 hr
Extraction Fraction	85%	65%
Uptake mechanism	Na-K ATPase	Mitochondrial
Gamma-ray photopeak	70–80 keV	140 keV
Redistribution	Yes	Minimal

The emission data are reconstructed into tomographic slices by a computer for analysis. Standard image orientation includes short axis, vertical, and horizontal long axis views. The standard 16- or 17-segment nomenclature as described earlier for echocardiography is used for interpretation of perfusion defects.

Several computer software programs are commercially available for quantification of perfusion defects by normalizing perfusion throughout the myocardium and comparing it to a "normal" reference database.

Gated SPECT

The acquisition of emission data during SPECT is synced to the cardiac cycle via continuous ECG monitoring. The R-R interval is divided into a number of frames where the acquired counts at each position are stored. This provides an accurate assessment of LV volume, global and regional cardiac function.

Very irregular rhythms, such as atrial fibrillation, preclude accurate ECG-gating. Endocardial borders are defined and end-diastolic (EDV) and end-systolic (ESV) volumes are determined.

Ejection fraction (EF) = (EDV − ESV/EDV) × 100.

Interpretation of myocardial perfusion

Thorough and accurate interpretation requires review of the planar and rotating images, tomographic slices, and ECG gated data as well as the clinical history and indication for the test. Defect severity and extent should be determined as mild, moderate, or severe and small, medium, or large, respectively. The use of software for defect quantification can be helpful in this regard, but should not be solely relied upon. It is also important to remember that SPECT measures relative perfusion and not absolute blood flow.

During stress, blood flow in myocardial regions distal to a physiologically significant stenosis (i.e., > 50%–70%) is reduced, leading to decreased radiotracer activity and count density. This is what is measured with SPECT.

Interpretation

Fixed defect

- Similar decrease in count density at rest and during stress
- Represents infarct or scar
- Should see associated regional wall motion abnormality on gated movies

Reversible defect

- Decreased count density during stress with normalization at rest
- Represents ischemia (see Fig. 12.13)
- May or may not see regional wall motion abnormalities

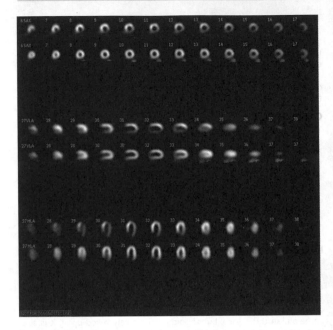

Figure 12.13 SPECT myocardial perfusion images during stress (top row) and at rest (bottom row) in the standard short axis (top), vertical long axis (middle), and horizontal long axis (bottom) views. In this example, there is inferior and inferolateral wall ischemia.

Partially reversible defect
- Decreased count density during stress with incomplete normalization at rest
- Implies peri-infarct ischemia

Artifacts
- Usually fixed, mild defects with normal regional function
- Due to photon attenuation/scattering, patient motion, instrumentation problems
- *Breast attenuation*—anterior, anterolateral defects
- *Diaphragmatic attenuation*—inferior wall defects
  - This can be reduced with prone imaging
  - Left lateral supine/decibutus imaging can aid in identification
- *Motion artifact* causes the "hurricane sign" and can be reduced or eliminated with motion correction software
- Attenuation correction algorithms can improve identification of artifacts and improve specificity of SPECT interpretation

Summed stress score (SSS)

This is a semiquantitative method of interpreting defect severity and extent. Each segment is assigned a score of 0 to 5, ranging from normal to absent uptake. The individual scores are added. The higher the SSS, the greater the annual cardiac event rate (see Table 12.7).

SPECT clinical applications

Coronary artery disease

Although exercise ECG is still the preferred initial test in evaluating inter-mediate-risk patients with chest pain, exercise perfusion imaging is indicated (ACC/AHA Guidelines) in the following situations:

• Pre-excitation/Wolf–Parkinson–White (WPW)
• Resting ST depression >1 mm (i.e., LVH, digoxin effect)
• Prior revascularization

Vasodilator stress perfusion imaging with adenosine or dipyridamole is recommended in patients with LBBB or ventricular pacemakers, as exercise SPECT often leads to false-positive septal defects. Patients who are unable to exercise should also undergo pharmacological (either adenosine/dipyridamole or dobutamine) stress perfusion imaging (Table 12.8).

Although exercise or vasodilator stress perfusion imaging is an AHA/ACC Class IIB indication as the initial test in patients with a normal resting

Table 12.7 Summed stress score

Score	Interpretation
0–3	Normal
4–8	Mild
9–13	Moderate
>13	Severe

Table 12.8 Indications for pharmacological stress agents

Indication	Preferred agent
Inability to exercise	Adenosine/dipyridamole
Asthma/COPD	Dobutamine
High grade AV block	Dobutamine
Caffeine/theophylline use	Dobutamine
LBBB	Adenosine/dipyridamole
Post-MI	Adenosine/dipyridamole

Specific α_{2a} receptor agonists are now available with fewer side effects.

ECG, this is an appropriate use according to the 2005 ACCF/ASNC Appropriateness Criteria.

Other useful applications of SPECT perfusion imaging in patients with coronary disease include the following:

- Determine lesion severity prior to planned revascularization
- Assess the response to medical therapy
- Risk stratification post-MI
- Risk stratification prior to noncardiac surgery

Results of SPECT perfusion imaging provide important prognostic information in patients with coronary disease, in addition to other clinical variables. The risk of future cardiac events is related to the extent and severity of perfusion defects.

Viability testing
- Thallium rest: 24-hour redistribution imaging. Normalization of perfusion on delayed imaging following reinjection implies viability.
- Technetium-99m. Tracer uptake >50% of normal implies viability.
- Normal regional function on gated SPECT imaging also suggests viable myocardium.

Acute chest pain
- Normal rest myocardial perfusion during active chest pain excludes ischemia/infarction with a negative predictive value of 99%.
- Stress myocardial SPECT perfusion imaging is a valuable diagnostic modality in the evaluation of low- to intermediate-risk patients with chest pain, a nondiagnostic ECG, and normal biomarkers in emergency department chest pain centers (ACC/AHA Class I indication).

High-risk findings on SPECT
Findings with 3%–5% risk of cardiac death or MI per year include the following:
- Transient ischemic dilatation due to global subendocardial ischemia during stress. There is increased risk even if there are no perfusion defects.
- Large reversible anterior wall defect
- LV systolic dysfunction post-stress
- Defects in multiple coronary territories
- Ischemic ECG changes during vasodilator stress
- Increased lung tracer uptake (>0.5 for thallium-201) due to increased pulmonary capillary wedge pressure

Balanced ischemia
Because SPECT imaging measures relative perfusion, a patient with multi-vessel coronary disease where perfusion is globally reduced with stress may have a relatively normal, though false-positive study.

Ancillary data from the stress protocol (especially abnormal exercise ECG or hemodynamics) and gated SPECT images (i.e., global or regional LV dysfunction) should be carefully reviewed for findings consistent with significant coronary disease.

PET scanning

Positron emission tomography (PET) is a nuclear imaging technique that uses short half-life radionuclides incorporated into radiopharmaceuticals allowing quantitative assessment of various aspects of cardiac function in different regions of the heart:

- Global and regional left ventricular function
- Myocardial blood flow
- Myocardial metabolism: glucose and fatty acid metabolism; myocardial oxygen consumption
- Pharmacology: β-adrenergic and muscarinic receptors; sympathetic innervation; myocardial ACE and angiotensin II receptors

Clinical applications

In current clinical practice, cardiac PET is used primarily for the assessment of myocardial viability and measuring myocardial perfusion in patients with equivocal SPECT imaging (i.e., obese patients) (see Fig. 12.14).

Myocardial perfusion

The radionuclides most commonly used in practice are Rb-82 and N-13 ammonia. The advantage of these PET tracers over SPECT tracers is the higher energy of the resulting photons (511 keV), which dramatically improves image resolution and test specificity by decreasing soft tissue attenuation and scatter.

The short half-life of these tracers, however, requires on-sight production and limits the application with exercise stress. Interpretation of tomographic PET imaging is similar to that described earlier for SPECT imaging.

Identification of myocardial viability

A valuable clinical application of PET scanning is the determination of *myocardial viability* in patients with ischemic cardiomyopathy who may benefit from surgical or percutaneous coronary revascularization. Studies have demonstrated that PET imaging has high sensitivity for predicting recovery of contractile function after revascularization and have also provided major insights into the mechanisms underlying left ventricular dysfunction in patients with coronary artery disease.

Perfusion is measured using either Rb-82 or N-13 as described above. Metabolism is assessed using 18-fluorine-labeled glucose (FDG), which is taken up by viable myocardial tissue. A perfusion–metabolism mismatch implies viable hibernating myocardium and predicts functional recovery following revascularization.

Research applications

The large variety of compounds available for study using PET permits interrogation of many facets of cardiac function, providing important in vivo mechanistic information (see Box 12.9). These measurements also allow analysis of the mechanisms underlying the benefit of established and novel therapies.

Examples include the following:

- Myocardial blood flow and microvascular function: ischemic heart disease, hypertrophic cardiomyopathy, dilated cardiomyopathy, aortic stenosis, syndrome X.

- Myocardial metabolism and cardiac energetics: ischemic cardiomyopathy, dilated cardiomyopathy.
- Cardiac autonomic function: hypertrophic cardiomyopathy, dilated cardiomyopathy, arryhthmogenic right ventricular dysplasia, autonomic neuropathy, long QT syndrome.

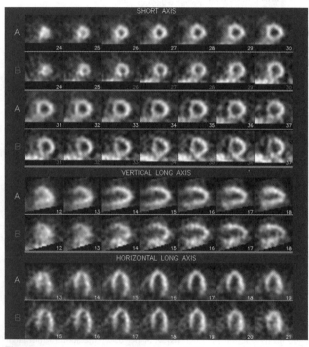

Figure 12.14 Example of an uninterpretable SPECT perfusion study in an obese patient due to significant attenuation, scattering, and poor spatial resolution (top). A Rb-82 PET study on the same patient clearly demonstrates normal myocardial perfusion (bottom).

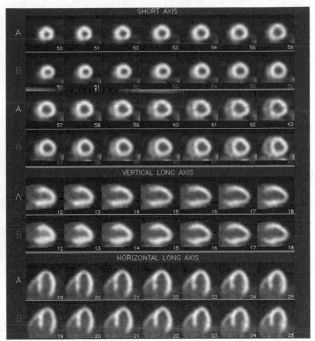

Figure 12.14 (*Cont'd.*).

Box 12.9 Comparison of PET with conventional SPECT imaging

Advantages
- Short half-life of radionuclides allows efficient same-day rest/stress protocols
  - Rb-82 $T_{1/2}$ is 75 seconds
  - N-13 $T_{1/2}$ is 10 minutes
  - O-15 water $T_{1/2}$ is 2 minutes
- Better spatial resolution
- Accurate attenuation correction, allowing absolute quantification of radiopharmaceutical concentration
- Can assess perfusion and metabolism

Disadvantages
- Expensive
- Limited availability
- Most tracers require cyclotron for production. Rb-82 is generator produced
- Difficult to perform with exercise stress because of short half-life of tracers

Equilibrium radionuclide angiography (ERNA)

ERNA, or multiple-gated (MUGA) blood pool imaging, is an accurate and reproducible noninvasive method for evaluating ventricular function using nuclear imaging techniques. Technetium-99m is the most commonly used radioisotope for this purpose.

A patient's red blood cells (RBCs) are labeled, either in vivo or in vitro, with reduced ^{99m}Tc and allowed to equilibrate in the blood pool. A gamma camera then obtains images (counts) gated to the ECG with each cardiac cycle divided into 16–32 frames where the counts are stored. Usually more than 2 million counts are acquired over hundreds of cardiac cycles for adequate image resolution.

As with gated SPECT, a regular rhythm is required for optimal performance. The standard views (see Fig. 12.15) are as follows:
- Anterior
- Left anterior oblique (LAO)
- Left lateral

A region of interest is drawn over the LV cavity, and LV ejection fraction is determined as

$$\frac{\text{End diastolic counts} - \text{End systolic counts}}{\text{End diastolic counts} - \text{Background counts}} \times 100$$

The most widely used application of this technique is measurement of LV systolic function. This modality is particularly valuable in serial assessment of LVEF in patients receiving cardiotoxic chemotherapy (i.e., doxorubicin). Other applications include the following:
- Ventricular volumes
- Regional wall motion
- RV function
- Diastolic function (peak filling rate, time to peak filling)
- Stress testing

An alternative to ERNA is first-pass radionuclide ventriculography. Instead of using radiolabeled RBCs, a bolus of ^{99m}Tc-labeled radiopharmaceutical is injected and tracer activity is measured in the superior vena cava, through the right heart and pulmonary circulation, and into the left heart and systemic circulation. This technique can be used to evaluate LV and RV function, as well as to detect right–left shunts.

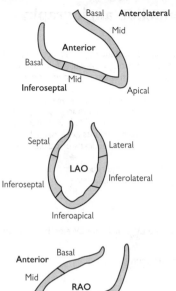

Figure 12.15 Standard ERNA views. LAO, left anterior oblique; RAO, right anterior oblique.

Cardiac CT

Cardiac CT has recently become a powerful tool to study cardiac anatomy. CT scanning involves measuring the attenuation of a fan-shaped X-ray beam projected around a patient, using multiple detectors. The 3-D projection data set is then reformatted to display images in any plane.

The most commonly used devices in practice today are multidetector or multislice CT scanners (MDCT). MDCT scanners use rotating gantries with a temporal resolution high enough to allow imaging of the beating heart as long as the cardiac rhythm is regular and fairly slow (i.e., <70 bpm). β-Blockers are often given to achieve this.

Newer single-source MDCT scanners acquire 256 or 312 slices per gantry rotation. Dual-source scanners have improved temporal resolution that does not necessitate slow heart rates.

Electron beam CT (EBCT) has been used extensively for calcium scoring. One of the advantages of CT over conventional noninvasive testing (i.e., SPECT imaging) is the rapidity of image acquisition. A comprehensive cardiac CT scan can be acquired in a matter of seconds.

Common applications of cardiac CT include the following:

- *Pericardial disease:* measurement of pericardial thickness and determine presence of calcification
- *Coronary artery calcium (CAC) scoring*
- *CT coronary angiography*

A concern with cardiac CT is incidental noncardiac findings. These images should be reviewed by or interpreted with a trained radiologist.

Another concern, particularly with newer multislice scanners, is the radiation exposure to the patient, which needs to be considered when ordering these tests. ECG-triggered tube current modulation and prospective gating can reduce the radiation dose administered.

Coronary calcium scoring

Because calcium highly attenuates X-rays, CT scanning can detect calcified atheromas with great sensitivity. The amount of calcium can be quantified using the *Agatson score*, which is proportional to the total burden of coronary atherosclerosis (Table 12.9).

Although the presence of coronary calcium does not necessarily imply obstructive coronary stenosis, a normal calcium score can exclude significant coronary disease with very high accuracy. Likewise, in symptomatic patients with chest pain, the presence of coronary calcium predicts significant coronary stenosis (>50%) with high sensitivity, albeit moderate specificity.

In asymptomatic patients, an abnormal coronary calcium score is a risk factor for future cardiac events and may aid in primary prevention strategies, especially in patients at intermediate risk based on traditional scores (i.e., Framingham).

Age- and gender-specific thresholds should be applied when interpreting a calcium score.

Table 12.9 CT coronary artery calcium scoring

Score	Plaque burden
0	None
1–99	Mild
100–399	Moderate
≥400	Severe

ACC/AHA 2007 Consensus
- Routine screening with CAC scoring is not recommended in asymptomatic patients with low or high risk for coronary disease based on Framingham risk score.
- In patients at intermediate risk, a CAC is reasonable if the results will reclassify the patient as low or high risk and alter management.

Coronary CT angiography

This technique evaluates coronary anatomy, unlike stress perfusion imaging with assesses the functional significance of a coronary stenosis. Current scanners can provide exquisitely detailed images of coronary anatomy, including bypass grafts.

Like invasive angiography, coronary CT requires the administration of iodinated contrast dye to enhance the vascular lumen and is thus contraindicated in patients with severe dye allergy or those at high risk for contrast nephropathy.

Significant coronary artery calcification and coronary stents can lead to reconstruction artifacts, which may limit the ability to accurately interpret the images. Vessel segments <1.5 mm in diameter may also be difficult to visualize.

Per-patient sensitivity and specificity for significant (>50%) stenosis are 98% and 88%, respectively. Hybrid CT/SPECT scanners are being studied with the advantage of allowing the physiological as well as anatomical extent of coronary disease to be measured.

Appropriate indications for CT coronary angiography are as follows:
- Congenital coronary anomalies
- Evaluate coronary bypass grafts not seen during cardiac catheterization in symptomatic patients
- As an alternative to cardiac catheterization in patients with typical symptoms or abnormal stress testing who either refuse an invasive procedure or are at high risk of complications
- Evaluate coronary anatomy in symptomatic intermediate-risk patients with nondiagnostic or equivocal stress test results

Coronary CT is not recommended for patients with a low or high pre-test likelihood of significant coronary disease.

Cardiac magnetic resonance imaging (CMR)

In the past decade, cardiac magnetic resonance imaging (CMR) has emerged as an important investigative and clinical tool in the diagnosis and management of a variety of cardiovascular diseases (see Box 12.10).

Technique
- It uses signals produced from protons (H^+ ions, abundant in vivo due to the large proportion of body being water).
- When a magnetic field is applied, the protons align both parallel (majority) and antiparallel to the field with a net vector between.
- Net vector can be altered by applying differing types of short radiofrequency pulses.
- On cessation of this secondary pulse, the vector returns or relaxes to its original position and releases energy in the form of radiowaves.
- There are two forms of net vector relaxation: longitudinal (T1) and transverse (T2).

Types of CMR
- *Spin-echo* is used to assess morphology. There is higher soft-tissue contrast, and flowing blood appears dark.
- *Gradient-echo* is used to assess shunts, valvular lesions, great vessels and LV function. Flowing blood (i.e., flowing protons) across magnetic gradient has magnetic vectors with phase shift proportional to flow velocity, thus allowing assessment of these dynamic lesions. It has lower soft-tissue contrast with blood flow shown by high signal intensity.

Box 12.10 Cardiac magnetic resonance imaging

Advantages
- Rapid scanning sequences
- Gives anatomical, hemodynamic and functional information from same scan
- Noninvasive
- High spatial resolution
- No ionizing radiation

Disadvantages
- Claustrophobia—tight, enclosed space within scanner
- Lack of adequate patient monitoring
- Expensive
- Metallic prosthetic implants—becoming less of a problem

Uses of CMR

Congenital heart disease
- Anatomical and hemodynamic assessment of complex abnormalities of the heart and great vessels.

Ventricular function
- Assessment of RV/LV function, volume, and mass
- Assessing response to novel therapies (e.g., stem cell therapy)

Aortic disease
- Aortic dissection—origin, extent, and organ involvement
- Aneurysms—serial scans to assess progression
- Intramural hematoma, aortic atheroma, penetrating ulcers

Valvular heart disease
- Echocardiography remains the mainstay of assessment.
- CMR use may be more common as specificity and sensitivity improve.

Cardiomyopathies
- Arrhythmogenic RV dysplasia (ARVD)—RV enlargement/aneurysms, RV dysfunction, fatty replacement of RV myocardium
- DCM, myocarditis, HOCM, sarcoidosis—mid-myocardial or subepicardial fibrosis and perfusion abnormalities

Cardiac tumors and pericardial disease
- Anatomical localization and extracardiac involvement
- Assess vascularity of tumor with gradient-echocardiogram

Coronary artery disease
- Coronary anatomy (inferior to CT)
- Pharmacological stress perfusion with first-pass gadolinium uptake
- Assessment of infarct size and viability by delayed myocardial enhancement with gadolinium (see Fig. 12.16)

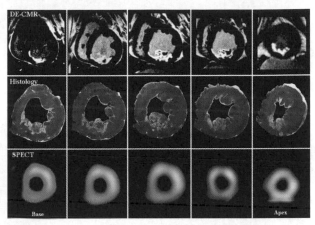

Figure 12.16 Comparison of in vivo delayed-enhancement CMR images (upper panel) to histopathology (middle panel) in a canine with subendocardial inferior wall infarction. Corresponding SPECT-sestamibi images are also shown for comparison (bottom panel). Adapted with permission from Wagner A, Mahrholdt H, Holly TA, et al. (2003). *Lancet* 361(9355):374–379.

Metallic prostheses and CMR

Ferromagnetism refers to metallic compounds attracted by a magnetic field; it initially referred to ferrous compounds and their properties in a magnetic field (i.e., attraction). Four other metals are also strongly magnetic: cobalt, dysprosium, gadolinium, and nickel. Alloys of these compounds will also exhibit magnetism to some degree.

Most human prosthetic implants are not strongly magnetic as they have impurities added to the iron to give them added strength and antioxidant properties.

Potential for causing injury with CMR and metallic objects

There are three main mechanisms for this (see also Table 12.10):

- *Projectile injury* refers to external adjunctive equipment, e.g., O_2 cylinders, forceps, scissors, etc., that is in the MR room. A strong magnetic field could launch these items across the room with obvious consequences. Ferrous compounds such as these must therefore be barred from the room or special "MR-safe" equipment used.
- *Implanted prostheses* Injury can result from internal movement of these prostheses. Potential for movement will depend on magnetic properties of the device and on the restraining tissue surrounding it. Thus hip prosthesis has less potential to cause damage than an intracranial arterial clip.
- *Electrical currents* CMR can induce electrical currents in devices with conductance properties, which can cause heating and thermal injury. Examples include pacing wires, guide wires, and PA catheters.

Table 12.10 Risk associated with CMR use in patients with metallic devices

Device	Risk*
Coronary stents	Currently available stents are safe and can be tested <3T any time after implantation
Other vascular stents	Similar to coronary stents
Guide wires	May cause thermal injury (newer CMR-safe ones developed for CMR intervention)
Prosthetic valves/rings	All valves appear safe.
Pacemakers and ICDs	Potential for movement, thermal injury, and electrical inhibition CMR use is associated with excess mortality, thus it is NOT currently recommended
Intracardiac catheters	Polyurethane and PVC ones are safe. Those with metallic component (e.g., PA catheters) will cause thermal injury and are NOT safe
IABP/LVAD	NOT safe due to thermal injury, movement, and mechanical malfunction
ECG leads	Standard metallic leads have been associated with burns. Newer carbon-based CMR-compatible leads are available
Sternal wires/ epicardial pacing wires	Safe, although may cause artifacts

*NB Always check with the MRI department if concerned.

Invasive electrophysiology

Mechanism of tachycardias

Knowledge of how arrhythmia are initiated and perpetuated is fundamental to understanding the techniques described in this chapter.

The electrical wavefront

The excitable impulse is generated at the cell membrane by the action potential (see Chapter 9). As one cell depolarizes, it causes a reduction in negativity of the resting potential in the adjacent cells, causing the adjacent cells to reach threshold potential and depolarize.

The shape, orientation, and presence of gap junctions between myocardial cells allow the rapid spread of depolarization, which can be described as an electrical *wavefront*. After a cell has depolarized, it cannot depolarize again until it repolarizes over a fixed period of time, the *refractory period*. Cells that are able to depolarize are *excitable*, and those that cannot are *refractory*.

In sinus rhythm (SR) the source of these wavefronts is the sinoatrial (SA) node, and they are conducted from the atria to ventricles via the atrioventricular node (AVN). SA nodal impulses are initiated at intervals largely regulated by the autonomic nervous system and circulating catecholamines. This control is lost in tachyarrhythmia and heart rates are inappropriate.

Conduction block

A wavefront will propagate as long as there are excitable cells in its path. Anatomical barriers such as the mitral valve annulus, vena cava, and aorta do not contain myocardial cells; therefore, the progression of wavefronts is halted there. This is described as *fixed conduction block*, as block is always present. Dead cells are another important source of fixed conduction block, e.g., the left ventricular scar of a myocardial infarction (MI).

Functional conduction block describes block that is only present under certain conditions. An example is myocardial ischemia, which may alter the electrical properties of myocytes such that they do not conduct.

It is also a functional block that prevents a wavefront from turning back on itself, as the cells behind the leading edge are temporarily refractory and force the wavefront to continue in one direction. Other causes of functional block are cyanosis, myocardial stretch, and the rate and direction of the wavefront.

Arrhythmia mechanisms

Three distinct mechanisms are described:
1. Enhanced automaticity
2. Reentry
3. Triggered activity

The first two mechanisms account for nearly all clinical tachycardias and their characteristics are compared in Table 13.1.

Table 13.1 Characteristics of automatic and reentry tachycardias*

	Automatic	Reentry
Autonomic sensitivity? (e.g., to exercise, emotion)	Often	Unusual*
Reproducible induction and termination by programmed stimulation	No	Yes
Entrainment of the tachycardia by pacing?	No	Yes
Induced by atropine/ isoproterenol infusion?	Yes	May augment induction by pacing
Related to metabolic causes	Often	Unusual
Onset/offset	May be gradual (warm up and down)	Sudden
Specific tachycardias caused	Inappropriate sinus tachycardia, focal atrial tachycardia, focal AF, junctional tachycardia	SNRT, macro-reentrant atrial tachycardia, AF, AVNRT, AVRT, VT

* The conduction properties of, e.g., the AV node, are influenced by autonomic tone. Spontaneous or drug-induced changes in this may then influence the development of reentry tachycardias such as AV-nodal reentry tachycardia (AVNRT). AF, atrial fibrillation; AVRT, atrioventricular reentrant tachycardia; SNRT, sinus node reentrant tachycardia; VT, ventricular tachycardia.

Mechanism of arrhythmias

Enhanced automaticity

If a nidus of myocardial cells depolarizes faster (rapid phase 4 of the action potential) than the SA node, it will act as the source of wavefronts that conduct through the heart. It may be atrial or ventricular, but if it occurs in the atria it will override the SA node. As it occurs from a single site it is often termed *focal*.

Common sites are where myocardial cells suddenly change shape or size or are under abnormal pressures, such as the junction of veins and atrium (SVC, PVs), crista terminalis, coronary sinus (CS), AV node area, mitral/tricuspid ring, and ventricular outflow tracts.

Reentry

Reentry accounts for >75% of clinical arrhythmias. It is caused by a perpetually propagating wavefront that it is constantly meeting excitable myocardium.

For reentry to occur, at least two distinct pathways must exist around an area of conduction block. This is best described using the example of VT due to reentry around a LV myocardial scar (see Fig. 13.1).

1. A myocardial scar acts as an area of block, around which a normal sinus wavefront passes via normal myocardium (A) and slowly through it via diseased myocardium (B)—hence two distinct pathways.
2. The sinus beat is followed closely by a ventricular ectopic, which is conducted around A normally but is blocked in B, which is still refractory following the last sinus beat.
3. The distal end of B, however, is now excitable and the wavefront passes backward up B, which has had time to fully recover by the time it reaches the proximal end. Conduction is sufficiently slow up B that now A is excitable again and the wavefront can pass down A.

Thus a reentrant wavefront has been formed that is constantly meeting excitable myocardium.

Triggered activity

This has features of both of the above mechanisms. It is caused by spontaneous (hence automatic) *after-depolarizations* (ADs) occurring late in phase 3 (*early ADs*) or in phase 4 (*delayed ADs*) of the action potential. These ADs, however, are often triggered by premature beats and thus are inducible (like reentry). If these ADs reach the threshold level, then a single or burst of action potentials is set off.

The ADs can be induced experimentally by ischemia, QT-prolonging drugs, cell injury, or low potassium. This mechanism underlies torsades de pointes and arrhythmias due to digoxin toxicity.

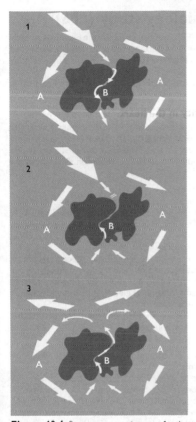

Figure 13.1 Reentry as a mechanism of tachycardia.
1 Normal sinus beat passing around and through scar.
2 Ectopic beat passing around but blocked through scar.
3 Reentry circuit of tachycardia.
Dark gray represents scar; light gray, normal myocardium; and white arrows represent electrical wavefronts.

The electrophysiology study (EPS)

The electrophysiology study (EPS) is most useful for the diagnosis of tachycardia. When tachycardia has been documented or is strongly suspected, it is generally the first part of a combined procedure with catheter ablation designed to cure the arrhythmia.

In EP it is usual to discuss cycle lengths (in ms) rather than heart rates, e.g., 60/min = 1000 ms; 100/min = 600 ms; 150/min = 400 ms.

Mapping electrical activity in the heart

The EPS is wrongly considered to be complex. Fundamentally, it is just recording of the heart's electrical signals during sinus rhythm, arrhythmia, or in response to pacing at specific sites. The ECG provides a great deal of this information and so a full 12 lead ECG is recorded throughout the procedure.

The intracardiac electrogram (Egram)

The ECG summarizes the entire cardiac activation. By placing 2-mm electrodes directly on the heart's endocardial surface, the electrical activity at precise locations is known. The Egram is therefore much narrower than the ECG and is best appreciated at 100 mms^{-1} sweep speed, four times faster than a standard ECG recording.

Either the potential difference between two closely spaced electrodes (a bipolar electrogram) or that between one electrode and infinity (a unipolar electrogram) can be recorded. The unipolar electrogram is more accurate regarding direction and location of electrical activity; however, it is subject to much greater interference.

A pacing current can be passed through any of these electrodes. Standard catheter location is shown in Figure 13.2.

Pacing protocols

Pacing in the EPS is done in a predefined manner, termed *programmed stimulation*. This has three forms:

1. *Incremental pacing*: the pacing interval is started just shorter than the sinus interval and lowered in 10-ms steps until block occurs or a predetermined lower limit (often 300 ms) is reached.
2. *Extrastimulus pacing*: following a train of eight paced beats at a fixed cycle length, a further paced beat (the extrastimulus) is introduced at a shorter coupling interval (the time between the last stimulus of the drive and the first extrastimulus). The stimuli of the drive train are conventionally termed S1, the first extrastimulus S2, the second extrastimulus S3, and so on. Extrastimuli can also be introduced after sensed heart beats *(singles in sinus* or *sensed extras)*.
3. *Burst pacing* is pacing at a fixed cycle length for a predetermined time.

Catheters have been passed into the right heart from sheaths in the femoral and subclavian veins under fluoroscopic guidance. These images from the right anterior oblique (above) and left anterior oblique (below) demonstrate the standard positions at the high right atrium (HRA) close to the SA node, on the His bundle (HIS), and at the RV apex (RVA), as well as a catheter passed through the os of the coronary sinus (CS), which wraps around the left posterior atrioventricular groove. From this position Egrams are recorded from the left atrium and ventricle. The CS catheter is often inserted via the left or right subclavian veins.

The intracardiac electrocardiograms conventionally ordered are HRA, His, CS, and RV (not displayed here), with an ECG lead at the bottom. On each catheter, bipolar electrode pairs are then ordered proximal to distal. In SR the activation starts at the HRA, passes across the His, and then along the CS catheter proximally to distally. Earliest ventricular activation is at the RVA (where the Purkinje fibers insert).

Normal *intervals* are PA 25–55 ms; atrium–His (AH) = 50–120 ms; His–ventricular (HV) = 35–55 ms; QRS <120 ms; and corrected QT <440 ms men, <460 ms women.

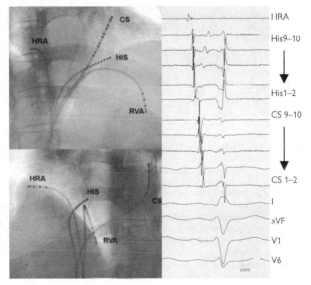

Figure 13.2 Standard positions of catheters in the EPS and intracardiac electrograms at those sites.

Uses of the EPS

Sinus node function

The *corrected sinus node recovery time (CSNRT)* and *sinoatrial conduction time (SACT)* are both measures of SAN function. Unfortunately, they are unreliable tests, as SAN function is greatly influenced by autonomic tone, drugs, and observer error. SAN dysfunction is best assessed with ambulatory monitoring and exercise testing.

EPS can be considered for patients who have symptoms consistent with bradyarrhythmia (syncope) and for whom noninvasive evaluations have been unrevealing. EPS for SAN function has higher specificity than sensitivity. Therefore, a positive test is much more informative than a negative one.

AV conduction (see Table 13.2)

Heart block

The degree of heart block is assessed via the ECG, which can also suggest the level (i.e., AV node or His Purkinje system). The true level of block is easily ascertained via EPS. The AH time is prolonged in nodal block and the HV interval, in infranodal block. The AH (but not the HV) time may be shortened by exercise, isoproterenol, or atropine and prolonged by vagal maneuvers.

AV nodal function

This is assessed in both the anterograde (A to V) and retrograde (V to A) directions, using both incremental pacing and extrastimuli. By incremental pacing in the HRA, conduction is observed in the His and RVA until block occurs. The longest pacing interval at which block occurs in the AVN is the anterograde Wenckebach cycle length (WCL).

Normal values are <500 ms; however, this increases with age and autonomic influences. The retrograde WCL is also measured, although absent VA conduction can be normal.

Extrastimulus pacing is also performed from the HRA. As the coupling interval between S1 and S2 is reduced, AV conduction is observed. The longest S1S2 interval at which AV block occurs is the anterograde AVN effective refractory period (ERP). This is usually measured at drive trains of 600 and 400 ms. If VA conduction is present, the retrograde AVN ERP is measured.

Decremental conduction

This is the key physiological property of the AV node. As the interval between successive impulses passing through the AV node decreases, the conduction velocity within the AV node also decreases. In AV conduction this is manifest as a prolongation of the AH (and AV) interval as the atrial pacing interval decreases.

This phenomenon can be observed during incremental and extrastimulus pacing. During extrastimulus pacing if the AH interval is plotted against the S1S2 (= A1A2), an anterograde conduction curve can be plotted.

Table 13.2 A standard basic electrophysiology study

Pacing protocol	Measure	Comments
1. Sinus rhythm	Basic sinus intervals (PA, AH, HV, QRS, corrected QT)	Is there AV conduction block?
2. Incremental ventricular pacing (IVP)	RWCL	Is VA conduction present? If so, is atrial activation normal and decremental?
3. Incremental atrial pacing (IAP)	AWCL	Is AV conduction decremental? Is pre-excitation manifest during pacing?
4. Extrastimulus pacing from atrium at 600 and 400 ms	Anterograde AVNERP at 600 and 400 ms	Is AV conduction decremental? Is pre-excitation manifest during pacing? Is there dual AV-nodal physiology?
5. Extrastimulus pacing from ventricle at 600 and 400 ms	Retrograde AVNERP at 600 and 400 ms	Is VA conduction present? If so, is atrial activation normal and decremental?
6. Arrhythmia induction from atrium. Use 2–4 extrastimuli, sensed extrastimuli, and burst pacing.	.	Note pacing protocol that induces arrhythmia. Is it reproducible? Compare arrhythmia induced to clinical arrhythmia
7. If VT suspected, perform PES with up to 3 extrastimuli	VERP at 600 and 400 ms	Observe induced arrhythmia
8. Repeat steps 2–7 during isoproterenol infusion.		Essential for tachycardias associated with enhanced automaticity

AVNERP, atrioventricular nodal effective refractory period; AWCL, anterograde Wenckebach cycle length; PES, programmed extra stimuli; RWCL, retrograde Wenckebach cycle length; VERP, ventricular effective refractory period.

Dual AV nodal physiology

It is possible in many patients (but not all) to identify two electrical connections between the atrial myocardium surrounding the compact AV node and the node itself, which have different conduction properties. The *slow pathway* has slower conduction velocity but a shorter ERP than the *fast pathway*, with faster conduction and a longer ERP. This is observed by plotting an anterograde conduction curve.

For longer A1A2 intervals AV conduction is preferentially via the fast pathway; however, once the fast pathway ERP is reached, conduction is via the slow pathway and consequently the AH time suddenly prolongs. This is called an AH interval *jump* and is defined as a lengthening of the AH by >50 ms, following reduction in the A1A2 interval by 10 ms (see Fig. 13.3).

Dual AV-nodal pathways are the substrate for AVNRT.

Identifying abnormal AV connections—accessory pathways

In normal hearts there is only one connection between the atrium and ventricle, the AV node. Activation of the atrium (during V pacing) or ventricle (during A pacing or SR) should therefore start at the AV node. Accessory pathways (AP) do not decrement. Their presence can be identified by both abnormal activation patterns and conduction physiology using incremental and extrastimulus pacing.

Atrial pacing

As the AV node decrements, a greater proportion of ventricular activation will occur via an AP if present. Thus, nondecremental AV conduction times and broadening of the QRS complex will be observed as the pacing interval shortens. If the ERP of the AP is longer than the ERP of the AV node, then the QRS will suddenly narrow and the AV time suddenly prolong when the AP blocks.

Ventricular pacing

The normal order of atrial activation is His, then CS (proximal to distal), and finally the HRA, termed *concentric* activation. If the atrium is activating via an AP, an *eccentric* activation pattern is usually observed. The site of the earliest atrial activation will localize the AP. Nondecremental VA conduction is also seen.

Induction of arrhythmia

The presence of an AP, dual AV-nodal physiology, or ventricular scar provides the substrate for a tachycardia but does not necessarily indicate that it will occur. A diagnosis can only be confirmed by inducing the tachycardia.

In addition to the pacing techniques described here, burst pacing, extrastimulus pacing with multiple extrastimuli, and sensed extras are used. If this fails, pacing maneuvers can be repeated during an isoproterenol infusion (1–4 μg/min) or boluses (1–2 μg). This is particularly important for tachycardias due to enhanced automaticity. "Aggressive" induction protocols increase the likelihood of inducing an unwanted, nonspecific arrhythmia such as AF or VF.

Once a tachycardia is initiated, it is useful to compare it with a 12 lead ECG of the tachycardia recorded during symptoms to ensure that this is the clinical arrhythmia. How individual tachycardias are diagnosed and treated is considered in subsequent sections.

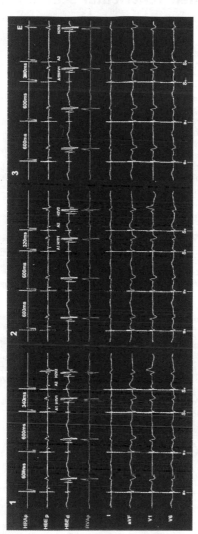

Figure 13.3 Example of AH interval jump during extrastimulation.

Programmed ventricular stimulation

An EP study focusing on induction of ventricular arrhythmias (the VT stimulation study) has been used to risk stratify for sudden cardiac death (SCD), to decide on the effectiveness of antiarrhythmic drugs and determine the need for ICD therapy. Evidence has now accumulated, however, that its predictive value is limited and that, in general, decisions regarding ICD therapy should be based on other risk factors, particularly LV function.

The EP study can be useful in the diagnosis and assessment of VT/VF and prior to ICD implant for other reasons:

- Does a patient with borderline LVEF (35%–40%) have inducible VT?
- To assess suitability for VT ablation (e.g., bundle branch VT)
- Are other arrhythmias present and easily induced?
- To aid programming of device:
  - Is VT well tolerated hemodynamically?
  - Is it easily terminated with overdrive pacing?
  - Is there VA conduction? During V pacing or VT?

Programmed ventricular stimulation is performed using the protocol devised by Wellens or a modification thereof (see Box 13.1).

Clinical indications

- Documented symptomatic tachycardia (as first stage of diagnostic and ablation procedure)
- Risk stratification for sudden cardiac death
- Suspected but not documented symptomatic tachycardia (diagnostic only)
- Wolff–Parkinson–White syndrome
- Unexplained syncope (suspicious of arrhythmic cause)
- Symptomatic SAN or AVN heart block suspected but not documented

Thus the pacing protocol becomes gradually more aggressive. The more aggressive the induction protocol, the more nonspecific the result may be. The most useful result is induction of a sustained monmorphic VT with one or two extrastimuli. This indicates a potential substrate for ventricular arrhythmias.

Nonsustained VT, polymorphic VT, and VF induced by an aggressive protocol are all nonspecific results and of little predictive value.

Box 13.1 Protocol for programmed ventricular stimulation

End points for the EPS
- >10 beats of inducible and reproducible ventricular tachycardia
- Completion of protocol without induction of ventricular tachycardia

Pacing sequences from RV apex
- *Step 1:* single extrastimulus at decreasing coupling intervals to ventricular refractoriness at 3 drive cycle lengths (600, 500, 400)
- *Step 2:* double extrastimuli at decreasing coupling intervals to ventricular refractoriness at 3 drive cycle lengths
- *Step 3:* triple extrastimuli at decreasing coupling intervals to ventricular refractoriness at 3 drive cycle lengths
- *Step 4:* 8–12 incrementally paced beats at decreasing coupling intervals to ventricular refractoriness

If no ventricular arrhythmia is induced, repeat from RV outflow tract.

If no ventricular arrhythmia is induced, isoproterenol can be infused and pacing repeated.

New technologies

EP procedures have become increasingly complex (e.g., for AF or congenital heart disease) and require greater radiation exposure. Both of these problems have been overcome by nonfluoroscopic, 3-D mapping systems. A computer-generated image of the cardiac chamber of interest is formed and onto this the electrical activation in the heart and the EP catheter location are superimposed (see Fig. 13.4).

In some cases it is now possible to perform a complete EP study and ablation without the use of X-ray. Also, 3-D CT or MR images of the patient can be imported and integrated with the electrical map to create a 3-D electroanatomical map of the chamber of interest.

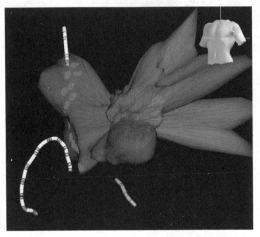

Figure 13.4 An Ensite NavX image of the left atrium. The torso demonstrates that this is an LAO projection. The catheter positions are located without the use of X-ray.

Catheter ablation

In medical terms, *ablation* is the removal of tissue. As many tachycardias depend on discreet foci or pathways to be sustained, they are amenable to cure by destruction of these areas.

Energy sources for ablation

Radiofrequency (RF) energy

Cells are destroyed by heating >50°C. The RF generator delivers an alternating current of 500–750 KHz between the active catheter electrode and a large indifferent electrode placed on the patient's skin. The ions within cells immediately adjacent to the catheter are agitated and generate heat (resistive heating). The heating power generated in this way dramatically decreases as the distance form the catheter increases. The remaining heat is conducted away to the surrounding tissue.

A lesion of ~5 mm depth is formed after 30–60 seconds, which is sufficient to destroy the full thickness of atrial myocardium. Catheters are 7 Fr with tip electrodes of 4 mm as standard or 8 to 10 mm where larger lesions are desired.

If the temperature approaches 100°C, boiling of cell water occurs, generating steam that escapes either by exploding through the endocardium, causing a large lesion (cavitation, "steam-pop"), or the pericardium (perforation + tamponade).

Temperature is monitored at the tip of the catheter and power delivery automatically limited to prevent such overheating. The generator allows the power, temperature, and duration of each RF delivery to be adjusted.

Cooled RF

The tip of the catheter is cooled during RF by the flow of blood, so the hottest part of an RF lesion is 1 mm beneath the surface. Stasis of flow occurs as the lesion is formed, hence the temperature rises, limiting the amount of power delivered and thus the size of the lesion.

Normal saline passed through a lumen (closed or open) in the tip of the catheter at a rate of 10–30 mL/hr continuously cools the catheter, allows higher powers and bigger lesions to be formed. This is needed where the myocardium is thick, e.g., left ventricle (VT) or Eustachian ridge (typical atrial flutter).

Low-flow (2 mL/hr) external irrigation with RF ablation may be useful for keeping the tip of the catheter free of thrombus, thus reducing stroke risk during RF in the LA or LV.

Cryoablation

Completely contained within the specialized ablation catheter, liquid nitrous oxide is released into the tip, rapidly vaporizes, and removes heat from the tissue in contact with the catheter. The gas is rapidly recycled back to the catheter console.

The tissue temperature (monitored at the tip of the catheter) falls to −30°C, at which stage there is reversible loss of cell function. If an appropriate response is seen (e.g., loss of pre-excitation during AP ablation), then the tissue is further cooled to −60°C for 4 minutes to cause permanent destruction. The formation of ice adheres the catheter to the tissue, making it very stable. If, however, an adverse change is seen (e.g., AVN block) at −30°C, the tissue can be rewarmed.

Other

Other energy sources under investigation are microwave, ultrasound, and laser.

Catheter ablation: complications

SVTs (other than AF) are cured in >90% of cases with ablation. For AVNRT, the rate is >97%. Registry data demonstrate that significant complications occur in <2%–3% of cases; however, this varies with specific procedures.

Major complications

- Death (0.1%–0.3%)
- *Stroke* (0.2%). Risk is higher for left-sided procedures. Minimize risk by: using preoperative TEE, intraoperative heparin guided by activated clotting time, postoperative anticoagulation (aspirin or warfarin), irrigated catheters, continuous pressured heparinized saline administration through left-sided sheaths, and cryoablation.
- *Cardiac tamponade* (0.5%–1%). Risk is higher with trans-septal puncture, but can occur even during the diagnostic procedure. BP is monitored throughout the procedure and in any hypotensive episode tamponade is suspected. The EP lab should have a readily available ECHO machine and emergency pericardial aspiration sets.
- *AV nodal block* (1%). High risk for septal accessory pathway (AP) or AVNRT (slow-pathway) ablation. During RF continuously image the catheter position and atrial and ventricular electrograms. If AV, VA block, or catheter movement occurs, STOP. Cryoablation may be preferred for high-risk cases.
- *Coronary artery spasm/MI:* Transient ST elevation and chest pain may occur without any long-term effect due to spasm.
- *Pneumothorax* occurs only if the subclavian approach is used for catheter placement.
- *X-ray exposure*. EP cases may be prolonged. Deterministic effects such as skin damage can be avoided with attention to fluoroscopy technique. Women of fertile age should be counseled and have pregnancy tests. Nonfluoroscopic catheter location (Carto, LocaLisa, Ensite NavX) is increasingly used.

Minor complications

- *Bruising/hematoma* is common at the puncture site if anticoagulation is used.
- *Chest pain* occurs transiently during energy delivery; IV opiates or benzodiazepines may be necessary.
- *Vasovagal episode* often occurs during initial percutaneous sheath insertion or at sheath removal. Ensure that patient has IV access prior to entering the lab.

Atrial tachyarrhythmias: mechanism

All regular atrial tachyarrhythmias should be named mechanistically, i.e., either focal atrial tachycardia or macro-reentrant atrial tachycardia (which includes atrial flutter).

Focal atrial tachycardia

The mechanism may be due to enhanced automaticity or micro-reentry. Common foci are the crista terminalis, PV–LA junction, vena cava–RA junction, and triangle of Koch.

Macro-reentrant atrial tachycardia

The most common form is *typical atrial flutter*. This is an ECG diagnosis, i.e., P wave rate >240/min. There is a reentry circuit contained within the RA, rotating counterclockwise around the tricuspid valve and dependent on conduction through the tricuspid isthmus (see Fig. 13.5). The opposite of this is *reverse typical flutter*.

Reentry circuits are also found in the left atrium, following cardiac surgery or ablation of atrial fibrillation, or in congenital heart disease. These have varying circuits that need to be carefully mapped before ablation can be performed.

Atrial fibrillation

The chaotic electrical wavefronts are seen because the atria do not activate uniformly. Two potential mechanisms account for this.

Focal

A single source of wavefronts emerges from cells with either enhanced automaticity (such as an atrial tachycardia located in a PV) or a single small reentry circuit (micro-reentry). These depolarize so rapidly that the rest of the atria cannot conduct them uniformly and the wavefronts break up to give multiple wavefronts (= fibrillatory conduction). This is usually the mechanism of paroxysmal AF, and these foci are considered triggers of AF.

Multiple reentry

This underlies permanent AF. Four to six separate reentry circuits or rotors of constantly varying course and velocity rotate around the atria, colliding with each other and anatomical structures such as veins and valves. They are self-perpetuating. The larger the atrium, the more room these wavefronts have to rotate and the more likely they will be sustained.

As any episode of AF persists, atrial dilation due to mechanical stunning increases (remodeling), which explains the natural progression of AF from paroxysmal to persistent to permanent: *AF begets AF*.

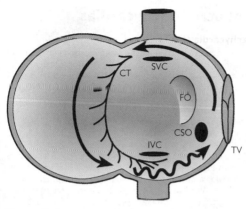

Figure 13.5 Mechanism of typical atrial flutter. A diagram of the right atrium with anterior surface cut open and swung out to the left. The arrow represents the wavefront passing up the septum, over the roof of the RA, anterior to the crista terminalis (CT), and then passing through the isthmus between the inferior vena cava (IVC) and tricuspid valve (TV). Conduction is slowed as it passes transisthmally. CSO, coronary sinus os; FO, fossa ovalis; SVC, superior vena cava.

Ablation of atrial tachycardias

Focal atrial tachycardia (FAT)

Tachycardia must be induced and sustained to map location in the atria of earliest activation (the focus) and this may require an isoproterenol infusion. The hallmark of AT is dissociation of the atrial and ventricular electrograms during tachycardia. This may occur spontaneously (AV block) or it may be necessary to pace the ventricle faster than the atrium to demonstrate this phenomenon.

ECG may indicate the origin (positive I and aVL, negative V1 = high lateral RA; negative II, III, and aVF = posteroseptal LA or RA; positive I, aVL, and V1 = right PVs; negative I and aVL, positive V1 = left PVs).

Catheters in the RA and CS will identify whether the LA or RA activates first. Beware: AT from the right superior pulmonary vein (RSPV) may give the appearance of having an RA origin. The RA is easily mapped with an ablation catheter via the IVC, but the LA requires a transseptal puncture.

A successful site usually has a local electrogram at least 30 ms ahead of the onset of the P wave. Success rates are >90%.

Typical atrial flutter

The reentry circuit can be interrupted by creating a series of ablation lesions creating a line of conduction block between the IVC and tricuspid valve that disrupts conduction through the RA isthmus (see Figs. 13.5 and 13.6). This is therefore a purely anatomical procedure that can be performed in SR or during tachycardia.

The TV annulus is usually mapped with a 20-pole catheter. Alternately, nonfluoroscopic catheter location systems can be used to map the RA and isthmus and guide the catheter during ablation.

Success is proven by demonstrating that there is conduction block in both directions across the RA isthmus (bidirectional block). Acute success occurs in 90% of cases with a 10% relapse.

Thirty percent of patients who undergo atrial flutter ablation later develop AF.

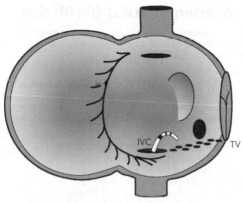

Figure 13.6 Ablation of typical atrial flutter. An ablation catheter is passed up from the IVC, and a series of burns is made in the RA isthmus to join the TV to the IVC with a line of scar. In this way, no activation can pass through and the reentry circuit of typical atrial flutter is broken. (See Fig. 13.5 for landmarks on the diagram.)

Catheter ablation of atrial fibrillation

There are two main catheter strategies to prevent recurrences of AF—abolishing the focal triggers, and changing the atrial substrate such that multiple reentry circuits cannot be sustained.

Single focal trigger

An example is focal AT from the PV. This is selectively ablated in the same way as described above. This is rarely a cure of AF, as there are often multiple triggers. In addition, ablation within the PVs increases the risk of developing pulmonary vein stenosis and is not generally a first-line approach.

Abolish potential triggers from affecting the atrial myocardium

All four PVs are isolated. This is done in two ways:

1. Create a line of conduction block outside the ostia of the veins (anatomical isolation, see Fig 13.7b), isolating not just the vein but also the LA tissue adjacent to the veins. The risk of PV stenosis is virtually eliminated. PVI is currently the preferred method for RFA of AF
2. Selectively ablate all the electrical connections between the LA and each PV (electrical isolation, see Fig. 13.7a). An important risk if ablating in the PV is PV stenosis (3%), which causes progressive dyspnea and is very difficult to manage.

In some centers it is common to also ablate electrical signals in the superior vena cava and coronary sinus. For paroxysmal AF, clinical success rates using this technique are 60%–70% in published series.

Newer approaches also include mapping the LA for complex fractionated electrograms (CFEs) and then ablating the CFEs that may serve as triggers or drivers of atrial fibrillation.

Linear ablation

The LA and RA can be compartmentalized by creating long lines of ablation within them. These interrupt the multiple reentry circuits and hence AF cannot be sustained. This treatment was pioneered by the cardiac surgeons performing the surgical Maze with great success; however, improvements in catheter technology and nonfluoroscopic localization systems (e.g., Carto or Ensite NavX) have made it feasible to do this percutaneously.

This treatment is suitable for symptomatic patients with persistent or permanent AF. In addition to isolating the PVs, lines are drawn across the roof of the LA, between the LIPV and MV, the RA isthmus, and between the SVC and IVC. Success rates are lower than for paroxysmal AF. Procedures are long (4 hours) and carry a higher risk of stroke than with standard ablation.

(a)

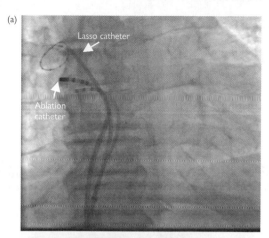

(b)

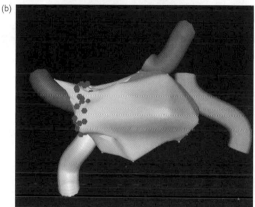

Figure 13.7 (a) Electrical isolation of the left superior pulmonary vein. A lasso catheter is placed well up inside the vein to record pulmonary vein potentials. The ablation catheter is back at the mouth of the vein. Where potentials are found linking the pulmonary vein to the surrounding LA, energy is applied. The procedure continues until no potentials are recorded in the vein or potentials are dissociated. (b) Anatomical isolation of the right superior pulmonary vein. This is a Carto image of the LA from the front with the four pulmonary veins posterior. Lesions can be seen well outside the vein, therefore not risking pulmonary vein stenosis.

Mechanism of AV reentry tachycardias

In young patients with paroxysmal regular narrow complex tachycardia, the diagnosis is either AVNRT or AVRT. The mechanism of both is reentry (see Fig. 9.7). The substrate for AVNRT is dual AVN pathways and for AVRT the presence of an AP. Occasionally, an atrial tachycardia may give an identical ECG appearance.

Diagnostic testing

Four standard catheters are positioned (see Fig. 13.2) and an EPS is carried out (see Table 13.2). Look for evidence of dual AVN physiology and presence of an AP. If tachycardia is induced, atrial activation is observed to see whether it is via the AVN (AVNRT) or an AP (AVRT).

Look closely for AVN block and BB block, especially at the onset and termination of tachycardia. HSVPBs (His synchronous premature beats) are introduced to identify whether an AP is mediating the tachycardia (AVRT).

AV block

If AVN block occurs, but tachycardia persists, it is almost always an atrial tachycardia.

Onset

• AVN jump immediately followed by tachycardia indicates AVNRT.
• Loss of pre-excitation followed by tachycardia indicates AVRT.

Termination

• Last tachycardia complex atrial (block in AVN): AVNRT or AVRT (almost certainly not atrial tachycardia)
• Last tachycardia complex ventricular: atrial tachycardia (AVNRT or AVRT still possible)

His synchronous ventricular premature beats (HSVPBs)

The aim is to introduce a ventricular paced beat exactly coincidental with the His potential during tachycardia, to see whether the ventricle is an essential component of the reentry circuit (Fig. 13.8).

To do this, the cycle length of the tachycardia is measured and a single sensed extrastimulus is delivered from the catheter in the RV at 20 ms less than the cycle length. This is repeated, reducing the coupling interval by 10 ms each time, until it is clear that the sensed extra is pre-His. Tachycardia is then terminated and the electrograms are analyzed.

Analysis (Fig. 13.8)

The HH and AA intervals are measured to ensure a stable tachycardia. The paced VPB must be synchronous with the His potential. The AA intervals before and after the HSVPB are measured. If the subsequent A is premature, this implies that the atrium *must* have been activated via an AP (as we know the His bundle is refractory due the presence of the anterograde potential) and that the ventricle is part of the reentry circuit, hence AVRT. If the A is not advanced, it suggests that this is AVNRT, but does not preclude AVRT.

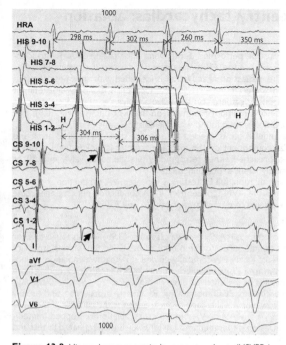

Figure 13.8 His synchronous ventricular premature beats (HSVPBs) resetting tachycardia. From top to bottom: intracardiac electrograms from high right atrium, His bundle catheter (proximal to distal), CS catheter (proximal to distal), and four surface ECG leads. The tachycardia cycle length is approximately 300 ms. During tachycardia, the earliest atrial activation is at the distal coronary sinus (lateral left atrium)—see arrows. A sensed extra (the HSVPB) is introduced just ahead of the His potential (H). The next atrial complex is advanced (see cycle lengths measured at the HRA). This strongly suggests an AVRT mediated by a left lateral pathway.

AV reentry tachycardias: ablation

AVRT

Ablation must be performed during ventricular pacing or AVRT to identify the location of the AP (unless it is manifest on the resting ECG i.e., WPW). The earliest atrial activation is identified with an almost continuous V-then-A electrogram. Its general location is found by bracketing it with a diagnostic catheter on the valve annulus, i.e., the CS catheter on the left side or a multipolar catheter on the right side (see Fig. 10.9). The precise location is then found with the ablation catheter.

A true annular site is needed for success, so an equal-sized atrial and ventricular component on the mapping catheter is looked for. Left-sided APs are approached either retrogradely (via the aortic valve and LV) or anterogradely (trans-septal puncture).

Following ablation, full EP testing is repeated. VA conduction should be absent or via the AVN (concentric). If VA conduction persists, adenosine boluses are given to demonstrate both VA and AV block.

AVNRT

The target is the slow AVN pathway (see Fig. 13.9b). This is found inferior to the His bundle, close to the mouth of the CS in the inferior aspect of the triangle of Koch. Anatomically guided slow pathway ablation is conducted in the area along the inferior part of Koch's triangle extending from the TV annulus to the anterior edge of the CS os.

With continuous ECG monitoring, RF energy is delivered, and usually transient slow junctional escape beats are seen as the cells die. If the catheter moves or any AV or VA block occurs, ablation is stopped immediately. If the lesion is therapeutic, a full EP study is then repeated to test and ensure that there is no AVNRT.

A successful procedural outcome is the inability to induce tachycardia and complete loss of dual AV-nodal physiology. Conventionally, the presence of a jump and a single echo beat is permitted, providing tachycardia cannot be induced. If isoproterenol was needed to induce tachycardia before the ablation, it should also be used during post-ablation testing.

Following ablation, full EP testing is repeated. VA conduction should be absent or via the AVN (concentric). If VA conduction persists, adenosine boluses are given to demonstrate both VA and AV block.

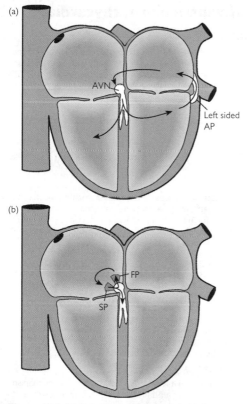

Figure 13.9 (a) Orthodromic AVRT via a left-sided accessory pathway (AP). Activation from A to V is down the atrioventricular node (AVN), then across the ventricular myocardium and back from V to A up the AP, thus completing the circuit. The ventricle therefore is an essential part of the circuit. Antidromic AVRT (not shown) would activate in the opposite direction. A left-sided AP as shown here would be accessed by a trans-septal puncture or retrogradely (via aortic valve and LV). (b) Typical AVNRT activates from the atrium to the AVN via the slow pathway (SP) and from the AVN to the atrium via the fast pathway (FP), thus completing the circuit. The ventricle is activated as a bystander via the bundle of His and is not an essential part of the circuit. Atypical AVNRT (not shown) activates in the opposite direction. Ablation targets the slow pathway.

Ablation of ventricular tachycardia

Clinical indications

Only a small percentage of patients with VT and structural heart disease are suitable for ablation. The VT needs to be relatively well tolerated (see Fig. 13.10) and ideally is monomorphic. In this group, success rates of 70% are expected. Ablation should be offered to patients whose VT is well tolerated and have one of the following features:

- Recurrent symptomatic paroxysms
- The number of therapies delivered by an ICD needs to be reduced
- Incessant VT
- VT in normal hearts: ablation offers a cure for these patients (>90% cure). RVOT and fascicular tachycardia are mapped during VT, looking for the earliest ventricular activation.

Mechanism of VT

In structural heart disease VT almost always has a reentry mechanism. Scarred ventricular myocardium (due to ischemia, cardiomyopathy, etc.) provides the substrate for reentry as described previously. A stable reentry circuit can break down into chaotic activation of fibrillation (VF), hence the link between VT and sudden death.

Mapping reentry VT

To successfully map the reentry circuit, the patient must be in VT (activation mapping). Thus the VT needs to be hemodynamically well tolerated. Remote defibrillation paddles are attached to the patient so that if VF or hypotensive VT occurs, it can be immediately cardioverted.

The aim is to identify the critical pathway at which the circuit is most susceptible to destruction. This is achieved by entrainment mapping. Alternately, 3-D noncontact scar mapping can be performed in SR and "escape pathways" can be eliminated by ablation.

Entrainment of VT

This can only be performed on tachycardias with a reentry mechanism. The ablation catheter is moved around the ventricle to sites where the circuit is expected (i.e., adjacent to areas of scar). By pacing with this catheter at a rate just faster than the tachycardia cycle length, a VT is entrained if it is following the same circuit but at a faster rate.

If the ECG during pacing is a 12/12 surface lead match to the clinical VT, then this is concealed entrainment. This implies that the pacing catheter is within the critical portion of the circuit. To confirm this when pacing is stopped, the return cycle length or post-pacing interval (the time from the final paced beat to the next activation at the catheter) should be almost identical to the tachycardia cycle length.

Ablation technique

The standard steps of a VT ablation are as follows:

- Induce VT. Ensure similar to clinical VT and well tolerated.
- Map VT to identify critical diastolic pathway:
  - Very early local electrogram occurring mid-diastole (50–150 ms ahead of ECG)

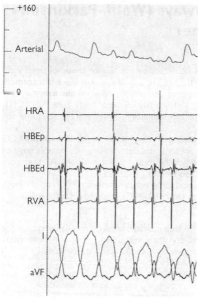

Figure 13.10 An induced VT at a cycle length of 320 ms (187/min). From top to bottom a tracing of arterial pressure, high right atrial Egram, proximal then distal His bundle Egram, RV Egram, then 2 surface ECG leads. There is no V-to-A conduction at this rate and the atrium is dissociated form the ventricle. Despite the rapid rate, the systolic BP is maintained at 100 mmHg, enabling the VT to be mapped if necessary.

- Concealed entrainment during pacing
- Return cycle length (= post-pacing interval) < tachycardia cycle length + 30 ms
• Deliver energy at site, meeting criteria above.
• If VT is terminated, attempt to reinduce again.

Failed ablation

If conventional ablation fails, alternative approaches are as follows:
• Arrhythmia cardiac surgery.
• Ablate the epicardial surface of the heart by delivering the catheter via the pericardium (as for a pericardial aspiration).
• Alcohol ablation via a small terminal coronary branch subtending the scarred area supporting reentry. This gives the patient a controlled, small MI that destroys the critical portion of the reentry circuit.

Accessory pathways (Wolff–Parkinson–White syndrome)

Definitions and ECG

The atria and ventricles are separated by the fibrous annuli of the TV on the right and MV on the left. The AV node is the only electrical connection in normal hearts. Abnormal accessory pathways can occur at any position along these annuli and are named accordingly (see Fig. 13.11). They may conduct in one or both directions. They are the substrate for AVRT to occur.

If an AP conducts anterogradely (A to V) it will be manifest on the ECG as pre-excitation (short PR interval and delta wave). The morphology of the delta wave helps to predict the location of the AP. An AP that conducts only retrogradely is described as concealed.

Wolff–Parkinson–White syndrome refers strictly to APs that are both manifest as pre-excitation on the resting ECG and cause tachycardia.

Tachycardias

An AP can be associated with tachycardia by several mechanisms:
- Orthodromic AVRT (most common, accounts for 95% of AP-mediated tachycardias)—*narrow complex tachycardia* with anterograde conduction over the AVN and retrograde conduction via the AP
- Antidromic AVRT—*wide complex tachycardia* with anterograde conduction via the AP and retrograde conduction via the AVN
- Bystander—SVT of another etiology that conducts down the AP

Prognosis

AF in the presence of an AP with anterograde conduction can be dangerous, as the ventricle is not protected by the decremental behavior of the AV node. This can precipitate VF and sudden death. If patients are discovered incidentally to have an AP and are truly asymptomatic, then sudden death is extremely rare (2 deaths in 600 patients followed for 3–20 years). Invasive EP can be used to risk stratify patients.

A worse prognosis is predicted by the following:
- Invasive EP testing
  - Anterograde ERP of the AP <250 ms (the longest interval that will not conduct down the AP during atrial extrastimulus pacing or AF)
  - Inducible AVRT
  - Multiple APs
- Symptomatic tachycardia
- Ebstein's anomaly

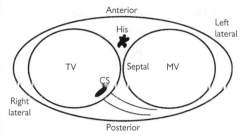

Figure 13.11 Tricuspid (TV) and mitral valve (MV) annuli. Accessory pathways can be positioned anywhere on the annuli. They are named anatomically, i.e., anterior, left anterolateral, left lateral, left posterolateral, etc. Anteroseptal pathways are close to the His bundle and AV node and are termed *parahisian*.

Accessory pathways: localization

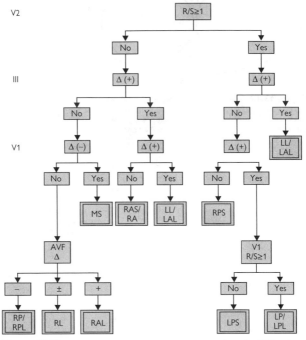

Figure 13.12 Algorithm to locate the accessory pathway from the ECG with pre-excitation. Δ = delta wave. Reprinted with permission from Chiang et al. (1996). *Am J Cardiol* 76(1):41–46.

Accessory pathways: management

Ablation

Accessory pathways (APs) can be inactivated by catheter ablation and this is first-line treatment for symptomatic patients. A catheter is moved around the MV or TV annulus until the AP is located by finding the exact point of

- Earliest ventricular activation during SR or atrial pacing.
- Earliest atrial activation during ventricular pacing.
- Earliest atrial activation during orthodromic AVRT.

Acute success is >90%. The complication rate is very low (death 0%–0.2%, AV nodal block <1%). For parahisian AP, the risk of AV nodal block is higher and cryoablation may be used if available.

Left-sided pathways can be approached via the femoral artery, aorta, and left ventricle, or from the RA by a transseptal puncture.

All symptomatic patients (with tachycardias) should be offered ablation. Asymptomatic young patients (<35 years) or those in a high-risk profession (pilots, divers, etc.) should be considered for invasive EP testing and ablation. However, risk of sudden death must be balanced against the 2% serious complication rate of ablating the pathway (particularly if left-sided or parahisian).

Pharmacological

Flecainide and propafenone slow conduction in the AP and the AV node and are the preferred agents. Drugs that slow AV-nodal conduction only (verapamil and digoxin) should not be used unless invasive EP has demonstrated that the AP does not conduct anterogradely (or conducts poorly).

Unusual pathways

Mahaim pathways

These are APs between the RA and RV (atrioventricular) or RA and right bundle branch (atriofascicular). Unlike ordinary APs, they exhibit AV nodal properties of decremental conduction and sensitivity to adenosine. They only conduct anterogradely and mediate an AVRT with a broad complex LBBB appearance. They are successfully treated by catheter ablation.

Implantable cardioverter defibrillators (ICDs)

Mirowski implanted the first defibrillator in 1980 to manage sudden cardiac death. Since then, there has been dramatic improvement in technology, and many randomized controlled trials provide evidence to support their use in both primary and secondary prevention of sudden cardiac death.

Initial implants used epicardial leads and required surgical implantation. The generators were large and placed in abdominal pockets. Currently, the devices are implanted transvenously and the generators placed in the pectoral region.

ICDs employ a series of complex sensing algorithms for arrhythmia detection and use tiered therapy of pacing and shocking to treat arrhythmia as well as to minimize myocardial injury.

Components

A typical pulse generator consists of a lithium silver vanadium oxide battery, an aluminum electrolytic capacitor, and sensing circuitry that can sense local electrograms and filter out noise like skeletal myopotentials. Defibrillators have at least one lead in the RV for pacing/sensing and defibrillation. There may be a second lead in the SVC or a dual coil lead to lower defibrillation threshold.

An atrial lead can be implanted for dual-chamber pacemaker indications or to help with detection or discrimination of arrhythmias.

Detection

Most leads sense between the tip of the lead and an electrode anywhere along the length of the shocking coil (integrated bipolar sensing). Potential problems are with noise, far-field sensing, or post-shock undersensing. True bipolar sensing between a ring and tip electrode is more reliable but requires the lead to have three conductors.

Basic detection of VT involves a heart rate, above which therapy will be delivered. Modern devices can be programmed to have multiple detection zones, each with its own specific therapies. Rate detection is very reliable but susceptible to inappropriate therapies for sinus tachycardia or poorly controlled atrial fibrillation. This is where medical therapy such as β-blockers is very important to help prevent inappropriate therapy.

To decrease inappropriate shocks, various *detection enhancements* are included in modern devices, such as rate stability (looking at variations in R–R intervals to recognize AF), electrogram morphology (to distinguish a normal QRS [SVT], including BBB, from the QRS when in VT), and sudden-onset criteria (gradual onset of sinus tachycardia).

The most useful algorithm, however, is to have an atrial lead so the device can analyze the timing of simultaneous atrial electrograms. The tradeoff of improved detection means that therapy for VT is inhibited. Most devices include "sustained rate duration" as a backup, which ensures delivery of therapy if the tachycardia is sustained. As a default, these detection algorithms do not apply in the programmed VF zone.

Indications for ICD implantation

Box 13.2 Indications for ICD implantation

Definite indications

- Survivors of cardiac arrest due to ventricular fibrillation or hemodynamically unstable sustained VT in the absence of a completely reversible cause
- Spontaneous sustained VT in a patient with structural heart disease, whether hemodynamically stable or unstable
- Syncope of undetermined origin with hemodynamically significant sustained VT or ventricular fibrillation induced at EPS.
- LVEF <35% due to prior MI in patients who are at least 40 days post-MI and are in NYHA functional Class II or III
- Patients with nonischemic dilated cardiomyopathy who have an LVEF ≤35% and who are in NYHA functional Class II or III
- Patients with LV dysfunction due to prior MI who are at least 40 days post-MI, have an LVEF <30%, and are NYHA functional Class I.
- Nonsustained VT due to prior myocardial infarction, LVEF <40%, and inducible ventricular fibrillation or sustained VT at EPS

Relative indications

- Unexplained syncope, significant LV dysfunction, and nonischemic dilated cardiomyopathy
- Sustained VT and normal or near-normal ventricular function
- Patients with hypertrophic cardiomyopathy who have one or more major* risk factor for SCD
- Prevention of SCD in patients with arrhythmogenic right ventricular dysplasia or cardiomyopathy who have one or more risk factor for SCD
- To reduce SCD in patients with long-QT syndrome who are experiencing syncope and/or VT while receiving β-blockers
- Nonhospitalized patients awaiting transplantation
- Patients with Brugada syndrome who have had syncope
- Patients with Brugada syndrome who have documented VT that has not resulted in cardiac arrest
- Patients with catecholaminergic polymorphic VT who have syncope and/or documented sustained VT while receiving β-blockers
- ICD implantation is reasonable for patients with cardiac sarcoidosis, giant cell myocarditis, or Chagas disease

*Risk factors for SCD with HCM: prior SCD, prior nonsustained VT, massive hypertrophy (>30 mm), family history of SCD, syncope.

Adapted from ACC/AHA/NASPE 2008 guidelines for device-based therapy. *J Am Coll Cardiol* 2008; 51;2085–2105.

ICD therapies

Antitachycardia pacing (ATP)

The two most common methods of ATP are rate-adaptive burst pacing and autodecremental or ramp pacing. With rate-adaptive burst pacing the device is programmed to deliver a set number of pulses (6–12) at a cycle length that is a programmed percentage of the tachycardia cycle length (TCL) (i.e., 81% of the TCL).

The sequences may be repeated with a decrementing cycle length. In ramp pacing the initial coupling interval is also a percentage of the TCL but each subsequent coupling interval decrements by a set amount (i.e., 10 ms). Again, this sequence can be repeated.

Generally, modern devices can be programmed to have one to three VT zones with multiple tiers of therapy. One manufacturer allows for a fast VT zone in the VF zone, which allows painless ATP to treat fast VT instead of cardioversion.

Defibrillation

Most ICDs deliver a maximum energy of 30–36 J via their capacitors as a biphasic waveform from the tip of the RV lead to the pulse generator, which is an "active can." The shocking vector travels superiorly from the RV including most of the IVS and LV.

Sometimes a third electrode is needed as either a separate SVC coil or a dual coil RV lead to improve the defibrillation threshold (DFT), and the device can shock either between both coils or between the can and either coil and sometimes the vector is reversed. Very rarely, a subcutaneous patch is needed and is placed in the left axillary region.

Low-energy defibrillation

Devices can also deliver low-energy cardioversions when the tachycardia is generally <180 bpm, which has some efficacy but patients feel shocks above 1 J. This has not been shown to be better than ATP.

Defibrillation threshold (DFT) testing

Unless contraindicated, DFTs should be tested at implant. The goal is for the DFT to be less than the maximum output of the device, ideally by 10 J. VF is induced via rapid burst pacing, T-wave shock, or AC current (unpleasant) while the patent is sedated.

Appropriate VF detection and device charge time as well as the DFT can be evaluated.

ICD: trouble shooting and follow-up

Follow-up
- *Oversensing* leading to therapy (e.g., T-wave sensing, electrical noise from lead fractures, atrial activity). Sensitivity settings can be adjusted to help prevent T-wave sensing. Lead fractures require replacement and atrial leads help distinguish atrial activity.
- *Undersensing* is more serious but less common. May not detect VT or VF. It is more likely with unipolar systems. It may indicate lead displacement, inflammation, or fibrosis at the lead tip.

Drug interactions
- Increased defibrillation threshold—Class I antiarrhythmics and amiodarone
- Decreased defibrillation threshold—sotalol
- Antiarrhythmics may slow VT below the detection threshold, affect the ability of ATP to terminate the tachycardia, or cause incessant VT. They may impair ventricular function and cause bradycardia requiring pacing. They may also affect the pacing threshold for bradycardia.

Table 13.3 Complications of ICD implantation

Early	Late
• Infection	• Infection
• Hemopneumothorax	• Pain
• Cardiac perforation	• Erosion
• Hemorrhage and pocket hematoma	• Lead/insulation break
• Vascular injury	• Lead displacement
• Venous thrombosis	• Twiddler's syndrome
• Lead displacement or damage	
• VT	
• Heart block	

Cardiac catheterization and coronary intervention

Radiation protection in the catheter laboratory

Staff working in the catheterization laboratory should be issued with radiation monitoring badges for the body and neck, which should always be worn while in the lab. These badges should be checked monthly to assess doses of radiation received by individual members of staff.

Minimizing patient dose

- Minimize screening time and minimize acquisition time.
- Keep distance between X-ray tube and image intensifier to a minimum.
- Use collimation and cones to minimize the irradiated area.
- Use lower magnifications when possible.
- Use the lowest number of frames/second to allow adequate imaging.
- For prolonged procedures, the intensifier should be moved regularly a few degrees to try to minimize the possibility of skin burns.

Minimizing operator dose

- Lead aprons and lead collars should be worn.
- A lead apron should be below the table.
- A mobile lead screen should go between the operator and the source.
- As above, minimize X-ray exposure by reducing screening and acquisition time.
- Some projections (e.g., left anterior oblique [LAO]) give much higher scatter of X-ray, and operators should be aware of this.

The dose for an interventional cardiologist has been calculated as 50 mSv (based on 150 working days per year and four interventions per day). The calculated effective dose if the operator wears the correct lead apron and thyroid collar is <5 mSv/year. The maximum allowed dose is 50 mSv/year.

Vascular access: the femoral artery

Procedure for femoral artery access

- The standard approach for left heart catheterization is the right common femoral artery.
- The artery is located by palpating below the inguinal ligament, the ideal position for puncture being approximately 3 cm below the inguinal ligament and slightly lateral to the position of the vessel (see Fig. 14.1).
- Shave area, and disinfect.
- The area should be anesthetized generously with of local anesthetic (usually 10 mL of 2% or up to 20 mL of 1% lidocaine). Warn the patient of "pins and needles" or transient numbness in the leg that may be caused by the effects of lidocaine on the femoral nerve.
- The procedure used to puncture the artery is known as the *Seldinger technique*. A hollow needle is introduced slowly; it is often possible to feel the pulsations of the artery via the needle before the vessel is punctured. When the needle is introduced into the vessel, pulsatile flow confirms its position in the arterial lumen. At this point, a 0.035" wire can be advanced into the vessel and toward the heart; this should be performed under fluoroscopic guidance.
- The needle is then withdrawn and a hemostatic sheath (usually 5 Fr–8 Fr diameter) is introduced over the wire. The hemostatic sheath allows the introduction of a guide wire and catheter into the femoral artery, while preventing excess bleeding from the femoral puncture site.

Sheath removal

- This can be performed immediately after diagnostic angiography or after an interval of 4–6 hours if heparin has been administered.
- Hemostasis can be achieved by manual compression or by using a compression device (e.g., Femstop™).
- Vascular closure devices (e.g., Angioseal™ or Perclose™) allow earlier removal of sheaths in anticoagulated patients and may reduce bleeding complications.

Complications

- Femoral artery dissection
- Femoral artery pseudoaneurysm
- Distal embolization
- Hematoma
- Retroperitoneal hemorrhage/hematoma (particularly with high punctures of the femoral artery above the inguinal ligament)

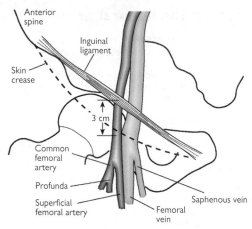

Figure 14.1 Anatomy of the inguinal canal: the femoral vein lies medial to the femoral artery. The arterial puncture should be made approximately 3 cm below the inguinal ligament.

Vascular access: the radial artery

The radial approach for coronary angiography is now widely accepted. There are several advantages, including a reduction in vascular complications and the ability to mobilize patients immediately following their procedure.

Patient selection for radial access should include palpation of the radial artery to confirm that pulsations are present and then an Allen's test (see Box 14.1). In the absence of robust supply via the ulnar artery, the radial approach should not be used.

Procedure for radial artery approach

- Perform Allen's test.
- Remove all jewelry from the arm, shave area, and disinfect.
- Local anesthesia: use 1–2 mL of 2% lidocaine instilled via a 25-gauge needle (i.e., enough to anesthetize, but not to distort the anatomy).
- The artery should be palpated with the index and middle fingers, the index finger lifted, and the artery punctured at 45°. The artery should be punctured as proximally as possible, and care should be taken to avoid the flexor retinaculum (Fig. 14.2).
- Once pulsatile flow is obtained, a guide wire can then be advanced through the needle and into the vessel.
- It is usual to make a small incision in the skin to allow passage of an arterial sheath. Care should be taken not to damage the radial artery while making this incision. Thus the blade should be used to incise in the longitudinal plane rather than transversely to reduce the risk of completely transecting the artery.

A variety of long and short sheaths are commercially available. The advantage of long sheaths is that they minimize trauma to the radial artery.

Complications

Radial artery spasm

This is the most common complication of radial artery puncture and sheath introduction. There are various techniques aimed at preventing radial artery spasm from occurring:

- Careful patient selection, avoiding small and difficult to palpate radial arteries.
- Adequate patient sedation if required (pain provokes spasm).
- The use of a cocktail of drugs introduced directly into the radial artery. A variety of different regimens have been described. We use 1 mg nitroglycerin, 2.5 mg verapamil, and 2500 U unfractionated heparin (UFH) made up to 10 mL with normal saline. Repeated doses of nitrates or verapamil (up to 5 mg) given directly into the sheath or in the catheter may be required.
- Shorter sheaths may be better tolerated.
- Some sheaths have a hydrophilic coating to reduce spasm and for less discomfort on removal.
- Always use the guide wire to straighten catheters prior to removal from the aortic arch through the radial sheath.

Box 14.1 Allen's test

Manual compression

- Compress radial and ulnar arteries.
- Ask patient to open and close their fingers making a fist (this will cause the hand to blanche).
- Release ulnar artery.
- Allen's test is POSITIVE if the color of the palm of the hand returns to normal within 10 seconds (confirming that the ulnar circulation is intact).

Plethysmography

- Attach plethysmography probe (pulse oximetry).
- Compress both the radial and ulnar arteries (the plethysmography trace will flatten).
- Release ulnar artery.
- The test is POSITIVE if the plethysmograph curve returns to normal (confirming that the ulnar circulation is intact).

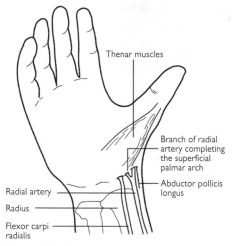

Thenar muscles

Branch of radial artery completing the superficial palmar arch

Abductor pollicis longus

Radial artery

Radius

Flexor carpi radialis

Figure 14.2 Radial artery anatomy.

Vascular access: site management

Femoral sheath removal

Femoral sheaths should be removed only by fully trained members of staff. After diagnostic coronary angiography, when no or little heparin is given, the sheath may be removed immediately. Direct pressure should be applied just proximal to the site of the skin puncture for 15 minutes.

After angioplasty, if unfractionated heparin was used, it is routine to wait for 4–6 hours and check an ACT (activated clotting time), if it is <150 seconds, it is acceptable for the sheath to be removed. In cases where bivalirudin was used, the sheath can be safely removed after 30 minutes.

Femoral clamps (FemoStop®, RADI Medical Systems) can be used to reduce bleeding complications in patients.

Radial sheath removal

Radial sheaths are removed immediately after both diagnostic angiograms and angioplasty, as the position of the artery renders compression simpler. Compression bands (RadiStop®, RadiMedical Systems USA, TR-Band™, and Terumo) can be used to achieve hemostasis.

Vascular closure devices

Until recently, mechanical compression was the only method for controlling bleeding from vascular access sites in the groin. Larger sheaths and the advent of the more widespread use of gpIIb/IIIa inhibitors have increased the risk of bleeding and made hemostasis more difficult.

Recently, various closure devices have been introduced, their aim being to increase patient comfort and reduce puncture related complications.

Suture-based closure devices

Perclose® (Abbot Vascular, USA) delivers a suture to the arterial puncture site. The device is sheath-like in nature; needles are positioned above the sheath in the handle and are deployed by a plunger. A "clincher" that performs a knot-tying function completes a sliding surgical knot.

Collagen-based closure devices

Devices that use a bioresorbable collagen plug that is deposited at the site of arteriotomy via a sheath include the VasoSeal® (Datascope Corp., USA) and Angio-Seal® (St Jude Medical, USA).

Other mechanical closure devices

StarClose® features a Nitinol® clip that is designed to promote the primary healing process to achieve a secure closure of femoral artery access sites following diagnostic or interventional vascular procedures. This clip provides 360° tissue apposition for rapid healing and hemostasis.

Drug-based closure devices

The Clo-Sur® P.A.D (Medtronic, USA), MINX (USA) device contains a naturally occurring biopolymer polyprolate acetate. This polymer has a coagulant property when brought into contact with heparinized blood. The device is placed over the puncture and the hemostatic sheath is removed. Direct continuous pressure is applied until hemostasis is achieved.

Coronary angiography

Preshaped coronary angiographic catheters

The catheters used in diagnostic coronary angiography come in a wide variety of preformed shapes. In the United States, the most commonly used preshaped catheters are the Judkins Left 4 and Judkins Right 4 (known as the JL4 and JR4, respectively), used to image the left and right coronary arteries, and the pigtail catheter used for left ventriculography.

The diameter of catheters is measured in French gauge (Fr); catheters between 4 Fr (0.053") and 8 Fr (0.105") are commonly used (Fig. 14.3).

Catheter advancement and manifold usage

A "J" tipped 0.035" guide wire is placed within the flushed catheter, which is then passed into the hemostatic sheath. The guide wire is advanced ahead of the catheter under fluoroscopic guidance, until it reaches the aortic root, just above the aortic valve. The catheter is then advanced to this position and the guiding wire is removed (see Box 14.2).

To ensure that no air or clot is within the catheter, a small volume of blood (5 mL) is aspirated from the catheter directly into a syringe and discarded. The catheter is then carefully connected to a two-way manifold that allows pressure monitoring, saline flushing, and contrast injection through a closed system.

Contrast injection

Great care must be taken at all times to ensure that air is not injected into the coronary arterial tree. The injection syringe should be filled with contrast from the reservoir and then the syringe held with the plunger elevated such that any air bubbles rise to the top of the syringe. Contrast should then be injected at a continuous rate, aiming to fully opacify the coronary vessel of interest.

Care should be taken that the pressure trace prior to injection is normal—damping suggests an ostial lesions, excessively deep intubation, or selective intubation of a branch.

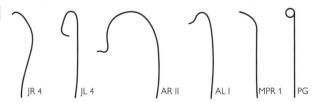

Figure 14.3 Commonly used cardiac catheter shapes. JL, JR: Judkins left and right coronary catheters; AL, AR: Amplatz left and right; MP: multipurpose coronary access catheter; PG: pigtail catheter.

Box 14.2 Coronary angiography/left ventriculography

Left coronary artery
- The 50° left anterior oblique (LAO 50) is the best projection for cannulation of both the left and right coronary ostia.
- The JL4 catheter will almost invariably cannulate the left coronary ostium without manipulation.
- In patients with large aortic roots (large, hypertensive patients), the JL5 (with a larger curve) may be needed, and conversely a smaller root may need a smaller catheter curve, the JL3.5.

Right coronary artery
- The LAO 50 projection is best used for cannulation of the right coronary ostium.
- The JR4 catheter is introduced to the aortic root, until it lies 1–2 cm above the aortic valve.
- The catheter is then rotated ("torqued") in a clockwise direction such that the catheter tip rotates toward the right coronary ostium. It may be necessary to reduce the torque to prevent the catheter from overshooting.
- There is often a noticeable lateral movement as the catheter enters the artery.
- Before contrast is injected, it must be ensured that the pressure tracing transduced from the tip of the catheter is not damped, which can suggest that the catheter has selectively intubated the conus branch of the right coronary artery, and injection of contrast into this vessel can induce ventricular arrhythmias.

Left ventriculography
- Position pigtail catheter a few centimeters above the aortic valve and pull wire back 5–10 cm to make catheter tip soft, and push gently (the catheter may cross at this point).
- If catheter does not cross, apply torque as it is gently withdrawn.
- Once catheter has been placed in a stable (free of ectopy) position in mid-LV cavity, connect to manifold and measure pressure.
- Disconnect manifold catheter connected to a power injector and expel all air.
- Set injection rate: typically 36 mL of contrast at a rate of 12 mL/sec. Warn patient about hot flush and the feeling of extra systoles.
- When the left ventriculogram has been performed, the catheter is reconnected to the manifold to allow pressure recording as the catheter is withdrawn across the aortic valve (the pullback pressure).

Interpreting the coronary angiogram

LCA angiographic views

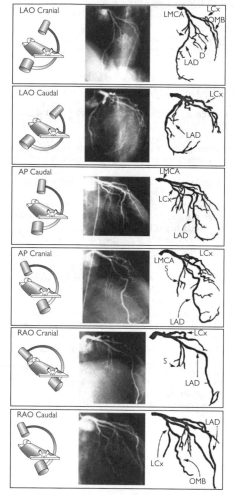

Figure 14.4 This figure was published in Libby P. *Braunwald's Heart Disease*, 8th ed. Saunders. Copyright Elsevier 2001.

RCA angiographic views

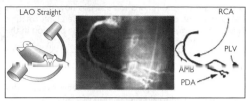

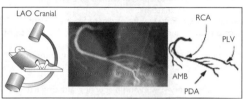

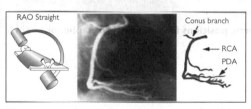

Figure 14.5 AMB, acute marginal branch; LAO, left anterior oblique; PDA, posterior descending coronary artery; PLV, posterior left ventricular branch; RCA, right coronary artery; RAO, right anterior oblique. This figure was originally published in Libby P. *Braunwald's Heart Disease*, 8th ed. Saunders. Copyright Elsevier 2007.

Angiographic study of grafts

It is important to study the surgical record to ascertain how many grafts were placed at the time of the operation. Sometimes, useful information (often from a surgeon's diagram) can be obtained as to the position in the ascending aorta that the grafts arise from.

As a rule, leftward-facing grafts are best cannulated from the RAO 50 projection, and rightward-pointing grafts are best cannulated in the LAO 50 projection. It may be necessary to perform an aortogram to visualize the position of grafts. Special catheters (e.g., the left coronary bypass catheter, or LCB) have been designed to aid cannulation of grafts.

There is usually a predictable anatomy:
- Posterior descending artery (PDA) grafts originate from the right anterior aspect of the aorta and run vertically to the inferior surface of the heart.
- Obtuse marginal branch (OM) grafts originate from the left anterior aspect of the aorta and arc toward the posterolateral surface of the heart.
- Left anterior descending artery (LAD) and diagonal grafts originate from an intermediate position and run laterally toward the anterior interventricular groove.

Common aortic positions for placement of saphenous vein graft (SVG)

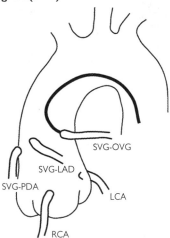

Figure 14.6 Vein graft anatomy. This figure was published in Braunwald E. *Heart Disease: A Textbook of Cardiovascular Medicine*, 5th ed. Copyright Elsevier 2001.

Complications of angiography

Peripheral vascular complications

Hematoma

The incidence of hematoma formation is related to the following factors:

- Length of time sheath is left in place
- Gauge (size) of sheath
- Anticoagulation
- Risk factors, e.g., hypertension, obesity, and pre-existing peripheral vascular disease
- Technique of sheath removal

Features suggesting that a hematoma may require further investigation are an overlying bruit, expanding mass, and a large, tense swelling.

Pseudoaneurysm

A *pseudoaneurysm* represents a rupture of the femoral arterial wall at the site of puncture, with the formation of a false aneurysm involving the media and adventitia (Fig. 14.7). They are best visualized on ultrasound examination (Fig. 14.8).

Small pseudoaneurysms can often be managed conservatively; however, large pseudoaneurysms may require thrombin injection, compression, or surgical intervention.

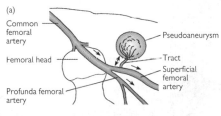

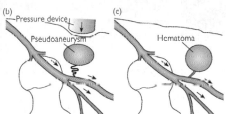

Figure 14.7 Anatomy of a pseudoaneurysm. (a) Bleeding along a small tract allows blood to collect within the extravascular tissues. Manual compression fails to obliterate the tract (b) and allows the hematoma to persist. Failure of thrombosis of the hematoma produces an extravascular collection with persistent connection and flow from the main artery (c). This can be visualized on ultrasound (see Fig. 14.8).

Hemorrhage

If prolonged, then direct pressure (either manually or using a clamping device) may be needed.

Limb ischemia

This is rare and usually occurs in patients with pre-existing limb ischemia. If limb ischemia is suspected, urgent vascular surgical team review should be sought.

Dissection

Dissection can occur at the time of sheath insertion and/or catheter manipulation; this can be diagnosed by dampening in the pressure tracing. If this is noted, an iliac angiogram should be performed and pressure gradient recorded. If significant dissection is noted, a percutaneous intervention (i.e., iliac stent) should be pursued.

Contrast reactions

Mild contrast reactions such as rash, urticaria, blurred vision, and rigors are relatively common. These symptoms may settle spontaneously but are often treated with a combination of IV diphenhydramine 25 mg and IV hydrocortisone 100–200 mg. Anaphylactic reactions are rare; these should be treated with diphenhydramine and hydrocortisone, but also plasma expanders and SQ adrenaline.

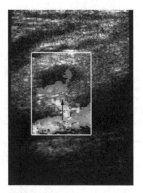

Figure 14.8 Ultrasound of femoral pseudoaneurysm demonstrating flow (arrow) in the aneurysm above the femoral artery.

Vasovagal reactions

These are common both during angiography and at the time of sheath removal. They are characterized by hypotension and bradycardia. They are treated with IV atropine and volume expanders.

Arrhythmia

Brief episodes of SVT are common and often transient. During catheter manipulation (especially in the LV), runs of VT are common. VF may occur during coronary artery injection and should be treated with rapid defibrillation.

Right heart catheterization

Indications for right heart catheterization

- Evaluation of cardiac shunts
- Evaluation of valvular heart disease
- Dyspnea not explained by noninvasive investigation

The acute settings in which right heart catheterization can be helpful (e.g., cardiogenic shock) are discussed in Chapter 1.

Access to the right heart is usually achieved via the right femoral vein (RFV). The RFV is located 0.5 cm to 1 cm medial to the femoral arterial pulsation (Fig. 14.1). An 18-gauge needle, attached to a syringe partially filled with saline, can be used to locate the position of the vein, followed by the larger-bore needle.

When venous blood is freely aspirated, a 0.035" guide wire is passed into the vein, using a technique similar to femoral artery cannulation, and a hemostatic sheath introduced.

Right heart catheterization protocol

- A balloon-tipped catheter (Swan–Ganz catheter) may be used.
- Ensure that the catheter is flushed and that the transducer is correctly zeroed.
- Advance catheter to the IVC, and with the balloon inflated, advance further to the right atrium. Record the phasic and mean pressures.
- It is customary to then advance the catheter to the pulmonary artery wedge position. Advance into the RV. A combination of rotation of the catheter and gentle traction will allow the catheter to flick upward into the RVOT. It can then be advanced into the main PA and out to the periphery. Occasionally a guide wire is necessary to achieve this.
- Advance the catheter to the pulmonary capillary wedge position and record phasic and mean pressures.
- With a pigtail catheter in the LV, measure and record the LV pressures. Record simultaneous PCWP and LV pressures, ensuring that the scale allows interpretation of the end diastolic pressures accurately (to assess for MV gradient).
- Withdraw the wedge catheter slightly; the balloon may be deflated, and record pulmonary artery phasic and mean pressure. Obtain oxygen saturations from the main PA (also RPA and LPA if a PDA is suspected).
- Withdraw the pulmonary catheter to the RV. Measure and record simultaneous RV and LV pressures.
- Withdraw the catheter to the RA and measure the pressures again.
- The LV catheter should be pulled back to the ascending aorta while the pressure is being monitored to record any pull-back gradient. Aortic saturations should be measured to allow calculation of cardiac output (see Fig. 14.9) and to compare with saturations from the right side if a shunt is suspected.
- For shunts a full saturation run should be performed (SVC, high to mid- and low RA, IVC, RV, MPA, RPA, LPA, etc.).

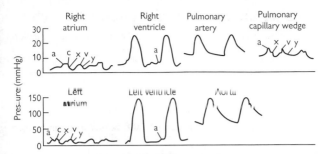

Figure 14.9 Cardiac catheterization—normal pressure waveforms.
a contraction in atrial systole
c closure mitral valve
x fall in left atrial pressure
v ventricular systole and passive atrial filling in diastole
y fall in left atrial pressure following opening of mitral valve and passive filling of the
left ventricle

Cardiac output and LV function

Cardiac output is most often measured using the thermodilution method with a pulmonary catheter.

Cardiac output can also be measured using the Fick principle, which assesses the difference between the pulmonary arterial and aortic O_2 saturation.

$$\text{Cardiac output (L/min)} = \frac{\text{Oxygen consumption (mL/min)}}{(\text{Ao SaO}_2 - \text{PA SaO}_2) \times \text{Hb} \times 1.34}$$

Ao SaO$_2$: systemic oxygen saturation; PA SaO$_2$: pulmonary artery oxygen saturation; Hb: hemoglobin.

Systemic and pulmonary vascular resistance

Pulmonary vascular resistance (PVR) is an important prognostic factor in patients with valvular heart disease, heart failure, and cor pulmonale or pulmonary hypertension. The measurement of PVR and SVR is especially important in patients being assessed for cardiac transplantation.

PVR and SVR are measured Woods units (mmHg/L/min) or dynes cm^{-5}, with 80 dynes cm^{-5} = 1 wood unit.

$$\text{Cardiac output} = \frac{\text{Mean aortic pressure} - \text{Mean right atrial pressure}}{\text{Systemic vascular resistance}}$$

$$\text{Cardiac output} = \frac{\text{Mean PA pressure} - \text{Mean left atrial pressure}}{\text{Pulmonary vascular resistance}}$$

Cardiac catheterization in valve disease

Valve stenosis

Several parameters can be assessed during cardiac catheterization.

Peak-to-peak gradient

Aortic and LV pressures are recorded during withdrawal of the pigtail catheter across the aortic valve. The gradient is the difference between peak aortic and peak LV pressure.

Peak instantaneous gradient

This is more accurately measured using a double-lumen pigtail catheter where one lumen measures pressure in the LV while the other measures pressure in the aortic root simultaneously. This is rarely done in practice.

Alternatively, simultaneous measurements may be made from the side port of the arterial sheath (in the femoral artery) and the pigtail in the LV. However, this method can lead to erroneous gradient measurements if there is significant peripheral vascular disease dampening the measured pressure in the femoral artery.

Mean gradient

The mean pressure gradient is measured using planimetry of the area between aortic and LV pressure traces. This can be used to calculate valve area using the Gorlin equation, and a similar method can be used to assess the mitral valve area (see Fig. 14.10).

Valve regurgitation

The severity of aortic regurgitation can be estimated by performing an aortogram. In severe aortic regurgitation the LV is seen to opacify within one or two beats after contrast injection.

Mitral regurgitation may be assessed by left ventriculography, with contrast seen to opacify the left atrium and pulmonary veins in severe regurgitation. In addition, mitral regurgitation may be associated with a prominent V wave in the pulmonary capillary wedge tracing.

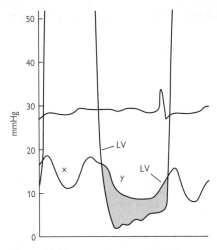

Figure 14.10 Simultaneous LV and PCWP tracing in mitral stenosis. The mean gradient across the mitral valve is calculated as the area of the region colored in gray. This figure was published in Braunwald E. *Heart Disease: A Textbook of Cardiovascular Medicine*, 5th ed. Copyright Elsevier 2001.

Intravascular ultrasound

Intravascular ultrasound (IVUS) is a technology that allows direct visualization of atherosclerotic plaque and the vessel lumen (Fig. 14.11). Ultrasound images are produced by passing an electrical current through a piezoelectric crystal that expands and contracts to produce sound waves when electrically stimulated. These sound waves are reflected from tissues, and return to the transducer where they are detected and converted to an electrical impulse that can be presented graphically.

A phased array of crystals (usually 64) is used, and these are sequentially activated to produce circumferential imaging.

The equipment required to perform an IVUS examination involves a miniaturized ultrasound transducer mounted on a catheter (usually 2.6–3.5 Fr gauge) and computer interface that carries out image reconstruction.

Examination technique

- Intracoronary nitroglycerin and IV heparin should be administered.
- The IVUS catheter should be carefully advanced distal to the area of interest.
- A motorized pullback device is then used to withdraw the IVUS catheter proximally at a fixed speed.
- Landmarks such as side branches can be useful, and positions may also be recorded angiographically.

Advantages of ultrasound

- Full circumference of vessel wall is seen, not just two surfaces as in angiography, and is thus the method of choice to determine vessel luminal area.
- IVUS is useful in imaging ambiguous lesions:
  - Intermediate lesions of unknown severity
  - Ostial stenosis
  - Left main stem disease
  - Bifurcation lesions
- It images the plaque, not just the lumen.
- It allows optimal results during angioplasty and stenting.

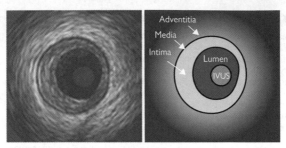

Figure 14.11 Example of image obtained by IVUS.

Angioplasty and coronary stenting

Currently, coronary stents are implanted in >85% of revascularization procedures in the United States.

AHA/ACC guidelines state that "stents should be used routinely for people with either stable or unstable angina or with acute myocardial infarction undergoing percutaneous intervention."

Angioplasty

Before stents became widely used in the mid to late 1990s, balloon angioplasty alone was the most common percutaneous treatment for significant coronary artery lesions (see Box 14.3). The two main designs of balloon catheters now commonly used are over-the-wire and rapid-exchange systems. Both types of catheter consist of three parts:

1. The shaft: there are two main varieties:
   • The hypotube, the advantage of which is a better balance between strength and flexibility
   • The core wire design, which is superior in terms of flexibility
2. The lumen: coaxial design (a tube within a tube) is the most common.
3. The balloon: these are constructed from varying plastics (e.g., polyethylene, nylon), the mix of which affects the balloon's compliance. The design of the tip is important, as tapered tips are less traumatic when crossing index lesions. The balloon may also have a hydrophilic coating.

"Plain old balloon angioplasty" (POBA) remains indicated in the treatment of some coronary artery lesions, particularly small vessels, vein grafts, and bifurcation side branches, in which the benefit of stenting has not been clearly demonstrated. It is also used for patients who need revascularization prior to noncardiac surgery, thus minimizing the bleeding risk of dual antiplatelet agents required after stent placement.

Coronary stenting

Stents can be made of stainless steel, cobalt-based alloy, titanium, nitinol, or polymer. Most stents used today are stainless steel and balloon mounted.

The primary function of a stent is to act as a scaffold to maintain vessel patency (see Fig. 14.12). Thus much of the success of stents is due primarily to their mechanical ability to produce large, acute gains in lumen dimensions.

Currently, there are two types of stents available for clinical practice: the bare metal stent (BMS) and the drug-eluding stent (DES). With the BMS, there is an increased risk of in-stent restenosis (ISR) as a result of intimal hyperplasia after stent deployment. By contrast, use of the DES decreases significantly the incidence of ISR because of the antiproliferative action of the agents that recover the stent.

The delayed healing of the vessel wall has led to the occurrence of acute and late episodes of stent thrombosis, which requires the continuous long-term use of double antiplatelet agents (1–2 years). In the case of BMS, 6 weeks of double antiplatelet therapy followed by continuous ASA use is the recommended approach.

Box 14.3 Angioplasty procedure

- Cannulate artery with the chosen guiding catheter. Ideally, the guiding catheter should be coaxial with the coronary ostium (thus allowing maximum support and minimizing trauma to the vessel).
- A steerable 0.014" guide wire is introduced to the catheter via the hemostatic valve. The tip of the guide wire may be preshaped; however, many operators prefer to take a straight guide wire and shape the tip by hand.
- Using fluoroscopy and contrast to delineate the coronary anatomy, the guide wire is advanced along the vessel, beyond the narrowing, and placed as distally as possible in the vessel.
- An appropriately sized balloon is then chosen; the guiding catheter can be used as a reference when sizing the vessel. For calcific lesions and in-stent restenosis, shorter balloons with higher rated burst pressure may be better.
- The balloon is advanced along the guide wire to the correct position. In some situations, it may be difficult to pass the balloon to the desired position, thus deeper insertion of the guide catheter or a more supportive guide catheter may be needed.
- Radio-opaque markers are used to position the balloon accurately. Inflation should be undertaken under X-ray screening to ensure that the balloon does not move.

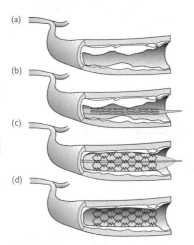

Fig 14.12 Coronary stenting: A guide wire is introduced across the stenotic segment of artery (a) and is used to position the stent (b). The stent is deployed by inflating the balloon (c). The balloon and guide wire are removed, leaving the stent in place (d).

Restenosis following PTCA

Pathophysiology
The restenotic process consists of a series of complex events:
- Vessel injury leads to platelet activation and **local thrombosis**.
- An **inflammatory reaction** is invoked, with neutrophil, monocyte, and lymphocyte migration to the site of injury.
- **Smooth muscle proliferation** is driven by activated platelets and inflammatory mediators.
- Finally, negative (inward) remodeling can occur, resulting in lumen compromise and restenosis.

These processes occur at different rates and may occur to different degrees depending on the nature of vessel injury and individual patient characteristics.

The problem
Large randomized trials have established that following percutaneous transluminal coronary angioplasty (PTCA), restenosis rates in the treated vessel are between 30% and 60% (following POBA) and 15%–30% (following stent implantation). They are higher still in selected high-risk patients (e.g., diabetics).

This relatively high incidence of **angiographic** restenosis, however, translates into revascularization in about 10% of patients, in whom **clinical** restenosis is said to have occurred.

Prevention of restenosis
Mechanical
Stent implantation
Stent implantation reduces restenosis rates by increasing the mean luminal diameter after angioplasty and preventing elastic recoil and adventitial constriction.

Optimization of stent deployment by IVUS guidance
Using intravascular ultrasound to establish whether a stent has been adequately deployed improves the results of percutaneous intervention.

Antithrombotic and antiplatelet treatment
Early aggressive antithrombotic and antiplatelet therapy with heparin, aspirin, gpIIb/IIIa antagonists, and clopidogrel reduces the incidence of acute stent thrombosis.

Drug-eluting stents

Implantation of stents has to a great extent overcome the problem of elastic recoil and negative remodeling following PTCA. It is thus evident that neointimal proliferation, resulting in stent restenosis, remains the major limiting factor for stenting procedures. Much research has focused on the role of antiproliferative agents in the reduction of restenosis, and recently drug-eluting stents have emerged as the preeminent solution to this problem.

Drug-eluting stents are coated stents, capable of releasing bioactive components into the local tissue and bloodstream (see Box 14.4). The advent of stents as a platform for the delivery of drugs, with subsequent reduction in rates of stent restenosis, is radically changing the treatment of patients with coronary artery disease.

The number of CABG procedures performed worldwide is falling, with more patients who previously would only have been candidates for CABG being treated by percutaneous coronary intervention (PCI). Increasingly, the favorable results obtained with DES mean that PCI is performed in complex cases such as LMCA stenosis, diffuse disease, and bifurcation anatomy.

Several large RCTs, which have demonstrated both the safety and efficacy of these stents, have supported the introduction of DES into routine clinical practice.

Sirolimus-eluting stents

The drug sirolimus has potent antifungal, immunosuppressive, and antimitotic properties. This agent was approved for rejection prophylaxis in renal transplantation in 1999, with trials of a sirolimus-coated coronary stent following soon thereafter.
- The first human experience of a sirolimus-coated stent (45 patients) illustrated a virtual absence of neoinitimal proliferation at follow-up.

Box 14.4 Drug-eluting stents

- Similarities between tumor growth and benign neointimal proliferation introduced the concept that immunosuppressant and cytotoxic agents might be beneficial for preventing in-stent restenosis.
- Incorporation of these agents into stent coatings, using a number of techniques, has now enabled delivery of the active agent directly to its site of action, while limiting systemic side effects.
- Crucially, the coatings allow sustained release of the agent such that the therapy is present at the time that the target mechanism is physiologically active.
- The commonly used agents are sirolimus, which has a cytostatic action, and paclitaxel, which is cytotoxic. Other agents include everolimus and zatorolimus.

- The seminal RAVEL study enrolled 238 patients, randomly allocated to BX velocity stent, or sirolimus-eluting BX velocity stent (the Cypher™ Stent). It reported 0% restenosis in the group treated with the DES.
- The large-scale SIRIUS study ($n = 1100$) confirmed the potent antirestenosis effects of Cypher™ stents.

Paclitaxel eluting stents

Paclitaxel has potent antitumor activity via its action as a microtubule-stabilizing agent. Coronary stents eluting paclitaxel have been extensively investigated.

- TAXUS I studied 61 patients randomly assigned to paclitaxel-coated stent or bare metal stent. This study both established the safety of the stent, but also showed a major adverse cardiac events (MACE) rate in the DES arm of 3%, compared with 10% in the BMS arm at 1-year follow-up.
- TAXUS II compared slow- and moderate-release formulations of paclitaxel with bare metal stenting, and found significantly lower MACE rates in both slow- and moderate-release DES (2.3%/4.7%) than those in BMS-treated control groups (20.2%).

SIRIUS and TAXUS, and each of their subsequent follow-up studies and registries, have established that Cypher™ and Taxus™ stents have similar, low rates of TLR (between 3% and 8%).

Box 14.5

AHA/ACC/ESC recommends the use of a DES in PCI for patients with symptomatic CAD in whom the target artery is <3 mm in caliber or the lesion is longer than 15 mm. In real-world practice this translates to coronary artery lesions in approximately 60%–70% of patients undergoing PCI.

Stent thrombosis

It should be appreciated that documentation of ST by angiography under-estimates the real incidence of this event, since some of the patients with stent thrombosis develop MI or die without angiographic documentation of stent thrombosis.

To address this issue, an Academic Research Consortium (ARC) com-posed of clinical investigators, industry representatives, and regulatory authorities (including the FDA) has proposed new definitions for ST in an attempt to establish uniformity and improve sensitivity for the diagnosis of ST.

There are three levels of evidence in defining ST:

1. Definite stent thrombosis

Angiographic confirmation is based on TIMI (thrombolysis in myocardial infarction) flow:
- TIMI flow 0 with occlusion originating in the stent or in the segment 5 mm proximal or distal to the stent region with presence of thrombus
- TIMI flow 1, 2, or 3 originating in the stent or the segment 5 mm proximal or distal to the stent region with presence of thrombus

AND at least one of the following criteria has been fulfilled within a 48-hours period:
- New acute onset of ischemic symptoms at rest
- New ischemic electrocardiogram changes that suggest acute ischemia
- Typical rise and fall in cardiac biomarkers as evidence for an acute MI

Pathologic confirmation
- Confirmation of recent ST either at autopsy or via examination of tissue retrieved after thrombectomy

2. Probable stent thrombosis

Considered to have occurred after intracoronary stent implantation in the following cases:
- Any unexplained death within the first 30 days
- Irrespective of the time after the index procedure, any MI that is related to acute ischemia in the territory of the implanted stent without angiographic confirmation of stent thrombosis and in the absence of any other obvious cause

3. Possible stent thrombosis
- Any unexplained death from 30 days after intracoronary stenting until end of trial follow-up

Based on the timing after implantation of DES, ST could be
- Acute: 0 to 24 hours post–stent implantation
- Subacute: 24 hours to 30 days post–stent implantation
- Late: 30 days to 1 year post–stent implantation
- Very late: >1 year post–stent implantation

Based on the design of the pivotal clinical trials that led to approval of DES, dual antiplatelet therapy was prescribed on an empirical basis for 2–3 months after implantation of sirolimus-eluting stents and for 6 months after implantation of paclitaxel-eluting stents, with lifelong aspirin.

However, concerns about long-term safety were first made public in 2005 after several case reports were published that suggested that even late after DES placement, discontinuation of antiplatelet therapy may allow stent thrombosis. This appears to be due to failure of DES to re-endothelialize.

These concerns were confirmed when 746 nonselected patients with 1133 stented lesions surviving 6 months without major events were followed for 1 year after the discontinuation of clopidogrel in the BASKET-LATE trial, which showed that documented late stent thrombosis and related death/target vessel MI were twice as frequent after DES vs. BMS (2.6% vs. 1.3%). Thrombosis-related events occurred between 15 and 362 days after the discontinuation of clopidogrel, presenting as MI or death in 88% of the cases.

Since then, multiple trials, registries, and meta-analyses have studied the incidence of DES ST with numbers that range from 0.1% to 2.9%. Based on these data, the FDA now recommends continuous use of dual antiplatelet therapy for 1–2 years if there are not major bleeding complications.

Physiological assessment of coronary flow

The shortcomings of coronary angiography in the *physiological* assessment of coronary stenosis are clear. Intravascular ultrasound can provide information on the size of the lumen and the composition of plaque, but again gives no information on the effect that an atheromatous plaque may have on coronary flow. The knowledge as to whether a narrowing seen on angiography is the culprit causing hemodynamic effects, and thus anginal symptoms, is valuable when guiding percutaneous intervention.

The fractional flow reserve (FFR) correlates distal coronary pressure to myocardial blood flow during maximum hyperemia (induced by infusion of adenosine, or papaverine). *FFR* is defined as maximum myocardial blood flow in the presence of a stenosis divided by the theoretical maximum flow in the absence of a stenosis (see Fig. 14.13).

Thus the information derived from FFR allows an "on-the-spot" diagnosis of the extent to which a given stenosis contributes to myocardial ischemia (and angina), and can guide decisions regarding revascularization. At present, the best established indication for coronary FFR estimation is as a diagnostic tool to assess "severe" coronary stenosis, and for this it is extremely sensitive when used with a cutoff point of 0.75. The technique has also been used to optimize the results of stent implantation.

Two technologies are currently available that provide hemodynamic information derived from FFR calculations; these are pressure wires (which consist of a pressure transducer mounted on a 0.014" guide wire), and Doppler flow wires (which examine coronary flow velocities using spectral analysis).

Pressure wire, e.g., the PressureWire™ (Radi Medical Systems, Volcano Medical Systems)
- The pressure transducer is located at the transition between the radiopaque wire tip and the nonradiopaque stem.
- The analyzer shows simultaneous aortic and intracoronary pressure, as well as instantaneous FFR.

Doppler wire, e.g., FlowWire™ (Endosonics)
- This obtains information on coronary flow velocity in the central area of the arterial lumen.
- Combining flow and ECG information, it calculates systolic and diastolic components of flow velocity at baseline.
- Following induction of hyperemia, the machine can calculate the coronary flow velocity reserve.

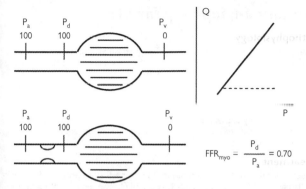

Figure 14.13 During maximal arteriolar vasodilatation, the resistance of the myocardium is minimal, and so maximum myocardial blood flow is proportional to hyperemic perfusion pressure. This equals P_d P_v. As there is no decline in pressure along a normal coronary artery, and neglecting P_v, this implies that in a normal epicardial artery, perfusion pressure at hyperemia equals P_a. In the presence of a stenosis, hyperemic perfusion pressure decreases to P_d (after the stenosis). Thus the maximum flow in the presence of a stenosis as a ratio (fraction) of normal maximum flow is represented by the ratio of perfusion pressures: P_d/P_a. This fraction of normal maximum flow, which is maintained despite the stenosis, is called the *fractional flow reserve* (FFR). Reproduced with permission from Pijls NH (2004). *Heart* 90(9):1085–1093.

Primary angioplasty for STEMI

Pathophysiology

In the context of cardiac chest pain, ST segment elevation on the 12 lead ECG usually signifies complete occlusion of a proximal epicardial coronary artery. This occurs as a result of rupture or erosion of a vulnerable atheromatous plaque, which leads to platelet activation and adhesion, formation of platelet-rich (white) thrombus, fibrin deposition, and red cell entrapment (forming red thrombus).

If untreated, myocardial necrosis commences within 30 minutes, affecting full myocardial thickness within 6 hours; 30% of patients die before reaching the hospital.

Treatment

Urgent restoration of coronary blood flow (reperfusion) prevents further LV damage and improves prognosis (Box 14.6). The amount of myocardium that can be salvaged falls exponentially with time, with the greatest benefit within 3 hours following symptom onset, and little benefit after 12 hours.

Primary angioplasty is the preferred reperfusion strategy, where angiography can be performed within 90 minutes of presentation.

Patients can be transferred safely (by a trained ambulance crew with an ACLS trained escort) from a community hospital to a cardiac center for primary angioplasty.

Box 14.6 Options for reperfusion

Primary angioplasty

Immediate coronary arteriography, culprit vessel angioplasty, and stent implantation *without antecedent fibrinolysis* achieves full arterial patency (TIMI grade 3 flow) in 90%–95%, treating the occlusive thrombus and the culprit plaque.

Intravenous fibrinolysis

Immediate administration of a fibrinolytic agent (also called *thrombolysis*) without planned coronary arteriography achieves full arterial patency (TIMI grade 3 flow) in 50%–60%. It is contraindicated in up to 30% of patients and does not treat the culprit plaque.

Rescue angioplasty

Urgent coronary arteriography, culprit vessel angioplasty, and stent implantation are performed when fibrinolysis has failed to achieve reperfusion (persistent ST-segment elevation 9 pain at 60–90 minutes).

Primary angioplasty: procedure

Indications
- Cardiac chest pain <12 hours (e.g., see Fig. 14.14)
- ST Elevation ≥1 mm in 2 contiguous leads and/or new LBBB

Contraindications
- Suspected aortic dissection
- Major contraindication to anticoagulation therapy

Relative contraindications
- Active bleeding (antiplatelet therapy may have to be avoided but may compromise outcome. These cases should be discussed directly with the operator).

Pre-procedure (work quickly—minutes matter)
- Consent
- Basic blood work including CBC, chemistries, type and cross, cardiac biomarkers
- Oxygen if saturations <94%
- Aspirin 325 mg (chewed)
- Systemic anticoagulation (i.e., heparin, bivalirudin)
- Platelet glycoprotein gpIIb/IIIa receptor antagonist (abciximab) is indicated when heparin alone is used and as a bailout option in cases where bivalirudin is used and there is a significant thrombus burden, non-reflow, and high risk of vessel closure.
- Access—femoral or radial. The femoral region should always be prepared in case of need for transvenous pacing or intra-aortic balloon pump (IABP) insertion.
- Diagnostic angiogram should be performed to identify the culprit vessel.
- Angioplasty should then performed.

Additional considerations
- Culprit-vessel PCI is a Class I indication. PCI to a non-infarct-related artery is Class III and should be deferred for a later time (typically >24 hours).
- Procedural success is defined by TIMI grade 2 or 3 flow with residual stenosis <30%.

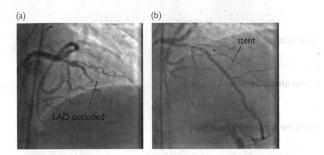

Figure 14.14 Angiographic images from a 54-year-old male presenting with chest pain and anterior ST elevation. (a) The left anterior descending (LAD) artery is occluded mid-vessel (arrow). (b) The same artery now widely patent following primary angioplasty; a 3.5 × 24 mm bare metal stent has been implanted (arrow). The patient sustained minimal left ventricular damage and was discharged 48 hours later.

Invasive assessment of vulnerable plaque

It has become apparent from intravascular ultrasound studies that non-obstructive and hemodynamically insignificant atherosclerotic plaques can be responsible for sudden death due to myocardial infarction. These high-risk, or "vulnerable," plaques are left untreated, as it is unclear which will progress to rupture. Angiography does not help differentiate between stable and vulnerable plaques, thus new technologies have been developed to assist in the identification of these plaques.

Histopathological correlates of vulnerable plaque

- Lipid-rich core
- Thin fibrous cap
- Necrotic core
- High degree of macrophage infiltration

Intravascular ultrasound

- Able to discriminate plaques with low (lipid) and high (fibrous) echodensity
- Able to identify the capsule
- Able to identify areas of rupture within the plaque
- In combination with image analysis, information regarding the tissue types imaged can be derived to provide a histological map of the plaque.

Optical coherence tomography (OCT)

- This is similar in principle to intravascular ultrasound, but uses light instead of sound waves.
- The system has high axial resolution, down to 20 µm.
- At present, useful anatomical information can be obtained by this technique, but this is yet to be correlated with functional data.

Intravascular elastography

- This technology uses sound waves in a similar way to IVUS.
- Images are based on radial strain, and the system is therefore able to help differentiate soft from hard material.
- Plaque rupture is often seen to occur in areas of increased strain, such as at the edge of plaques.

Complex coronary angioplasty

Chronic total occlusion

Chronic total occlusion (CTO) is defined as a completely occluded coronary artery, with the occlusion being known to have been present for >3 months. The age and length of the occlusion are the main determinants of success of PCI (e.g., see Box 14.7). The objectives in treating CTOs percutaneously are as follows:

- Crossing of the total occlusion with a guide wire and advancement of this wire into the distal vessel (inability to cross with the guide wire is the reason for failure in 50% of attempts at CTO PCI)
- Dilatation of the underlying occlusion
- Preservation of the newly recanalized lumen by the implantation of a stent and by pharmacological means

Techniques that may improve success

- Aggressive guide catheter support, including deep cannulation of the coronary artery
- Over-the-wire balloon to support the guide wire as it is advanced against the CTO
- Stiffer guide wires that require greater forces to deflect the tip and may be more successful in penetrating the "cap" of the CTO. Great care must be taken with guide wires of this nature, as there is risk of perforation of the target vessel.

Unfortunately, if the lumen is recanalized, the rates of reocclusion are high, even when the CTO is stented.

Bifurcation lesions

A simple definition of bifurcation lesions can be the involvement of a side branch with a reference diameter >2 mm in the stenosis. IVUS studies show that plaque in the main vessel almost invariably extends some distance into side branches that arise within the plaque. Furthermore, angioplasty to a plaque will often cause plaque shift (the so-called snow plow effect) into the daughter vessel.

Unless flow in the side branch was severely impaired, or the ostium severely narrowed, during the treatment of the main vessel, a single-stent technique is preferable to the use of two stents. This is the so-called *provisional stenting* technique (see Fig. 14.15).

Dilating with a balloon through the stent struts carries the risk of deforming the distal parts of the stent and failure of adequate apposition of stent to vessel wall. This carries a high risk of thrombosis and restenosis, thus a final "kissing" balloon should be employed.

Recent data on the use of DES in the treatment of bifurcations suggest that implantation of DES reduces the restenosis and reintervention rates after bifurcation lesion treatment.

Box 14.7 What makes angioplasty complex?

• Increased risk of procedural failure
• Suboptimal result likely
• Complication rate higher
• Worse long-term outcome (death, MI, repeat procedure)

Patient characteristics
• Clinical presentation—acute vs. stable
• Diabetes
• Body habitus
• Significant comorbidity
• Access problems—peripheral vascular disease

Lesion characteristics
• Lesion characteristics, e.g., long, calcified, bifurcation, left main stem, chronic total occlusions
• Difficult anatomy

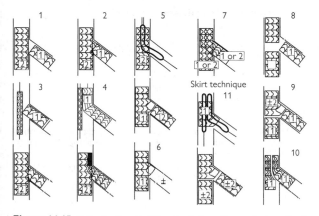

Figure 14.15 Methods of treating bifurcation lesions. The numbering refers to the order in which the stents are deployed. All of these methods have been tried, but recent data suggest that the provisional stent technique (part 5) produces the best results. Adapted with permission from Louvard Y, et al (2004). *Heart* 90(6):713–722.

Left main stem angioplasty

AHA/ACC/ESC guidelines suggest that patients with stenosis of the left main coronary artery should be offered bypass graft surgery. However, the registry data for both bare metal stents and, more recently, drug-eluting stents have suggested that PCI to the left main stem (LMS) in patients with suitable LMS anatomy achieves acceptable results with low rates of procedural complication and long-term vessel patency. Nonetheless, it remains a Class III indication to perform LM PCI.

The advent of drug-eluting stents and the reality of lower rates of in-stent restenosis with DES than with BMS have further changed the approach of many interventional cardiologists to this previously taboo subset. In patients treated electively for LMS stenosis, reference vessel size and left ventricular function appear to be the strongest predictors of favorable outcome.

Patient groups in whom LMS PCI may be appropriate

Emergency LMS PCI
- Bailout PCI after complications involving the LMS

Elective LMS PCI
- Patients considered to high risk to undergo CABG, but with continuing angina
- Patients who refuse surgery
- Younger patients with favorable LMS anatomy (i.e., not ostial disease, not short LMS)

Optimization of results of LMS PCI

Nothing less than an excellent angiographic result should be accepted. Intravascular ultrasound may be used both pre-procedure to ascertain the true vessel diameter and post-procedure to ensure that stents have been adequately deployed.

LMS bifurcations may be approached using the techniques described before. There is emerging evidence that the use of DES in the LMS bifurcation results in improved clinical outcomes.

Most operators routinely reexamine the LMS by angiography 6–9 months after PCI to look for restenosis.

Adjunctive therapy for angioplasty and stenting

Aspirin

The beneficial effect of aspirin during PCI has been shown in multiple trials, in which treatment with aspirin and dipyridamole was superior to placebo in the prevention of periprocedural Q-wave MI.

Subsequent studies have shown that dipyridamole added nothing to the beneficial effects provided by aspirin. Aspirin (usually 325 mg once daily), initiated at least 24 hours prior to procedure, is recommended in patients undergoing elective PCI.

Thienopyridines

Clopidogrel and ticlopidine are thienopyridine derivatives that inhibit platelet function independent of aspirin by interference with the platelet ADP receptor. Early studies showed that a dual antiplatelet therapy with aspirin and ticlopidine was superior to aspirin alone. The use of ticlopidine is limited by its side effects, including severe neutropenia.

Clopidogrel, a newer thienopyridine, with a safer side-effect profile, has thus become the agent of choice. The PCI-CURE study showed that pre-treatment with clopidogrel (300 mg loading dose, followed by 75 mg daily) in addition to aspirin for a median of 10 days before percutaneous coronary intervention, compared with aspirin alone, reduced the composite of cardiovascular death, myocardial infarction, or urgent target vessel revascularization by 30% after 1 month.

Most centers have adopted the policy of high loading dose clopidogrel (600 mg 2–4 hours pre-PCI) if the patient has not been preloaded.

Heparin

Although there is general agreement that patients undergoing PCI should receive heparin before the intervention, there remains controversy regarding the issue of optimal heparin dosage. An inverse relation between the level of anticoagulation (measured by activated clotting time [ACT]) and the occurrence of acute ischemic complications has been observed. However, longer ACTs are associated with higher bleeding risks.

Currently, an ACT of 250–300 seconds is recommended for patients undergoing PCI. Low-molecular weight heparin (enoxaparin) has been shown to be effective in PCI, although it has not yet replaced unfractionated heparin in routine use.

Glycoprotein IIb/IIIa inhibitors

The final common pathway for platelet aggregation is mediated by the platelet glycoprotein (gp) IIb/IIIa receptor. Trials in both diabetics and nondiabetics undergoing percutaneous transluminal coronary angioplasty have found that the combination of stenting and a gpIIb/IIIa inhibitor reduces cardiovascular morbidity and mortality compared with stent plus placebo.

Bivalirudin

Bivalirudin is a direct thrombin inhibitor that exerts its activity by specifically and reversibly interacting with circulating (inactive) and clot-bound (active) thrombin.

Clinical trials in patients with stable or unstable angina or acute myocardial infarction (Replace, Acuity, Horizons) who received bivalirudin in PCI have demonstrated similar benefits to the combination of abciximab and heparin, with a reduced risk of clinically significant blood loss.

Embolic protection devices

The distal embolization of particulate matter that lodges in the microcirculation (e.g., plaque debris, thrombus, and fibrin) during balloon inflation and stent deployment is becoming increasingly recognized as a cause of suboptimal results after PCI. Distal embolization leads to poor flow in the proximal vessel undergoing intervention due to occlusion of distal microvasculature, the "no-reflow" phenomenon.

Vein grafts, and thrombotic lesions are now recognized as being particularly prone to complications arising from distal embolization, which is seen in up to 30% of vein grafts (these often contain thrombus at the time of PCI). Hence the use of distal protection devices should be considered in these angioplasty subsets.

Devices for distal protection

Devices can be broadly split into those that occlude the conduit distally and then allow aspiration of debris, or distal filters that capture debris downstream.

Balloon occlusion devices

- PercuSurge GuardWire. This consists of three parts:
  1. The GuardWire temporary occlusion catheter, which is placed distally in the vessel to allow occlusion.
  2. The MicroSeal adapter, which allows control over the inflation and deflation of the balloon.
  3. The Export aspiration catheter, which allows collected debris to be aspirated into a 20 mL syringe.

One of the main disadvantages of this system is that the target vessel is temporarily occluded, thus the distal myocardium may be rendered ischemic.

Filter devices

- AngioGuard. This device consists of an angioplasty guide wire with an expandable filter at the distal tip. The filter can be expanded once the target lesion has been crossed. Anterograde blood flow in the vessel is maintained, and displaced debris should theoretically be collected in the filter. The filter is then collapsed and withdrawn into the retrieving catheter.
- FilterWire EZ™ (Fig. 14.16). This device consists of a "fish mouth" opening distal filter, mounted on an angioplasty guide wire. The "mouth" of the filter in theory expands to fill the entire lumen of the vessel. The filter is deployed by withdrawing a delivery sheath, and collected into a retrieval sheath.

Limitations of distal protection devices

- Crossing profile may cause distal embolization
- Incomplete filter apposition or incomplete conduit occlusion
- Lack of protection of side branches
- Distal ischemia in balloon occlusion devices

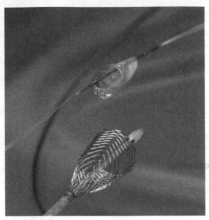

Figure 14.16 FilterWire EZ™. Reproduced with permission from Boston Scientific.

Thrombectomy

In the context of the limitations of distal protection devices, devices that can aspirate particulate debris and thrombus proximally have been developed.

Transluminal extraction catheter (TEC)

This is a rotational cutting device. However, the blades are not protected, thus limiting use in native coronary arteries.

Export catheter

This aspiration catheter allows collected debris to be aspirated into a 20 mL syringe.

The Angiojet

This device relies on the Venturi effect produced from backward-directed fluid jets. These jets create vortices and areas of low pressure that cause debris distal to the catheter to be drawn in and aspirated.

Mitral valvuloplasty

In carefully selected patients with mitral stenosis, percutaneous balloon mitral valvuloplasty (PMV) (see Fig. 14.17) is now the treatment of choice, according to the American Heart Association and American College of Cardiology:

In centers with skilled, experienced operators, PMV should be considered the initial procedure of choice for symptomatic patients with moderate to severe mitral stenosis who have favorable valve morphology in the absence of significant mitral regurgitation or left atrial thrombus. In asymptomatic patients with favorable valve morphology, PMV may be considered if there is evidence of a hemodynamic effect on left atrial pressure (new-onset atrial fibrillation) or pulmonary circulation (pulmonary artery pressure >50 mmHg at rest or 60 mmHg with exercise).[1]

Case selection

Careful case selection is paramount. The factors that must be considered are described below.

Age

Older patients seem to have poorer outcomes in PMV. This outcome is likely related to valve morphology in this group instead of age per se. In patients in whom surgery of the mitral valve is contraindicated (e.g., extreme age, significant comorbidity), adequate results can be obtained even in the presence of suboptimal valve morphology.

Valve morphology

A valve scoring system (an echocardiogram-based evaluation of valve calcification and anatomy) is used to assess the valves suitability for PMV: leaflet mobility, leaflet thickening, valve calcification, and involvement of the subvalvular apparatus. Each parameter evaluated receives from 0 (none) to 4 (severe).

Studies have shown that patients with a valve score of ≤8 consistently achieve superior and more sustained results from the procedure than patients with scores >8.

Mitral regurgitation

The presence of significant mitral regurgitation is a contraindication to PMV.

Left atrial thrombus

This is a contraindication to PMV. Patients in AF should have been fully anticoagulated for a period of 4–6 weeks prior to the procedure.

Pregnancy

PMV can be performed in pregnancy. Radiation risk to the fetus is reduced after 14 weeks.

---

1 Bonow RO, et al. (2008). *J Am Coll Cardiol* 52(13):e1–142.

Complications of mitral valvuloplasty

- Mitral regurgitation
- Pericardial tamponade
- Thromboembolic events
- Iatrogenic ASD

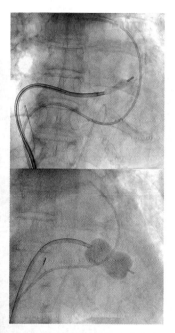

Figure 14.17 Balloon mitral valvuloplasty. The upper panel shows the balloon partly inflated across the mitral valve, demonstrating the typical dumb-bell shape. As the inflation pressure and volume are increased, the stenosed valve dilates (lower panel).

Glossary of terms and abbreviations

Bifurcation: A bifurcation lesion involving a main vessel and a side branch or a main vessel.

Binary angiographic restenosis (BAR): Greater than 50% luminal narrowing on follow-up angiogram.

Canadian Cardiovascular Society (CCS) Angina Classification
1. No chest pain. No limitation of physical activity by pain. Ordinary physical activity, such as walking and climbing stairs, does not cause angina. Angina with strenuous, rapid, or prolonged exertion at work or recreation.
2. Slight limitation of ordinary activity. Walking or climbing stairs rapidly, walking up hill, walking or stair climbing after meals, in cold, in wind, or when under emotional stress or during the first few hours after awakening may cause pain. Walking more than two blocks on the level and climbing more than one flight of stairs at a normal pace and in normal conditions.
3. Marked limitation of ordinary physical activity. Walking 1–2 blocks on a level and climbing one flight of stairs at normal pace results in angina.
4. Inability to carry on any physical activity without discomfort. Anginal syndrome may be present at rest.

Chronic occlusion: An occlusion presumed to have been present for at least 1 month prior to the procedure.

Culprit (target) lesion revascularization (CLR/TLR): Repeat revascularization of a culprit lesion in the target vessel.

In-segment: The portion of coronary artery located either within the margins of the stent or 5 mm proximal or distal to the stent.

In-stent: The portion of coronary artery located within the margins of the stent.

IVUS: Intravascular ultrasound.

Late lumen loss: Post-procedural minimum lumen diameter minus follow-up minimum lumen diameter.

Minimum luminal diameter (MLD): The average of two orthogonal views (when possible) of the narrowest point within the area of assessment—in lesion, in-stent, or in-segment.

National Heart Lung and Blood Institute (NHLBI) Dissection Classification System
- **A** Minor radiolucencies within the lumen during contrast injection with no persistence after dye clearance.
- **B** Parallel tracts or double lumen separated by a radiolucent area during contrast injection with no persistence after dye clearance.
- **C** Extraluminal cap with persistence of contrast after dye clearance from the lumen.

D Spiral luminal filling defects.
E New persistent filling defects.
F Non-A–E types that lead to impaired flow or total occlusion.

Percutaneous coronary intervention (PCI): Refers to all interventional cardiology methods for treatment of coronary artery disease.

QCA: Quantitative coronary analysis.

QIVUS: Quantitative intravascular ultrasound.

Reference vessel diameter (RVD): The mean of two angiographic measurements that are derived by interpolation at the target lesion.

Subtotal occlusion: TIMI grade I, and with collateral filling of the distal segment.

Target lesion revascularization (TLR): Repeat PCI or CABG to the target lesion (culprit lesion).

Target vessel revascularization (TVR): Repeat PCI or CABG to the target vessel (culprit vessel), inclusive of target lesion.

TIMI flow grade
0 No contrast flow through the stenosis.
1 A small amount of contrast flows through the stenosis but fails to fully opacify the vessel beyond.
2 Contrast material flows through the stenosis to opacify the terminal vessel segment. However, contrast enters the terminal segment perceptibly more slowly than more proximal segments.
3 Antegrade flow into the terminal coronary vessel segment through a stenosis is as prompt as antegrade flow into a comparable segment proximal to the stenosis.

Total occlusion: An occlusion with no antegrade filling of contrast to the distal segment (TIMI grade 0).

Further reading

Andersen HR, Nielsen TT, Rasmussen K, et al. (2003). A comparison of coronary angioplasty with fibrinolytic therapy in acute myocardial infarction. *N Engl J Med* 349:733–742.

Keeley EC, Boura JA, Grines CL (2003). Primary angioplasty vs. intravenous thrombolytic therapy for acute myocardial infarction: a quantitative review of 23 randomized trials. *Lancet* 361:13–20.

Widimsky P, Budesinsky T, Vorac D, et al. (2003). Long distance transport for primary angioplasty vs. immediate thrombolysis in acute myocardial infarction. Final results of the randomized national multicentre trial-PRAGUE-2. *Eur Heart J* 24:94–104.

Major trials in cardiology

ACUITY

Bivalirudin for Patients with Acute Coronary Syndromes

Purpose: To evaluate treatment with heparin plus glycoprotein (gp) IIb/IIIa inhibition compared with bivalirudin with or without gpIIb/IIIa inhibition among patients with acute coronary syndromes.

Follow-up: 1 year

Results: Treatment with bivalirudin alone was associated with a reduction in the net clinical benefit end point compared with UFH/Enox plus gpIIb/IIIa inhibitors, driven primarily by a reduction in bleeding. Major bleeding was significantly lower in the bivalirudin alone group than in the heparin plus gpIIb/IIIa group (3.0% vs. 5.7%, *p* < 0.001 for superiority), and was noninferior but not superior for the comparison of bivalirudin plus gpIIb/IIIa inhibitor with the UFH/Enox plus gpIIb/IIIa group (5.3% vs. 5.7%, *p* = 0.001 for noninferiority).

Reference: Stone GW, et al. (2006). *N Engl J Med* 355: 2203–2216.

ADMIRAL

Abciximab before Direct angioplasty and stenting in Myocardial Infarction Regarding Acute and Long-term follow-up

Purpose: To demonstrate the superiority of abciximab over placebo in primary PTCA with stenting in 300 patients with acute myocardial infarction of <12 hours symptom onset. Patients were given unfractionated heparin, aspirin, and ticlopidine prior to randomization. Coronary angiography was performed at the time of randomization, 24 hours later, and at 6 months.

Follow-up: 30 days and 6 months

Results: Abciximab in conjunction with primary stenting improved early TIMI 3 flow rate, left ventricular function and 30-day mortality, recurrent MI, and rates of any revascularization. There was excess minor bleeding in the abciximab group.

Reference: ADMIRAL Investigators (2001). *N Engl J Med* 344: 1895–1903.

AFCAPS/ TexCAPS

Airforce/Texas Coronary Atherosclerosis Prevention Study

Purpose: To determine if lovastatin 20–40 mg/day has a role in the primary prevention of acute coronary events (MI, unstable angina, sudden cardiac death) in 5608 men and 997 women with normal or mildly elevated total or LDL cholesterol, low HDL cholesterol, and no clinically evident atherosclerotic disease, in a randomized, placebo-controlled trial.

Follow-up: 5.2 years

Results: Lovastatin reduced LDL cholesterol by 25% and increased HDL cholesterol by 6%. The incidences of first major acute coronary events, MI, unstable angina, coronary revascularization, and cardiovascular events were all significantly reduced. There were too few fatal cardiovascular and fatal coronary heart disease events to perform a survival analysis.

Reference: Downs JR, et al (1999) *JAMA* 279:1615–1622.

AFCAPS/ TexCAPS

Atrial Fibrillation Follow-up Investigation of Rhythm Management (AFFIRM) Investigators

AFFIRM

Purpose: To evaluate two management strategies in treating AF: 1) cardioversion followed by drugs to maintain sinus rhythm (a choice of amiodarone, disopyramide, flecainide, moricizine, procainamide, propafenone, quinidine, sotalol); 2) rate-control drugs, allowing AF to persist (a choice of β-blockers, verapamil, diltiazem, digoxin). Anticoagulation was recommended for both groups. 4060 patients with recent-onset AF and a high risk of stroke or death were randomized. The primary end point was overall mortality. 71% had hypertension, and 38% had coronary artery disease. 3311 had echocardiograms, and of these, 65% had enlarged left atria, and 26% had impaired LV function.

Follow-up: 5 years

Results: Mortality at 5 years was 23.8% in the rhythm-control group and 21.3% in the rate-control group (hazard ratio 1.15, $p = 0.08$). More patients in the rhythm-control group were hospitalized and had more adverse drug effects. In both groups, most strokes occurred after warfarin had been stopped or if INR was subtherapeutic; this occurred more often in the rhythm-control group. During the course of the study, 594 patients assigned to the rhythm-control group crossed over to the rate-control group, mainly because of inability to maintain sinus rhythm and drug intolerance.

Reference: The AFFIRM Investigators (2002). *N Engl J Med* 347:1825–1833.

African American Heart Failure Trial

AHEFT

Purpose: To evaluate treatment with fixed-dose isosorbide dinitrate plus hydralazine compared with placebo among black patients with heart failure. 1050 patients were randomized to either fixed-dose hydralazine and isosorbide dinitrate vs. placebo. Randomization was stratified by β-blocker use. Initial dosing was 20 mg isosorbide dinitrate and 37.5 mg hydralazine and titrated up to 120 mg isosorbide dinitrate and 225 mg hydralazine. Most patients were NYHA Class III, with a mean age of 57 years and a mean ejection fraction of 24%.

Follow-up: Mean 18 months

AHEFT

Results: Mortality was lower in the combination-therapy group, 6.2% vs. placebo 10.2%. The survival difference began at 6 months after randomization and continued to diverge through follow-up. The primary composite score was significantly improved in the combination-therapy group compared with placebo (-0.1 ± 1.9 vs. -0.5 ± 2.0, $p = 0.01$). Target dose was given in 68.0% of patients in the combination-therapy group and 88.9% of patients in the placebo group ($p < 0.001$). Blood pressure (BP) was lower in the combination-therapy group than in the placebo group (systolic BP -1.9 mmHg vs. $+1.2$ mmHg for placebo, $p = 0.02$; diastolic BP -2.4 mmHg vs. $+0.8$ mmHg for placebo, $p < 0.001$). Adverse events of headache (47.5% vs. 19.2%, $p < 0.001$) and dizziness (29.3% vs. 12.3%, $p < 0.001$) were higher in the combination-therapy group, but exacerbations of CHF were lower, including all exacerbations (8.7% vs. 12.8%, $p = 0.04$) and severe exacerbations (3.1% vs. 7.0%, $p = 0.005$).

Reference: Taylor AL, et al. (2004). *N Engl J Med* 351:2049–2057.

AIRE

Acute Infarction Ramipril Efficacy Study

Purpose: To evaluate the effect of ramipril on total mortality of AMI survivors with early clinical evidence of heart failure, and to assess progression to severe or resistant heart failure, nonfatal reinfarction, and stroke, compared to placebo. 2006 patients aged ≥ 18 years with confirmed AMI 3–10 days prior to randomization with clinical evidence of heart failure were given ramipril at a starting dose of 2.5 mg or placebo.

Follow-up: Mean 15 months

Results: All-cause mortality was significantly lower at 30 days and maintained at the end of follow-up in the ramipril group (27% risk reduction), with 30% reduced risk of sudden death. 38% of the reduction in overall mortality was in the sudden-death subgroup that had developed severe resistant heart failure. There was no alteration in risk of stroke or reinfarction in the ramipril group. The study was continued in the AIREX study.

Reference: Cleland J, et al. (1997). *Eur Heart J* 18:41–51.

AIREX

AIRE Extension Study

Purpose: To assess the long-term (3 years after the end of AIRE) benefit of ramipril in the 603 UK patients from the AIRE study retrospectively, 302 initially on ramipril, 301 on placebo.

Follow-up: 3 years

Results: All-cause mortality occurred in 27% of ramipril-treated patients compared to 39% of placebo controls, representing a relative risk reduction of 36%.

Reference: Hall AS, et al. (1997). *Lancet* 349:1493–1497.

Antihypertensive and Lipid-Lowering Treatment to Prevent Heart Attack Trial

ALLHAT

Purpose: To compare outcomes in high-risk hypertensive patients >55 years old in a prospective, randomized trial using standard antihypertensive drugs and newer agents as initial monotherapy. Initially, more than 42,000 patients were randomized, but this number dropped to 33,357 after the doxazosin arm was halted because of increased morbidity (mainly stroke and heart failure) in this group compared to the chlorthalidone arm. The remainder was randomized to receive chlorthalidone, amlodipine, or lisinopril. 50% were women, and 35% were black. The primary end point was combined incidence of fatal CHD or nonfatal MI by intention to treat. Secondary outcomes were all-cause mortality, stroke, combined CHD (fatal CHD, nonfatal MI, coronary revascularization, or angina with hospitalization), or combined cardiovascular disease (combined CHD plus stroke, treated angina without hospitalization, heart failure, and peripheral arterial disease).

Follow-up: Mean 4.9 years

Results: All-cause mortality was not different between groups. Systolic pressures were higher with both amlodipine and lisinopril than with chlorthalidone, but diastolic pressures were slightly better with amlodipine. Secondary outcome measures were also better with chlorthalidone than with lisinopril.

Reference: The ALLHAT Officers and Coordinators for the ALLHAT Collaborative Research Group (2000). *JAMA* 283:1967–1975.

Anglo-Scandinavian Cardiac Outcomes Trial—Lipid Lowering Arm

ASCOT-LLA

Purpose: To assess benefits of cholesterol lowering in the primary prevention of coronary disease in hypertensive patients not conventionally deemed dyslipidaemic. 19,342 hypertensive patients with at least three other cardiovascular risk factors were randomized to one of two antihypertensive regimens (β-blocker plus diuretic, or calcium channel blocker plus ACE inhibitor). Of these, 10,305 had cholesterol of >6.5 mmol/L (250 mg/dL) and were randomized to atorvastatin 10 mg or placebo. The primary end point was death from coronary disease and nonfatal MI.

Follow-up: Median 3.3 years

ASCOT-LLA

Results: There was a significant reduction in the primary end point in the atorvastatin group (hazard ratio 0.64, $p =$ 0.0005), with the benefit being seen by the first year of follow-up. There was a significant reduction in fatal and nonfatal stroke, total cardiovascular events, and total coronary events in the atorvastatin group. Atorvastatin lowered cholesterol by 1.1 mmol/L after 3-year follow-up compared to controls. Risk reduction in primary events was unrelated to baseline cholesterol levels.

Reference: Sever P, et al. (2003). *Lancet* 361:1149–1158.

ASSENT-1

Assessment of the Safety and Efficacy of a New Thrombolytic-1

Purpose: To evaluate the safety of different doses of TNK-tPA (tenecteplase) as a single bolus for AMI patients. 3235 patients with a mean age of 61 years were randomized to receive 30 mg ($n - 1705$), 40 mg ($n - 1457$), and 50 mg ($n - 73$) of TNK-tPA over 5–10 seconds. Aspirin and IV heparin were given concomitantly.

Follow-up: On hospital discharge, and at 30 days

Results: Total stroke incidence at 30 days was 1.5%. Intracranial hemorrhage occurred in 0.77% at 30 days, with most of these occurring in the 30 mg group. The incidence of intracranial hemorrhage was lower in those treated within 6 hours of symptom onset. The incidence of death, nonfatal stroke, and severe bleeding were 6.4%, 7.4%, and 1.6% for the 30 mg, 40 mg, and 50 mg groups respectively, without significant differences between groups.

Reference: Van de Werf F, et al. (1999). *Am Heart J* 1737: 786–791.

ASSENT-2

Assessment of the Safety and Efficacy of a New Thrombolytic-2

Purpose: To compare single bolus tenecteplase (TNK-tpA) and alteplase (t-PA) infusion in treatment of AMI. 16,949 patients with symptom onset within 6 hours and median age 61 years were randomized to receive either drug. Aspirin and IV heparin were given concomitantly.

Follow-up: 30 days

Results: 30-day mortality, nonfatal stroke, and rates of intracranial hemorrhage were similar in the two groups, but there were fewer bleeding complications and less need for blood transfusion in the TNK-tpA group.

Reference: Assessment of the Safety and Efficacy of a New Thrombolytic (ASSENT-2) Investigators (1999). *Lancet* 354:716–722.

Assessment of the Safety and Efficacy of a New Thrombolytic–3, Assessment of the Safety and Efficacy of a New Thrombolytic–3 PLUS

ASSENT-3 and ASSENT-3 PLUS

In ASSENT-3 the aim was to determine the safety and efficacy of full-dose TNK-tPA in combination with enoxaparin, half-dose TNK-tPA plus abciximab plus low-dose unfractionated heparin, or full-dose TNK-tPA plus weight-adjusted unfractionated heparin in the treatment of 6095 patients with STEMI presenting within 6 hours of symptom onset. This was the first large-scale trial to investigate the use of low-molecular-weight heparin in thrombolysis. The combined end points of 30-day mortality, recurrent ischemia, recurrent MI, major bleeding, and intracranial hemorrhage were significantly lower in the enoxaparin and abciximab group. However, if 30-day mortality was considered separately, there was no significant difference between the groups. Major bleeding, mortality, and intracranial hemorrhage were higher in the abciximab group, and this effect was more pronounced in patients >75 years of age and in diabetics.

In ASSENT-3 PLUS, TNK-tPA was given to 1639 STEMI patients presenting within 6 hours with either enoxaparin or unfractionated heparin. Prehospital treatment with enoxaparin plus TNK provided no significant benefit over treatment with unfractionated heparin, although intracranial hemorrhage was greater in the enoxaparin-treated patients who were >75 years old, female, and weighed <60 kg. 50% of patients were treated within 2 hours compared to just 29% in ASSENT-3. Earlier treatment was associated with better 30-day mortality.

Reference: The ASSENT-3 Investigators (2001). *Lancet* 358:605–613.

Bypass Angioplasty Revascularization Investigation

BARI

Purpose: To compare percutaneous and surgical revascularization strategies in patients with multivessel disease suitable for either procedure, working on the hypothesis that an initial PTCA strategy does not result in a poorer 5-year clinical outcome than CABG. Patients with multivessel disease were randomized to an initial treatment strategy of CABG (n = 914) or PTCA (n = 915).

Follow-up: Mean 5.4 years

Results: 5-year survival rates for CABG and PTCA were 89.3% and 86.3%, respectively (p = 0.19), and the respective rates free from QWMI were 80.4% and 78.7%. 8% of patients in the CABG group vs. 54% in the PTCA group underwent further revascularization procedures. 69% of the PTCA group did not undergo subsequent CABG.

BARI

In diabetic patients, 5-year survival was 80.6% in the CABG group and 65.5% for the PTCA group. The conclusion was that PTCA initially did not compromise 5-year survival compared to CABG in patients with multivessel disease, except in diabetics. PTCA-treated patients underwent more frequent revascularization after initial randomization.

Reference: Aldermann E, et al. (1996). *N Engl J Med* 335: 217–225.

CADILLAC

Controlled Abciximab and Device Investigation to Lower Late Angioplasty Complications

Purpose: To examine the impact of the platelet glycoprotein IIb/IIIa inhibitor abciximab as an adjunct in treating acute MI (AMI). 2082 patients with AMI were randomized in an open-label 2x2 factorial design trial of primary stenting vs. angioplasty, and abciximab treatment (n = 1052) vs. no abciximab treatment (n = 1030). Baseline characteristics were balanced between groups.

Follow-up: 30 days and 1 year

Results: At 30 days, abciximab treatment vs. no abciximab significantly reduced the composite end point of death, MI, ischemia-led target vessel revascularization (TVR), or disabling stroke (4.6% vs. 7.0%, $p = 0.01$). However, at 12 months, there was no significant difference in composite end point. In an angiographic substudy (n = 656), restenosis, myocardial salvage, and infarct-artery reocclusion were unaffected by abciximab.

Reference: Tcheng JE, et al. (2003). *Circulation* 108: 1316–1323.

CAMIAT

Canadian Amiodarone Myocardial Infarction Trial

Purpose: To evaluate the impact of amiodarone vs. placebo on risk of VF or death due to arrhythmia in 1202 patients who had MI in the previous 6–45 days with frequent ventricular depolarizations ($\geq$10/hr or $\geq$1 run of sustained VT). Amiodarone was given initially at 10 mg/kg daily for 2 weeks, then as a maintenance dose 300–400 mg daily for 3–5 months, 200–300 mg daily for 4 months, then 200 mg for 5–7 days per week for 16 months. Patients had concomitant therapy with aspirin, β-blockers, calcium antagonist, warfarin, digoxin, and ACE inhibitors.

Follow-up: Mean 1.79 years

Results: There was a relative risk reduction in the end points of 48.5% in the amiodarone group. Death occurred in 6.0% of the placebo group and 3.3% of the amiodarone group.

Reference: Cairns AJ, et al. (1997). *Lancet* 349:675–682.

Clopidogrel versus Aspirin in Patients at Risk of Ischemic Events

CAPRIE

Purpose: To evaluate the relative effect of 75–325 mg aspirin and 75 mg clopidogrel in reducing the risk of a composite end point of ischemic stroke, MI, or vascular death in 19,185 patients with recent ischemic stroke, recent MI, or symptomatic peripheral vascular disease.

Follow-up: Mean 1.9 years

Results: Compared to aspirin, clopidogrel reduced the combined risk of ischemic stroke, MI, or vascular death by 8.7% ($p = 0.043$). There were no major differences in terms of safety or bleeding risk.

Reference: Harker LA, ct al. (1999). *Drug Safety* 4: 325–335.

Chimeric 7E3 Antiplatelet Therapy in Unstable angina Refractory to standard treatment

CAPTURE

Purpose: To evaluate the effect of abciximab in mortality, incidence of AMI and urgent intervention for recurrent ischemia in 1265 patients with refractory unstable angina scheduled for PTCA in a randomized placebo controlled trial. Patients in the abciximab group were given a bolus and infusion beginning 18–24 hours before the PTCA and continuing 1 hour after PTCA. The primary end point was death, AMI, or urgent intervention within 30 days of enrolment.

Follow-up: 30 days and 6 months

Results: At 30 days the primary end point occurred in 11.3% of the abciximab group and 15.9% of the placebo group ($p = 0.012$). The rate of MI was lower in the abciximab group than in the placebo group both before and during PTCA. Major bleeding occurred more frequently in the abciximab group than in placebo. At 6 months, there was no significant difference in the rates of death, MI, or repeat intervention, however.

Reference: The CAPTURE Investigators (1997). *Lancet* 349:1429–1435.

Cholesterol And Recurrent Events

CARE

Purpose: To evaluate the effect of 40 mg pravastatin on fatal and nonfatal MI in patients with average cholesterol levels. 4159 patients were recruited in a randomized, double-blind, placebo-controlled trial who were aged 21–75 years and had MI 3 20 months before randomization. Plasma cholesterol was <240 mg/dL, LDL 115–274 mg/dL, and triglycerides <350 mg/dL. If LDL cholesterol increased during the study, dietary counseling was offered as well as cholestyramine.

CARE

Follow-up: At least 5 years

Results: The pravastatin group had 24% lower risk of fatal and nonfatal MI, and the risk of CABG was reduced by 26% and risk of PTCA reduced by 23%. There was no reduction in coronary events if baseline total cholesterol was <125 mg/dL.

Reference: Sacks FM, et al. (1996). *N Engl J Med* 335: 1001–1009.

CARE HF

The effect of Cardiac Resynchronization on morbidity and mortality in Heart Failure

Purpose: To evaluate the addition of cardiac resynchronization therapy (CRT) to optimal pharmacological therapy in patients with advanced heart failure and cardiac dyssynchrony despite standard pharmacological therapy. A total of 813 patients were enrolled. Mean age was 67 years and mean left ventricular ejection fraction (LVEF) was 25%.

Follow-up: Mean 29.4 months

Results: Treatment with CRT was associated with a reduction in the primary end point of all-cause mortality and hospitalization for major cardiovascular events compared with standard pharmacological therapy in this patient population. The reduction in mortality in the CRT was significantly lower than with standard medical therapy alone in this study.

Reference: Cleland JG, Daubert JC, Erdmann E, et al. (2005). *N Engl J Med* 352(15):1539–1549.

CARMEN

Carvedilol ACE inhibitor Remodelling Mild heart failure Evaluation trial

Purpose: To evaluate the effects of carvedilol and enalapril, either alone or in combination, on 572 patients with LVEF <40% in a randomized, double-blind parallel group study. Primary outcome was measuring left ventricular end systolic volume index (LVESVI) using Echo at baseline and at 6, 12, and 18 months to represent changes in LV remodeling.

Follow-up: 18 months

Results: Combination therapy significantly reduced LVESVI compared to enalapril alone, and carvedilol significantly improved LVESVI compared to baseline, while enalapril did not.

Reference: Remme WJ, et al. (2004). *Cardiovasc Drugs Ther* 18(1):57–66.

Candesartan in Heart Failure

CHARM

Purpose: 7601 patients with symptomatic heart failure were entered into 3 individual component randomized trials in which candesartan was used at 4 or 8 mg a day, titrated to target dose 32 mg vs. placebo: 1) CHARM added—patients with LVEF ≤40% and treated with an ACE inhibitor; 2) CHARM alternative—patients with LVEF ≤40% and ACE inhibitor intolerant; 3) CHARM preserved—patients with LVEF ≤40% with or without ACE inhibitor. Primary outcome results were all-cause mortality for the trial as a whole, or cardiovascular mortality/CHF hospitalization for component trials.

Follow-up: Minimum 2 years

Results: CHARM overall: lower cardiovascular mortality compared to placebo (23.3% vs. 24.9%, $p = 0.055$) and lower cardiovascular mortality/CHF hospitalizaton (30.2% vs. 34.5%, $p < 0.0001$). CHARM added: lower cardiovascular mortality compared to placebo (23.7% vs. 27.3%, $p = 0.02$) and lower heart failure hospitalizations. CHARM alternative: lower mortality compared to placebo (21.6% vs. 24.8%, $p = 0.072$) and lower heart failure hospitalizations. CHARM preserved: non significant reduction in death and fewer heart failure hospitalizations.

Reference: Pfeffer MA, et al. (2003). *Lancet* 362: 759–766.

Cardiac Insufficiency Bisoprolol Study

CIBIS

Purpose: To evaluate effects on mortality in 641 of patients with NYHA Class III and IV heart failure and LVEF <40% using bisoprolol in a randomized double blind placebo-controlled trial.

Follow-up: 2 years.

Results: There was significant reduction in hospitalization for heart failure in the bisoprolol group, and significant improvement in functional class, but no significant difference in mortality, sudden death, or death related to VF or VT.

Reference: CIBIS Investigators and Committees (1994). *Circulation* 90:1765–1773.

Cardiac Insufficiency Bisoprolol Study II

CIBIS II

Purpose: To evaluate bisoprolol in reducing mortality in 2647 patients with NYHA Class III and IV heart failure in a randomized, double-blind, placebo controlled trial, and to determine safety and efficacy using cardiovascular death and hospitalization.

Follow-up: Mean 1.3 years

CIBIS II

Results: All-cause mortality, hospital admission, and death were significantly lower in the bisoprolol group. All-cause mortality at 2 years was significantly lower in women.

Reference: Simon T, et al. (1999). *Circulation* 100 (Suppl I):1–297.

COMET

Carvedilol Or Metoprolol European Trial

Purpose: To determine if the β_2 receptor and α_1 blocking effect of carvedilol (target dose 25 mg bid), in addition to its effect of increasing insulin sensitivity, confers a greater benefit in heart failure compared to metoprolol tartrate (target dose 50 mg bid), with which it shares a β_1 blocking effect, in a randomized, double-blind, parallel group trial. 3028 patients had NYHA Class II–IV, LVEF <35%, on optimum therapy with ACE-I and diuretics. Primary end point was all-cause mortality, composite end point was all-cause mortality or all-cause admission.

Follow-up: Mean 58 months

Results: There was 17% reduction in all-cause mortality in the carvedilol group.

Reference: Poole-Wilson PA, et al. (2003). *Lancet* 362 (9377):7–13.

COM-PANION

Comparison of Medical Therapy, Pacing, and Defibrillation in Heart Failure Trial

Purpose: To compare rates of hospitalization or death of >1600 patients with heart failure and evidence of conduction delay on surface ECG. Patients had NYHA Class III or IV, LVEF ≤35%, QRS ≥120 ms, PR>150 ms. They had been hospitalized at least once in the previous year. They were treated with optimal drug therapy alone (β-blockers, ACE inhibitors, angiotensin receptor blockers, spironolactone), drug therapy plus a biventricular pacemaker (cardiac resynchronization), or drug therapy plus a defibrillator with resynchronization capability.

Follow-up: 12 months

Results: The combination of all-cause death and all-cause hospitalization was reduced in both resynchronization groups, with a greater benefit observed for the defibrillator arm than the pacemaker arm (43.4% and 23.9% mortality reduction, respectively). No significant difference in effect was found between patients with ischemic and nonischemic cardiomyopathy.

Reference: Pinski SL (2003). *JAMA* 289(6):754–756.

Carvedilol Prospective Randomized Cumulative Survival Trial

COPERNICUS

Purpose: To evaluate the impact of carvedilol on mortality in 2289 patients with severe heart failure, LVEF <25% in a randomized, double-blind, placebo-controlled trial.

Follow-up: Mean 10.4 months

Results: There was a 35% decrease in mortality in the carvedilol group compared to placebo.

Reference: Packer M, et al. (2001). *N Engl J Med* 344: 1651–1658.

Optimal medical therapy with or without PCI for stable coronary disease

COURAGE

Purpose: To evaluate the efficacy of percutaneous coronary intervention (PCI) compared with optimal medical therapy among patients with stable coronary artery disease. 2287 patients were enrolled with a mean age of 62 years.

Follow-up: Mean 4.6 years

Results: Among patients with stable coronary artery disease, treatment with PCI was not associated with a difference in death or MI compared with treatment with medical therapy through 5 years of follow-up. PCI was performed in 94% of the PCI cohort, with successful PCI in 93%. At 5 years, use of ACE inhibitors was in 64% of patients, statins in 93%, aspirin in 95%, and β-blockers in 85%. LDL levels were reduced to a median of 71 mg/dL. Compliance with life style modification was also high. Angina was significantly reduced in both groups during follow-up. There was no difference in the reduction between PCI and medical therapy at 5 years in both groups (freedom from angina in 74% of the PCI group and 72% of the medical therapy group, $p = 0.35$); however, there was a slightly higher rate of freedom from angina in the early time frame with PCI (at 1 year: 66% for PCI vs. 58% for medical therapy, $p < 0.001$; at 3 years: 72% for PCI vs. 67% for medical therapy, $p \equiv 0.02$). The majority of PCI patients did not receive drug-eluting stents.

Reference: Boden WE, O'Rourke RA, Teo KK, et al. (2007). *N Engl J Med* 356:1503–1516.

CREDO

Clopidogrel for Reduction of Events During Observation

Purpose: To evaluate the benefit of long-term clopidogrel after PCI combined with aspirin, and to evaluate the benefit of initiating clopidogrel with loading dose before the procedure. 2116 patients with symptomatic coronary artery disease and objective evidence of ischemia who were undergoing elective PCI or were deemed highly likely to undergo PCI were enrolled in 99 centers in North America. Patients were randomized to receive a 300 mg clopidogrel loading dose (n = 1053) or placebo (n = 1063) 3 to 24 hours before PCI. After the procedure, all patients received clopidogrel 75 mg/day for 28 days. From day 29 to 12 months, the loading-dose group received clopidogrel 75 mg/day, whereas placebo was given to the control group. The 1-year primary end point was a composite of death, myocardial infarction (MI), and stroke in the intent-to-treat population.

Follow-up: 28 days, 6 months, and 1 year

Results: At 1 year, there was a 26.9% risk reduction in the combined end point of the clopidogrel-treated group. Pretreatment did not significantly reduce the end point, but in a subgroup of patients receiving the loading dose more than 6 hours beforehand there was a significant risk reduction.

Reference: Steinhubl SR, et al. (2002) *JAMA* 288: 2411–2420.

CTOPP

Canadian Trial Of Physiological Pacing

Purpose: To assess the potential benefits (measured by risk of cardiovascular death or stroke) of physiological (dual chamber) pacemakers compared with those of nonphysiological (single chamber) pacemakers over an extended period. 1474 patients requiring pacemakers for symptomatic bradycardia were randomized to receive one of the two modes of pacemaker.

Follow-up: Initially 3 years, extended to a mean 6.4 years

Results: There was no difference between groups in the primary outcome measures of cardiovascular death or stroke, or total mortality. However, there was a significant reduction in the risk of developing atrial fibrillation in the physiological pacing group (relative risk reduction 20.1%, *p* = 0.009).

Reference: Kerr CR, et al. (2004). *Circulation* 109:357–362.

Clipidogrel in Unstable angina to prevent Recurrent Events **CURE**

Purpose: To evaluate the impact of clopidogrel on 12,562 patients presenting within 24 hours of onset of acute coronary syndrome symptoms, either unstable angina (75%) or non-ST elevation MI (25%). Patients were randomized to receive 75 mg clopidogrel or placebo, preceded by 75–325 mg aspirin. There were similar rates of use of IV heparin, low-molecular-weight heparin, ACE inhibitors, β-blockers, and lipid-lowering agents in the two groups.

Follow-up: Mean 9 months

Results: The clopidogrel group had a 20% overall reduction in the primary composite end point of cardiovascular death, nonfatal MI, and nonfatal stroke, and this benefit was seen within 30 days. There was also a reduction in the incidence of refractory ischemia by 14% and severe ischemia by 24% in the clopidogrel group. All subgroups benefited from clopidogrel treatment. The incidence of major bleeding was 34% higher in the clopidogrel group (3.6% vs. 2.7%, $p = 0.003$), but life threatening bleeding did not differ between the groups.

Reference: CURE Study Investigators (2000). *Eur J Cardiol* 21:2033–2041.

Danish trial in Acute Myocardial Infarction **DANAMI**

Purpose: To compare a deferred invasive strategy of PCI or CABG ($n = 503$, within 2–5 weeks of discharge) with a conservative strategy ($n = 505$) in patients with inducible myocardial ischemia (on exercise testing) within the first few weeks after receiving thrombolysis for a first AMI. Primary end points were death, AMI, and admission with unstable angina.

Follow-up: 2.4 years

Results: In the invasive group, PCI was given to 53% and CABG to 29%. Mortality was not significantly different at 2.4 years between the invasive and conservative groups. However, the invasive group had a lower incidence of AMI, unstable angina, and stable angina. Therefore, the recommendation was to refer patients with inducible ischemia following AMI for a coronary angiogram ± revascularization.

Reference: Madsen JK, et al. (1997). *Circulation* 96: 748–755.

DANAMI II   Danish trial in Acute Myocardial Infarction II

Purpose: To compare coronary angioplasty with thrombolysis in AMI in patients who require transport from a community hospital to a center capable of PCI. 1572 patients with AMI were randomized to alteplase or angioplasty; of these, 443 were at an invasive-treatment center. Platelet gpIIb/IIIa inhibitors were given at the discretion of the physician performing PCI; ticlopidine or clopidogrel was given to all patients undergoing PCI for at least 1 month. The primary end point was a composite of death, clinical evidence of infarction, or disabling stroke at 30 days.

Results: In those patients randomized from community hospitals, the primary end point was reached in 8.5% of the invasive group compared to 14.2% the thrombolysis group ($p = 0.002$). In invasive centers, the end point rates were 6.7% and 12.3% for invasive and thrombolysis groups, respectively (attributable mainly to lower rates of reinfarction). There was no significant difference in death or stroke rates. 96% of patients were transferred from a community hospital to an invasive center within 2 hours. An invasive strategy is better than thrombolysis in patients at community hospitals if the transfer takes <2 hours.

Reference: Henning R, et al. (2003). *N Engl J Med* 349: 733–742.

DAVID   Dual chamber And VVI Implantable Defibrillator

Purpose: To evaluate efficacy of dual chamber (DDDR) pacing compared with backup ventricular pacing (VVI) in 506 patients with standard indications for ICD implantation but without indications for antibradycardia pacing. All had LVEF <40%, no bradycardia indications for pacing, and no persistent atrial arrhythmias. They were randomized to VVI at a backup rate of 40/min or DDDR at a backup rate of 70/min. Optimum medical therapy was continued. Primary composite end point was time to death or first hospitalization for CCF.

Follow-up: 1 year

Results: The VVI group had 1-year survival-free rate of 83.9% vs. 73.3% for the DDDR group. The composite end point, mortality (6.5% in VVI vs. 10.1% DDDR), as well as hospitalization for heart failure was also better in the VVI group. This suggests that in patients without bradycardia indications for pacing but with indications for ICD and LVEF <40%, the DDDR mode may have no advantage and may prove detrimental over VVI.

Reference: Wilkoff BL, et al. (2002). *JAMA* 288:3115–3123.

Danish Investigations of Arrhythmia and Mortality On Dofetilide

DIAMOND

Purpose: To evaluate the prophylactic use of dofetilide in 3028 patients at high risk of sudden death. There were two arms: the CHF arm (n = 1518) and the AMI arm (n = 1510), with patients having had AMI within 7 days. Dofetilide was given at 250 mg once daily initially, titrating to 500 mg twice daily, and reduced or withdrawn if creatinine clearance fell or QTc was >20% baseline or >550 ms. There was placebo. A substudy examined the effect of dofetilide in the CHF arm on rates of cardioversion to sinus rhythm in patients who had AF.

Follow-up: ≥12 months

Results: The 1-year mortality was 28% in the CHF arm and 22% in the AMI arm. There were fewer hospitalizations for heart failure than with placebo, but there was no significant difference in mortality between the dofetilide group as a whole and placebo. In the CHF arm, there was a significantly greater conversion rate of patients to sinus rhythm compared to placebo.

Reference: Torp-Pederson C, et al. (1999). *N Engl J Med* 341:857–865; *Circulation* 2001; 104:292–296.

Digitalis Investigation Group

DIG

Purpose: To evaluate the effect of digoxin vs. placebo on all-cause mortality in 7788 patients in sinus rhythm with symptoms of heart failure and with LVEF ≤45%.

Follow-up: Maximum 5 years

Results: Overall mortality was not reduced by digoxin compared to placebo. There was a significant reduction in hospitalization for worsening heart failure ($p < 0.001$).

Reference: The Digitalis Investigation Group (1997). *N Engl J Med* 336:525–533.

Diabetes mellitus Insulin-Glucose infusion in Acute Myocardial Infarction

DIGAMI

Purpose: To determine if insulin-glucose infusion in diabetic patients with AMI reduces initial high mortality rate, and if strict metabolic control during the early post-infarction period improves prognosis. 620 diabetic patients with suspected AMI and glucose >11 mmol/L were randomized to receive insulin-glucose infusion and, subsequently, subcutaneous insulin for ≥3 months.

Follow-up: 12 months

Results: At 12 months there was a relative mortality reduction of 29% in the insulin-glucose group. This risk reduction was most pronounced in patients with a low cardiovascular risk profile who were not previously on insulin, with a relative risk reduction of 52% at 3 months ($p = 0.046$) and 52% at 1 year ($p = 0.2$).

Reference: Malmberg K, et al. (1995). *J Am Coll Cardiol* 26:57–65.

DINAMIT

Defibrillator In Acute Myocardial Infarction Trial (DINAMIT)

Purpose: To evaluate the effects of prophylactic implantable cardioverter defibrillator (ICD) early in high-risk patients after acute MI with the hypothesis that mortality would be lower in the ICD therapy group. A total of 674 patients were followed with a mean age of 62 years and mean EF of 28%.

Follow-up: Mean follow-up 2.5 years

Results: Anterior MI was present in 72% of patients, and 48% of patients had chronic heart failure (CHF) associated with the index MI. Acute reperfusion therapy (percutaneous transluminal coronary angioplasty, thrombolytic, or both) was performed in 62% of patients. The primary end point of all-cause mortality was not different between the ICD therapy and medical therapy. Prophylactic implantable defibrillator therapy was not associated with a reduction in the primary end point of all-cause mortality compared with optimal medical therapy. The frequency of arrhythmia deaths was lower in the prophylactic ICD therapy arm. Nonarrhythmic deaths were higher in the ICD arm.

Reference: Hohnloser SH, et al. (2004). *N Engl J Med* 351:2481–2488.

EMIAT

European Myocardial Infarction Amiodarone Trial

Purpose: To evaluate the effect of amiodarone on mortality in 1486 patients enrolled 5–21 days post-MI with LVEF <40% in a randomized, double-blind, placebo-controlled manner.

Follow-up: Median 21 months

Results: All-cause mortality and cardiac mortality did not differ between groups, but there was a 35% risk reduction in arrhythmic deaths in the amiodarone group ($p = 0.05$).

Reference: Julian DG, et al. (1997). *Lancet* 349:667–674.

EPILOG

Evaluation in PTCA to Improve Long-term Outcome with abciximab GpIIb/IIIA blockade

Purpose: To determine the effect of the glycoprotein receptor blocker cF7E3 (abciximab) on mortality and morbidity when used during percutaneous coronary intervention. In a randomized, double-blind, placebo-controlled trial, 2792 patients were given IV unfractionated heparin as a bolus, and were randomly assigned to receive either placebo or abciximab. Within the abciximab group, patients could receive either an additional bolus of heparin alone or an additional bolus plus an infusion of heparin.

Follow-up: 30 days

Results: There was a significant reduction in the composite event rate in the abciximab group, with no significant difference between the high- or low-dose heparin subgroups within the abciximab group. There was no difference in the risk of major bleeding, although minor bleeding was more frequent in the abciximab group. The trial was stopped after the interim analysis showed a reduction in death and MI that exceeded the predetermined stopping level in the abciximab group.

Reference: The EPILOG investigators (1997). *N Engl J Med* 336:1689–1696.

Evaluation of Platelet gpIIb/IIIa Inhibition in Stenting

Purpose: To evaluate the influence of platelet glycoprotein inhibitor cF7E3 on coronary disease treated with PTCA or stenting. Study design was randomized, double blinded, part placebo controlled. 2399 patients who were to undergo elective or urgent intervention, either balloon angioplasty alone or stenting, were randomized to receive abciximab or placebo. Aspirin and heparin were given to all patients, with ticlopidine given at physician's discretion.

Follow-up: 6 months

Results: Death, MI, or need for urgent revascularization was lower within 30 days in both abciximab groups than with placebo. Within the abciximab group, these rates were lower in the stenting group than in the PTCA group alone. These trends were also observed at 6 months.

Reference: Lincoff et al. (1999). *N Engl J Med* 341:319–327.

Simvastatin with or without ezetimibe in familial hypercholesterolemia

Purpose: To compare the mean change in the intima-media thickness (IMT) measured at three sites in the carotid arteries between patients with heterozygous familial hypercholesterolemia (HeFH) treated with ezetimibe-simvastatin 10/80 mg vs. patients treated with high-dose simvastatin 80 mg alone, over a 2-year period. A total of 720 patients were enrolled with a mean age of 45.9 years. This was a randomized, double-blinded study.

Follow-up: 24 months

Results: They suggest that in patients with very high baseline LDL levels, such as those with HeFH, the combination of ezetimibe-simvastatin 10/80 mg does not result in significant changes in mean carotid IMT at 2 years compared with high-dose simvastatin 80 mg alone. There was no difference in incidence of cardiovascular mortality, nonfatal MI, nonfatal stroke, and need for revascularization, although the study was not powered to study clinical outcomes. The incidence of adverse events was similar. The LDL-lowering effect of ezetimibe-simvastatin was greater than that with high-dose simvastatin alone.

Reference: Kastelein JJ, et al. (2008). *N Engl J Med* 358: 1431–1443.

EPILOG

EPISTENT

ENHANCE

EUROPA

European trial on Reduction Of cardiac events with Perindopril in stable coronary Artery disease

Purpose: To evaluate the effect of perindopril on cardiovascular risk in a low-risk population and no overt heart failure. 12,218 patients with previous MI, angiographic evidence of coronary disease, coronary revascularization, or a positive exercise test were randomized to receive perindopril 8 mg once daily or placebo. Concomitant treatment was with antiplatelet therapy (92%), β-blockers (62%), and lipid-lowering agents (58%). The primary end point was cardiovascular death, MI, or cardiac arrest.

Follow-up: Mean 4.2 years

Results: The primary end point was reached by 8% of the perindopril group and 10% of placebo ($p = 0.0003$), representing a 20% risk reduction. Perindopril was well tolerated.

Reference: The EUROPA Investigators (2003). *Lancet* 362:782–788.

FRISC

Fragmin during Instability in Coronary Artery Disease

Purpose: To determine whether the addition of the low-molecular-weight heparin Fragmin (dalteparin) influences the recurrence of cardiac events in patients with unstable angina if added to aspirin and antianginal drugs. The study design was randomized, double blind, placebo controlled, parallel group. 1506 patients who were in the hospital with unstable angina within 72 hours of having chest pain were given either placebo or Fragmin 120 U/kg every 12 hours for the first 6 days, then 7500 U once a day for 35–45 days thereafter. All patients were on aspirin and β-blockers (unless contraindicated), with calcium antagonists and nitrates as required.

Follow-up: Up to 7 months

Results: Mortality, need for revascularization, reinfarction, and need for IV heparin were lower in the first 6 days in the Fragmin group. There was also a significant reduction in the composite end point (death, revascularization, IV heparin use, MI), which persisted for up to 40 days for nonsmokers (80% of the sample), but this effect was not carried 4 to 5 months after the end of treatment in the group as a whole. If the dose of Fragmin was decreased, there was a risk of reinfarction that was greater in smokers.

Reference: Fragmin during Instability in Coronary Artery Disease (FRISC) Study Group (1996). *Lancet* 347: 561–568.

Fragmin and Revascularization during Instability in Coronary Artery Disease

FRISC II

Purpose: To evaluate the impact of 3 months continuous Fragmin (dalteparin, a low-molecular-weight heparin) in patients with unstable angina, and to compare a direct invasive strategy with a stepwise approach, preferably non-invasive. The study design was randomized, double blind, placebo controlled. 2457 patients with anginal symptoms within 48 hours were randomized to have an initial invasive or noninvasive strategy. Within these two groups, patients were randomized to Fragmin or placebo for 3 months. All patients received aspirin and β-blockers (unless contra-indicated), as well as nitrates, calcium antagonists, statins, and ACE inhibitors, although these were optional.

Follow-up: 6 months

Results: There were significantly fewer deaths and MI in the early-revascularization group at 6 months in the invasive group, independent of Fragmin treatment. There was a nonsignificant decrease in deaths when considered separately. At 6 months, 23% of the noninvasive group had had an invasive procedure.

Reference: Invasive compared with non-invasive treatment in unstable coronary-artery disease: FRISC II prospective randomised multicentre study (1999). *Lancet* 354:708–715.

Gruppo Italiano per lo Studio della Streptochinasinell 'Infarto miocardio

GISSI-I

Purpose: To evaluate whether 1) streptokinase (SK) reduces in-hospital and 1-year mortality after AMI; 2) the effect of reduction, if present, depends on the interval between pain onset and treatment; and 3) the risks of treatment are acceptable. 11521 patients with AMI were randomized to SK 1.5 MU over 1 hour or to control.

Follow-up: 1 year

Results: At 21 days there was an 18% reduction in mortality in the SK group as a whole ($p = 0.0002$). In those treated within 3 hours, mortality was reduced by 23% ($p = 0.0005$). At 12 months, total mortality was 17.2% in the SK group vs. 19.0% in controls (relative risk 0.9, $p = 0.0008$).

Reference: GISSI Study Group (1987). *Lancet* ii:871–874.

Gruppo Italiano per lo Studio della Sopravviven-zanell'Infarto miocardico

GISSI 2

Purpose: To compare streptokinase (SK) and alteplase (rt-PA) in 12,490 AMI patients and to evaluate the effects of heparin after thrombolysis with either agent on survival and postischemic events in a randomized, open-label, controlled 2x2 factorial design.

Follow-up: 6 months

GISSI-2

Results: There was no significant difference in the combined end point of death and severe left ventricular damage, rates of in-hospital complications (15 days post thrombolysis), or rates of reinfarction in all groups, with or without heparin. Major bleeding occurred more frequently in the SK plus heparin group, but stroke rates were similar in all groups (1.14%); rt-PA was associated with a small but excess risk of stroke. Major bleeding was more frequent with SK than with rt-PA. Hypertensive patients had higher mortality throughout the follow-up period.

Reference: GISSI 2 Study Group (1996). *J Hypertens* 14: 743–750.

GISSI-3

Gruppo Italiano per lo Studio della Sopravviven-zanell'Infarto miocardico

Purpose: To evaluate the independent and combined effects of lisinopril and nitrates on survival and LV function after AMI in 18,895 patients presenting within 24 hours of symptoms in a randomized, open-label, controlled factorial trial. Nitrates were given initially as an NTG infusion, then as a patch or oral isosorbide mononitrate after 24 hours. Oral lisinopril was started at a dose of 2.5–5 mg once daily and titrated up to 10 mg after 24 hours. Controls were given neither drug. Trial drugs were continued for 6 weeks.

Follow-up: 6 weeks and 6 months

Results: Overall mortality and LV dysfunction at 6 weeks were significantly reduced by lisinopril, although NTG did not influence outcome. At 6 months, overall mortality was 18.1% in the lisinopril groups compared to 19.3% in those without lisinopril ($p = 0.015$); NTG produced no difference in mortality.

Reference: GISSI 3 Study Group (1996). *J Am Coll Cardiol* 27:37–44.

GISSI-Prevenzione

Gruppo Italiano per lo Studio della Sopravvivenza nell'Infarto miocardico Prevenzione

Purpose: To evaluate the impact of the dietary supplements n-3 polyunsaturated fatty acids (PUFA) and vitamin E within 3 months of MI in 11,324 patients in a randomized, open parallel group trial. Patients had concomitant therapy with aspirin, β-blockers, and ACE-I.

Follow-up: 3.5 years

Results: Vitamin E had no impact, either alone or in combination, on the risk of death, nonfatal MI, or nonfatal stroke, but there was a significant reduction in these end points with PUFA (20% reduction in CVS death, nonfatal MI or nonfatal stroke), mainly attributable to decrease in the risk of death and cardiovascular death.

Reference: GISSI-Prevenzione Investigators (1999). *Lancet* 354:447–455.

Global Utilization of Streptokinase and t-PA for Occluded coronary arteries   **GUSTO-1**

Purpose: To compare in a randomized parallel group the effect of treatment with a) streptokinase (SK) and SC heparin vs. b) SK and IV heparin vs. c) rt-PA with IV heparin (accelerated regimen) vs. d) rt-PA and SK and IV heparin simultaneously in the treatment of AMI in 41,021 patients <6 hours after symptom onset. Concomitant therapy included aspirin and atenolol.

Follow-up: 30 days and 1 year

Results: At both 30 days and 1 year, there was a 14% reduction in mortality in the accelerated t-PA group compared to the two SK-only regimens. Combination of SK and t-PA led to no significant difference in 1-year mortality compared to SK only, and a marginal difference when compared to t-PA only. Although the accelerated t-PA group had significantly more hemorrhagic strokes than the SK groups and the combination groups, overall there were fewer complications in the accelerated t-PA group, as well as significantly lower end point of death and disabling stroke at 1 year. However, in patients >75 years of age, those treated by accelerated t-PA had higher mortality at 30 days than that of younger patients but still had a greater absolute net benefit. Older patients generally had a greater risk of mortality, stroke, bleeding, and reinfarction.

Reference: White et al. (1996). *Circulation* 94:1826–1833.

Global Use of Strategies To Open occluded coronary arteries IV—Acute Coronary Syndrome   **GUSTO IV-ACS**

Purpose: To investigate long-term effects of abciximab in patients with ACS without ST elevation who were not scheduled for coronary intervention. 7800 patients with positive troponin or persistent ST depression were randomized to abciximab bolus and 24-hour infusion, abciximab bolus and 48-hour infusion, or placebo.

Follow-up: 1 year

Results: There was no survival benefit in the abciximab group. In subgroups with low troponin or high CRP, abciximab was associated with a higher mortality.

Reference: Ottervanger JP, et al. (2003) *Circulation* 107: 437–442.

HOPE

Heart Outcomes Prevention Evaluation Trial

Purpose: To assess the role of the ACE inhibitor ramipril and vitamin E in patients at high risk of cardiovascular events who did not have LV dysfunction or heart failure. 9297 patients >55 years old with evidence of vascular disease (previous MI, angina, multivessel PTCA or CABG, multivessel coronary artery disease, peripheral vascular disease, cerebrovascular disease) or diabetes plus one other risk factor but not known to have a low LV EF or heart failure were randomly assigned to receive 10 mg ramipril (titrated up from 2.5 mg) or placebo, plus vitamin E 400 U/day or placebo. Primary outcome was composite of MI, stroke, or death from cardiovascular events. Secondary end points were death from any cause, need for revascularization, hospitalization for unstable angina or heart failure, and complications of diabetes. Patients had approximately similar usage of aspirin, β-blockers, lipid-lowering agents, diuretics, and calcium channel blockers in the two groups.

Follow-up: Mean 5 years

Results: More people in the ramipril group stopped treatment due to cough, hypotension, or dizziness. However, there was a significant reduction in the primary end points of MI, stroke, and death compared to placebo (14% vs. 17%), as well a reduction in total mortality. There was no significant reduction in noncardiovascular death. In the ramipril group there was significantly less need for revascularization, fewer complications of diabetes, less heart failure or worsening angina, and smaller incidence of new-onset diabetes. The reduction in the primary end point and cardiovascular death was even more striking in diabetics (15.3% vs. 19.6%). There was a clear benefit in the ramipril group in patients with or without evidence of coronary artery disease, with or without history of MI and EF >40%. Benefits were also seen whether or not patients were taking aspirin, β-blockers, lipid-lowering agents, or anti-hypertensive drugs. In the vitamin E group there were no significant differences in primary or secondary end points. The study was stopped 6 months early due to consistent observed benefits in primary end points.

Reference: Yusuf S, et al. (2000). *N Engl J Med* 342: 145–153.

HORIZONS-AMI

Bivalirudin during primary PCI in acute myocardial infarction

Purpose: To evaluate treatment with bivalirudin compared with heparin plus gpIIb/IIIa inhibitors among patients undergoing primary PCI for acute ST-elevation myocardial infarction (STEMI). A total of 3602 patients were enrolled.

Follow-up: 1 year

Results: Among patients undergoing planned primary PCI for acute MI, use of bivalirudin was associated with a reduction in the composite end point of death, MI, target vessel revascularization, stroke, or major bleeding at 30 days compared with heparin plus gpIIb/IIIa inhibitors. This finding was driven by a reduction in major bleeding, with no difference in MACE. There was still a significantly reduced incidence of the composite end point at 12 months, but in addition to bleeding, a significant reduction in mortality and non–Q-wave MI was also noted. There was an increase in early (<24 hours) stent thrombosis with the use of bivalirudin; however, there was no difference between study arms at the end of 1 year.

Reference: Stone GW, et al. (2008). *N Engl J Med* 358: 2218–2230.

Heart Protection Study

Purpose: To evaluate whether the lowering of blood concentrations of low-density lipoprotein cholesterol (LDL-C), irrespective of the initial cholesterol measure, is associated with a lower cardiovascular risk. 20,536 patients with coronary disease, other occlusive arterial disease, or diabetes were randomized to 40 mg simvastatin once daily or placebo. The average compliance in the statin group was 85%, and in the placebo group the average non-study statin use was 17%. Primary outcome measures were death, and fatal or nonfatal vascular events.

Follow-up: 5 years

Results: All-cause mortality was significantly reduced in the simvastatin group (12.9% vs. 14.7%, p = 0.0003) mainly due to an 18% reduction in the coronary death rate. There was a marginal reduction in other vascular deaths, and no significant reduction in nonvascular deaths. There was a significant reduction in the first-event rate for nonfatal MI or coronary death, nonfatal or fatal stroke, and for coronary revascularization. The proportional reduction in event rate was similar in each subcategory— that is, those with diagnosed coronary artery disease, cerebrovascular disease, peripheral vascular disease, diabetes; and separately, in women; in those whose presenting LDL-C was <3.0 mmol/L or total cholesterol <5 mmol/L. The benefits of simvastatin were in addition to existing treatments. There was a 0.01 annual excess risk of myopathy, and there were no significant adverse effects on cancer incidence or hospitalization for any nonvascular causes.

Reference: Heart Protection Study Collaborative Group (2002). *Lancet* 360:7–22.

HORIZONS-AMI

HPS

ICTUS

Invasive versus Conservative Treatment in Unstable Coronary Syndromes (ICTUS)

Purpose: To evaluate the use of early invasive strategy compared with a more conservative, selective invasive strategy in troponin-positive patients with non-ST elevation myocardial infarction or acute coronary syndromes. A total of 1200 patients were randomized. The early invasive strategy included coronary angiography within 24–48 hours and percutaneous coronary intervention (PCI) within 48 hours or coronary artery bypass grafting (CABG) as soon as possible.

Follow-up: 3 years

Results: Treatment with an early invasive strategy was not associated with a difference in the primary end point compared with a selective invasive strategy. Revascularization was performed by hospital discharge in 76% of patients in the early-invasive group and 40% of patients in the selective-invasive group, with a shorter median time to revascularization in the early-invasive group (19 hours vs. 142 hours). The rate of MI was higher in this trial than in other similar trials, which likely reflects periprocedural MI given the definition of MI of creatine kinase-MB >1 times the upper limit of normal.

There was no difference in the primary composite end point of death, MI, or rehospitalization for ACS at 1 year (22.7% in early invasive vs. 21.2% in selective invasive, relative risk [RR] 1.07, $p = 0.33$) between the two groups. There was no difference in mortality at 1 year (2.5% each, $p = 0.97$). At 3-year follow-up, the composite of death, MI, or rehospitalization for ACS did not significantly differ for the invasive group compared with the conservative group (30.0% vs. 26.0%, HR 1.20, $p = 0.10$). There was no difference in all-cause mortality (7.9% vs. 7.7%, RR 1.11, $p = 0.63$) or cardiac death (5.0% vs. 4.5%, $p = 0.92$). The present trial results differ from the TACTICS-TIMI 18 trial and the FRISC-2 trial, which showed benefit of an early invasive strategy over a conservative strategy in a similar patient population.

Reference: de Winter RJ, et al. (2005). *N Engl J Med* 353: 1095–1104.

ISAR REACT

A clinical trial of abciximab in elective percutaneous coronary intervention after pretreatment with clopidogrel

Purpose: To evaluate whether treatment with gpIIb/IIIa inhibitor abciximab reduces postprocedure ischemic complications in low-risk patients pretreated with clopidogrel who undergo coronary stenting. A total of 2159 patients were enrolled with a mean age of 66 years.

Follow-up: Mean 30-day follow-up

Results: In low-risk patients with coronary disease pretreated with high-dose clopidogrel and undergoing elective coronary stenting, treatment with the gpIIb/IIIa inhibitor abciximab was not associated with a reduction in the primary composite end point of death, MI, or urgent TVR at 30 days. The trial patient population was at very low risk, excluding patients with insulin-dependent diabetes, acute coronary syndrome (ACS), and positive biomarkers. There was no difference in any component of the composite: death 0.3% in each arm; Q wave MI 0.4% vs. 0.5%; non-Q wave MI 3.3% in each arm; urgent TVR 0.9% vs. 0.7% for abciximab vs. placebo, respectively, all p = NS.

Reference: Kastrati A, et al. (2004). *N Engl J Med* 350: 232–238.

ISAR REACT

First International Study of Infarct Survival

ISIS-1

Purpose: To assess the impact on mortality of early use of β-blockers (atenolol 5–10 mg IV over 5 minutes followed by 100 mg orally once daily for 7 days) randomized in 16,027 patients with acute MI (<12 hours), in the first week and after longer follow-up.

Follow-up: Mean 20 months

Results: In the first 7 days, there was a 15% reduction (p < 0.02) in vascular deaths in the atenolol group, with greatest benefit on day 1, due to reduction in acute myocardial rupture. A further reduction in deaths was observed after 1 year.

Reference: Randomized trial of intravenous atenolol among 16027 cases of suspected acute myocardial infarction: ISIS-1. *Lancet* 1986; ii:57–66.

Second International Study of Infarct Survival

ISIS-2

Purpose: To assess effects of IV streptokinase and oral aspirin either alone or in combination in patients with suspected AMI (symptoms <24 hours, median 5 hours). 17,187 patients were randomized.

Follow-up: Up to 34 months

Results: There was a reduction in 5-week mortality with streptokinase alone or aspirin alone. There was a 25% odds reduction in death with streptokinase and 23% odds reduction with aspirin. There was a 42% odds reduction in death with aspirin and streptokinase combined, compared to the placebo group. Streptokinase was associated with more bleeding requiring blood transfusion (0.5% vs. 0.2% in placebo group) but fewer strokes (0.6% vs. 0.8% in placebo group). Aspirin significantly reduced nonfatal reinfarction and nonfatal stroke.

Reference: The ISIS-2 Collaborative Group (1988). *Lancet* ii:349–360.

ISIS-3

Third International Study of Infarct Survival

Purpose: To compare streptokinase vs. rt-PA vs. anistreplase (APSAC), plus aspirin or aspirin plus heparin in 41,299 patients with definite or suspected AMI (symptom onset <24 hours), in a randomized, double-blind, parallel-group factorial design.

Follow-up: 6 months

Results: The addition of heparin resulted in slightly fewer deaths and more major noncerebral bleeds, but no significant increase in cerebral hemorrhage; there was no significant difference in mortality after 2 months. The APSAC group had more reports of allergy and cerebral bleeds than the streptokinase group, with similar survival rates after 6 months. In the rt-PA group, there were more cerebral bleeds, but fewer reinfarctions than in the streptokinase group, without any significant difference in mortality between the groups.

Reference: The ISIS-3 (Third International Study of Infarct Survival) Collaborative Group (1992). *Lancet* 339:753–770.

ISIS-4

Fourth International Study of Infarct Survival

Purpose: To assess the effect on 5-week mortality of oral isosorbide mononitrate, oral captopril or IV magnesium, separately or in combination, on 58,050 patients with definite or suspected AMI (symptom onset <24 hours) in addition to standard therapy. The study design was randomized, partly placebo controlled, partly open, 2x2x2 factorial.

Follow-up: 5 weeks

Results: In contrast to magnesium and nitrate, the captopril group had a small but significant survival benefit that was maintained after 1 year, with greatest benefit in those at highest risk.

Reference: Fourth International Study of Infarct Survival Collaborative Group (1995). *Lancet* 345:669–685.

JUPITER

Rosuvastatin to prevent vascular events in men and women with elevated C-reactive protein

Purpose: To assess whether apparently healthy persons with levels of low-density lipoprotein (LDL) that do not mandate statin treatment, as per current guidelines (<130 mg/dL), but with levels of high-sensitivity C-reactive protein (hs-CRP) ≥2 mg/L, would benefit from taking rosuvastatin. A total of 17,802 patients were enrolled.

Follow-up: Mean 1.9 years (terminated early, planned 5-year follow-up)

Results: Rosuvastatin is associated with a significant reduction in major cardiovascular events, including death, in apparently healthy persons with LDL cholesterol <130 mg/dL, but hs-CRP ≥2 mg/L. Rosuvastatin was associated with a significant reduction in the incidence of the primary end point of nonfatal myocardial infarction (MI), nonfatal stroke, unstable angina, arterial revascularization, or cardiovascular death, compared with placebo (0.77 vs. 1.36 events per 100 person-years [PY] of follow-up, hazard ratio [HR] 0.56; 95% confidence interval [CI] 0.46–0.69, *p* < 0.00001). The number needed to treat based on these data with rosuvastatin is 95 patients for 2 years, and 31 patients for 4 years. Rosuvastatin was associated with a significant reduction in the levels of hs-CRP (median: 1.8 vs. 3.3 mg/L, *p* < 0.0001), LDL (median: 55 vs. 109 mg/dL), and triglycerides (99 vs. 118 mg/dL, *p* < 0.0001), but not HDL (50 vs. 50 mg/dL, *p* = 0.34). There was a higher incidence of physician-reported diabetes in the rosuvastatin arm (3.0% vs. 2.4%, *p* = 0.01) and a higher median glycated hemoglobin at 2 years with rosuvastatin (5.9% vs. 5.8%, *p* = 0.001).

Reference: Ridker PM, et al. (2008). *N Engl J Med* 359: 2195–2207.

JUPITER

Losartan Intervention For Endpoint Reduction in Hypertension

LIFE

Purpose: To evaluate the long-term effects of once-daily losartan compared with those of atenolol in patients with diabetes, hypertension, and ECG-documented LVH, with respect to the incidence of cardiovascular morbidity and mortality (cardiovascular death, stroke, or myocardial infarction). 1195 patients with mean blood pressure 177/96 mmHg after placebo run-in were randomized to losartan or atenolol on the basis of treatment.

Follow-up: Mean 4.7 years

Results: All-cause mortality and cardiovascular death were significantly lower in the losartan group. However, there was no difference in the risk of stroke or myocardial infarction. Losartan decreased ECG LVH better than atenolol. Losartan seemed to have benefits beyond BP reduction alone.

Reference: Lindholm LH, et al. (2002). *Lancet* 359:1004–1010.

LIPID Long-term Intervention with Pravastatin in IHD

Purpose: To evaluate the impact of long-term treatment with 40 mg pravastatin on mortality and morbidity in patients with a history of AMI, and unstable angina within 3–36 months of starting the trial with baseline cholesterol 4–7 mmol/L. A total of 9014 patients aged 31–75 years were enrolled in the trial, which was randomized, double blind, and placebo controlled.

Follow-up: Mean 6.1 years

Results: In the pravastatin group there was a relative risk reduction of 24% in death from coronary disease, and 22% relative risk reduction in all-cause mortality. There was also a significant reduction in incidence of nonfatal MI, stroke, and coronary revascularization.

Reference: The LIPID Study Group (1998). *N Engl J Med* 339:1349–1357.

MADIT Multicenter Automatic Defibrillator Implantation Trial

Purpose: To determine if patients at high risk of sudden cardiac death would have reduced mortality if they had an AICD implanted, compared with conventional drug therapy. 300 patients with a history of ventricular tachycardia or QWMI (>1 month previously) and LVEF <35% were randomized to receive either AICD or drug therapy (most commonly amiodarone).

Follow-up: Mean 27 months

Results: There was a 54% reduction in all-cause mortality in the AICD group compared with the non-device group.

Reference: MADIT Executive Committee (1991). *Pacing Clin Electrophysiol* 14:920–927.

MADIT II Multicenter Automatic Defibrillator Implantation Trial II

Purpose: To evaluate the impact of prophylactic ICD therapy in patients with MI at lest 30 days prior to enrollment and poor LV EF (≤30%). 1232 patients were randomized to receive conventional drug therapy alone (490 patients) or a combination of both ICD and drug therapy (742 patients).

Follow-up: Mean 20 months

Results: Mortality rates were 19.8% and 14.2% in the conventional and ICD groups, respectively, and there was a 31% reduction in death at any interval in the ICD group.

Reference: Moss A, et al., for the MADIT II Investigators (2002). *N Engl J Med* 346:877–883.

Metoprolol CR/XL Randomized Intervention
Trial I—Heart Failure

MERIT-HF

Purpose: To evaluate the impact of metoprolol succinate when added to standard therapy for chronic heart failure in 3991 patients with LVEF ≤40% and NYHA Class II–IV, when compared to placebo. Metoprolol was started at 12.5 or 25 mg once daily aiming to titrate up to 200 mg once daily.

Follow-up: 1 year

Results: At 1 year, the trial was terminated early because of the significant reduction in all-cause mortality with metoprolol compared to placebo (7.2% vs. 11.0%, $p = 0.00009$), including reductions in cardiovascular death, sudden death, and death from worsening heart failure.

Reference: Hjalmarson A, et al. (2000) *JAMA* 283: 1295–302.

Microalbuminuria, Cardiovascular and Renal Outcomes in the Heart Outcomes Prevention Evaluation

MICRO-HOPE

Purpose: To evaluate the impact of Ramipril and vitamin E in the development of diabetic nephropathy in patients with microalbuminuria, or the development of new-onset microalbuminuria in the diabetic subset of patients from the HOPE study. Of the HOPE cohort, 3577 were diabetic, and 1129 had microalbuminuria.

Follow-up: Mean 4 years

Results: 7% of the ramipril group and 8% of the placebo group ($p = 0.027$) developed proteinuria. There was a trend for reduction in risk of new-onset microalbuminuria, although this was not statistically significant ($p = 0.17$). Ramipril reduced the risk of overt nephropathy, dialysis, or laser therapy by 16%.

Reference: Heart Outcomes Prevention Evaluation (HOPE) Study Investigators (2000). *Lancet* 355:253–259.

Myocardial Ischemia Reduction with Aggressive Cholesterol Lowering

MIRACL

Purpose: To determine whether atorvastatin 80 mg once daily initiated 24–96 hours after an acute coronary syndrome (ACS) reduces death, nonfatal MI, cardiac arrest, or recurrent symptomatic myocardial ischemia requiring emergent hospitalization (the primary end points) in 3086 patients in a randomized, placebo-controlled trial.

Follow-up: 16 weeks

MIRACL

Results: The primary end point occurred in 14.8% of the atorvastatin group and 17.4% of the placebo group (*p* = 0.48). There were no significant differences in risk of death, nonfatal MI, or cardiac arrest between the two groups. However, the atorvastatin group had a lower risk of recurrent ischemic events requiring hospitalization.

Reference: Schwartz GG, et al. (2001). *JAMA* 285: 1711–1718.

MIRACLE

Multicentre Insync Randomized Clinical Evaluation Trial

Purpose: To evaluate whether cardiac resynchronization therapy (CRT) through atrial-synchronized biventricular pacing produces clinical benefit in patients with heart failure and IV conduction delay. 453 patients with NYHA Class III and IV heart failure, LVEF ≤35%, and QRS >130 ms were randomized to a CRT group (*n* = 228) or a control group (*n* = 225), while continuing optimal medical therapy. Primary end points were 6-minute walk distance and NYHA functional class.

Follow-up: 6 months

Results: Patients in the resynchronization group had significantly improved walking distance, quality of life score, and NYHA class after 1 month, which was maintained throughout the study, compared to nonpaced controls. Significant improvements were also seen in secondary end points of LVEF, peak oxygen consumption, total exercise time, and duration of the QRS interval. The risk of major clinical events (death and hospitalization for heart failure) was also significantly lower.

Reference: Abraham WT, et al. (2002) *N Engl J Med* 346: 1845–1853.

MIRACLE ICD

Multicentre   Insync   ICD   Randomized   Clinical Evaluation

Purpose: To evaluate the safety and efficacy of combined cardiac resynchronization therapy (CRT) through biventricular pacing and implantable cardiac defibrillator (ICD) in 369 patients with NYHA Class III (*n* = 328) or IV (*n* = 41) despite appropriate medical management. LVEF was ≤35%, and QRS 130 ms. Of these 369 patients, 182 were controls (ICD on, CRT off), while 187 were in the CRT group (ICD on, CRT on). Primary end points were quality of life, 6-minute walk distance, and functional class compared to baseline.

Follow-up: 6 months

Results: The CRT group had greater improvement in quality-of-life score and functional class compared to controls. There was no difference in 6-minute walk distance, but peak exercise oxygen consumption and treadmill exercise duration increased in the CRT group. There was no difference in survival (15 deaths in control arm, 14 deaths in CRT arm), LV size or function, overall heart failure status, and rates of hospitalization.

Reference: Young JD, et al. (2003). *JAMA* 289:2719–2721.

MIRACLE ICD

Mode Selection Trial in sinus-node dysfunction

MOST

Purpose: To evaluate whether dual-chamber pacing would provide better event-free survival and quality of life than single-chamber pacing for sinus node dysfunction. 2010 patients were randomized to dual-chamber or ventricular pacing. The primary end point was all-cause mortality or nonfatal stroke. Secondary end points included the composite of death, stroke- or heart failure–related hospitalization, AF, heart failure score, the pacemaker syndrome, and quality of life.

Follow-up: Mean 33.1 months

Results: Incidence of the primary end point did not differ between groups. The risk of AF was lower in the dual-chamber group (hazard ratio 0.79, $p = 0.0008$) and heart failure scores were better, as were quality of life scores. Rates of hospitalization for heart failure, death, and stroke were not different. 16.5% of the ventricular pacing group experienced pacemaker syndrome and were crossed over to dual-chamber pacing.

Reference: Lamas GA, et al. (2002). *N Engl J Med* 346: 1854–1862.

Multisite Stimulation in Cardiomyopathies Trial

MUSTIC

Purpose: To evaluate the impact of biventricular pacing on 67 patients with severe heart failure (NYHA III) and QRS >150 ms in a single-blind, controlled, randomized cross-over study. The primary end point was distance walked in 6 minutes, with secondary end points of quality of life measures, peak oxygen consumption, patients' treatment preference (active vs. inactive pacing), hospitalizations due to heart failure, and mortality.

Follow-up: 6 months

Results: Mean distance walked in 6 minutes was 23% longer in the active pacing group. 85% preferred the active pacing period. Quality-of-life score and peak oxygen uptake were both significantly improved, and hospitalizations were 66% less when paced. Longer follow-up was required to determine impact on mortality.

Reference: Cazeau S, et al. (2001). *N Engl J Med* 344: 873–880.

MUSTT Multicenter Unsustained Tachycardia Trial

Purpose: To identify individuals at greatest risk of sudden cardiac death using signal-averaged ECG and electrophysiological studies, and then optimizing antiarrhythmic therapy on the basis of the data to reduce sudden death and mortality. 2139 patients ≤80 years old were enrolled with coronary heart disease, or MI more than 4 days previously, with LVEF ≤40% and asymptomatic non-sustained VT. 704 patients had inducible sustained VT after electrophysiological testing and were entered into the randomized trial (184 drug therapy, 167 ICD, 353 no therapy). β-Blockers were recommended for all patients, but drug therapy varied and included sotalol, amiodarone, procainamide, dispyramide, propafenone, quinindine, and mexiletine. The remaining 1435 patients were entered into a registry.

Follow-up: 5 years

Results: β-Blockers reduced all-cause mortality in the whole cohort but did not influence death from arrhythmia or cardiac arrest. In patients with inducible sustained VT, incidence of death from cardiac arrest or arrhythmia was significantly lower in the EP-guided treatment group than in the no-treatment group; benefit occurred only in those receiving ICDs. Similarly, the ICD group had significantly reduced risk of arrhythmic death, cardiac arrest, and overall mortality compared to the other groups.

Reference: Buxton AE, et al. (1999) *N Engl J Med* 341: 1882–1890.

OPTIMAAL Optimal Therapy In Myocardial infarction with the Angiotensin II Antagonist Losartan

Purpose: To compare the effects on all-cause mortality of losartan 50 mg once daily and captopril 50 mg twice daily in 5477 patients with confirmed acute MI, acute anterior QWMI, or reinfarction, and heart failure during acute phase. Patients were randomized in a double-blind, parallel method. Primary end point was all-cause mortality.

Follow-up: 2.7 years

Results: There was a nonsignificant difference in total mortality for captopril, but losartan was better tolerated.

Reference: Dickstein K, et al. (2002). *Lancet* 360:752–760.

PASE Pacemaker Selection in the Elderly

Purpose: To assess the effect of pacing mode (DDDR or VVIR) on long-term health-related quality of life of 407 elderly patients (65–96 years, mean age 76 years) with pacemakers, randomized to one of these two modes. All patients were in sinus rhythm requiring pacing for bradycardia. Primary end point was quality of life; secondary end points: all-cause mortality, hospitalization for heart failure, nonfatal stroke, new AF, or pacemaker syndrome.

Follow-up: 30 months

Results: Quality of life improved significantly for both groups after implantation, but there was no significant difference between groups in this end point, or in cardiovascular events or death. 26% of the VVIR group crossed over due to the pacemaker syndrome. Patients with sinus node disease, however, had an improved quality of life with dual-chamber compared to single-chamber pacing (explored more fully in MOST trial).

Reference: Lamas GA, et al. (1998). *N Engl J Med* 338: 1097–1104.

Percutaneous Coronary Intervention and Clopidogrel in Unstable angina to prevent Recurrent Events

Purpose: To evaluate the effect of pretreatment of patients undergoing PCI with clopidogrel followed by long-term therapy, in addition to concomitant use of aspirin. 2658 patients with NSTEMI undergoing PCI in the CURE study were randomly assigned double-blind treatment with clopidogrel or placebo. Patients were pretreated with aspirin and clopidogrel for a median of 10 days. After PCI, >80% of patients in both groups received open-label clopidogrel for 4 weeks. After this, clopidogrel was restarted in the randomized individuals for a mean of 8 months (up to 1 year). Primary composite end point was cardiovascular death, MI, or urgent target vessel revascularization within 30 days of PCI.

Follow-up: Up to 1 year

Results: There was a 30% reduction in cardiovascular death or MI in the clopidogrel group, as well as a lower rate of revascularization, without any significant difference in major bleeding.

Reference: Mehta SR, et al. (2001). *Lancet* 358:527–533.

Primary Angioplasty in AMI patients from General community hospitals transported to PCI Units versus Emergency thrombolysis

PRAGUE 1: Long-term outcomes of three reperfusion strategies in 300 patients with acute STEMI presenting to community hospitals were compared: 1) thrombolysis alone in a community hospital; 2) thrombolysis during immediate transportation for angioplasty; 3) immediate transportation for angioplasty without thrombolysis. After 1 year, there were no significant differences in total mortality in the 300 patients, but in a subset of patients randomized within 2 hours of symptoms, total mortality was lower in the angioplasty group. Primary angioplasty patients had a lower combined end point of total mortality and nonfatal reinfarction rate. Combining thrombolysis and PCI was not superior to PCI alone.

PASE

PCI-CURE

PRAGUE Trials

PRAGUE Trials

PRAGUE 2: 850 patients with STEMI <12 hours were randomized to thrombolysis in a community hospital without PCI, or immediate transport for PCI. PCI strategy decreased mortality in patients presenting >3 hours after symptom onset, but in those presenting within 3 hours, thrombolysis had similar results to PCI (primary end point was 30-day death, secondary end points were death, reinfarction, or stroke at 30 days).

PRAGUE 4: 400 patients scheduled for CABG were randomized to off-pump and on-pump surgery by a cardiologist. The surgeon was allowed to change technique after randomization. Primary end point at 30 days was death, MI, stroke, or new renal failure needing dialysis. There was no significant difference in the primary end point. The off-pump group had lower postoperative CKMB levels, lower total hospital costs, less blood loss, and fewer distal anastomoses, suggesting that the off-pump technique was at least as clinically safe and effective as on-pump surgery.

References: Bednár F, et al. (2003). *Can J Cardiol* 19(10): 1133–7. Widimsky P, et al. (2003). *Eur Heart J* 24:21–3. Straka Z, et al. (2004). *Ann Thorac Surg* 77:789–793.

PRISM

Platelet Receptor Inhibition Ischemic Syndrome Management

Purpose: To compare tirofiban with unfractionated heparin in 3232 patients with unstable angina (last chest pain <24 hours, documented coronary artery disease) on aspirin in a double-blind, randomized control trial.

Follow-up: 48 hours and 30 days

Results: At 48 hours, the incidence of death, MI, and refractory ischemia was lower in the tirofiban group, but at 30 days theses rates were not significantly different. In 2240 patients who were troponin T positive at 24 hours, mortality and the incidence of MI were lower at 30 days for the tirofiban group. This benefit was not seen in troponin-negative patients.

Reference: Hamm CW, et al. (1999). *Circulation* 100 (Suppl I):1–775.

PRISM PLUS

Platelet Receptor Inhibition in Ischemic Syndrome Management in Patients Limited by Unstable Signs and Symptoms

Purpose: To evaluate the effect of tirofiban in the treatment of unstable angina and NQWMI. 1915 patients were randomized to tirofiban, heparin, or tirofiban and heparin. The study drugs were infused for a mean of 71.3 hours, during which coronary angiography and intervention were performed when indicated after 48 hours.

The drug infusion was maintained for 12–24 hours after an intervention The composite primary end point was death, MI, or refractory ischemia within 7 days' randomization. All patients were given aspirin unless there were any contraindications.

Follow-up: 6 months

Results: The study was stopped prematurely for the group who received tirofiban alone because of excess mortality at 7 days. The composite end point was reached by fewer people in the tirofiban plus heparin group than those who had heparin alone (12.9% vs. 17.9%, *p* = 0.004). The composite end point rates, as well as rates of death and MI, were lower in the tirofiban plus heparin group than in the heparin-alone group at 30 days and at 6 months. There was no significant difference in rates of bleeding between the tirofiban plus heparin group and the heparin-alone group.

Reference: The PRISM-PLUS Study Investigators (1998). *N Engl J Med* 338:1488–1497.

PRISM PLUS

Perindopril Protection against Recurrent Stroke Study

PROGRESS

Purpose: To evaluate the effects of BP reduction on risk of stroke in 6105 patients, normotensive or hypertensive, with a proven TIA or stroke in the previous 5 years. Patients were randomized to perindopril 4 mg/day plus 2.5 mg indapamide if required, or placebos.

Follow-up: 3.9 years

Results: BP was reduced by 9/4 mmHg in the treatment group compared to placebo. There was a relative risk reduction in stroke of 28% in the treatment group (*p* < 0.0001), and the risk of total vascular events was also lower in the treatment group. Risk of stroke was reduced in both normotensive and hypertensive patients. The combination of perindopril and indapamide reduced BP by 12/5 mmHg and stroke risk by 43%, but in the perindopril-alone group BP was reduced by 5/3 mmHg and did not lead to a reduced stroke risk.

Reference: PROGRESS Collaborative Group (2001). *Lancet* 358:1033–1041.

Platelet gpIIb/IIIa Underpinning the Receptor for Suppression of Unstable Ischemia Trial

PURSUIT

Purpose: To evaluate the effects of integrelin on the frequency and duration of ischemia in 227 patients with unstable angina in a randomized, double-blind, placebo-controlled trial. PCI was performed in 11.2% of patients during a period of medical therapy with integrelin that lasted for 72 hours in total and for 24 hours after the intervention. All patients received IV heparin.

Follow-up: 72 hours

PURSUIT

Results: Holter monitoring measured ischemic episodes, and their frequency and duration were lower in the integrelin group, as were refractory ischemia and MI. There was no excess bleeding risk in the integrelin group.

Reference: Schulman SP, et al. (1996). *Circulation* 94: 2083–2089.

RACE

Rate control versus electrical cardioversion for persistent atrial fibrillation

Purpose: To evaluate whether ventricular rate control in AF is inferior to maintenance of sinus rhythm. There were 522 patients with persistent AF after electrical cardioversion in the rate control or rhythm control group. The end point was a composite of death from cardiovascular disease, heart failure, thromboembolism, bleeding, permanent pacemaker implantation, and adverse drug effects. Rate control was achieved by digoxin, calcium channel blockers (non-dihydropyridine), and β-blockers, either alone or in combination, to achieve a target heart rate <100/min. All patients were orally anticoagulated unless contraindicated. The rhythm control group underwent DCCV without prior treatment with antiarrhythmics. Then they were placed on sotalol. If AF recurred within 6 months, DCCV was repeated and sotalol was replaced by flecainide or propafenone. If further AF recurred, a loading dose of amiodarone was given at 600 mg daily for 4 weeks, then DCCV was repeated and the antiarrhythmic drug continued. Patients were orally anticoagulated until 1 month of sinus rhythm was maintained, after which the anticoagulant was stopped or changed to aspirin. Aspirin was allowed in the rate control group if <65 years old without underlying cardiac disease.

Follow-up: Mean 2.3 years

Results: 39% of the rhythm control vs. 10% of the rate control group were in sinus rhythm, The primary end point occurred in 17.2% of the rate control vs. 22.6% of the rhythm control group, indicating that rate control was not inferior to rhythm control for preventing death and morbidity from cardiovascular causes in patients with recurrent AF after DCCV.

Reference: Van Gelder IC, et al. (2002). *N Engl J Med* 347:1834–1840.

RALES

Randomized Aldactone Evaluation Study mortality trial

Purpose: To evaluate the effect of adding 25 mg spironolactone in 1663 patients with LVEF <35%, already on ACE inhibitors and loop diuretic, and most also on digoxin. The primary end point was all-cause mortality.

Follow-up: Mean 24 months

Results: There was a 30% risk reduction in the spironolactone group, *p* < 0.001, due to lower deaths from both sudden cardiac death and progressive heart failure. There was also 35% less frequent hospitalization in the spironolactone group; this group had a significant improvement in NYHA functional class. There was a 10% incidence of gynecomastia and breast pain in men treated with spironolactone. There was minimal risk of serious hyperkalemia in either group. The trial was discontinued early after an interim analysis showed spironolactone to be efficacious.

Reference: Pitt B, et al. (1999). *N Engl J Med* 341:709–717.

RALES

A randomized (double blind) study with the sirolimus coated BX velocity balloon expandable stent (CYPHER) in the treatment of patients with de novo native coronary lesions

RAVEL

Purpose: 237 patients with single de novo lesions <18 mm in length and 2.5–3.5 mm in diameter received clopidogrel for a 2-month period and were randomized to receive either a Cypher or bare-metal stent. All patients underwent angiography at the end of the study.

Follow-up: 6 months

Results: Event-free survival was 97% at 6 months compared to 72% in the bare-metal stent group. There was no restenosis in the Cypher group compared to 26% in the control group. There were no reported cases of subacute thrombosis in the Cypher group.

Reference: Regar E, et al. (2002). *Circulation* 106: 1949–1956.

Reversal of Atherosclerosis with Aggressive Lipid Lowering

REVERSAL

Purpose: To evaluate the effect of two different lipid-lowering drugs on coronary atheroma burden and progression. Patients who were enrolled required coronary angiography for a clinical indication and demonstrated at least 1 obstruction with angiographic luminal narrowing of ≥20%. Lipid criteria required a low-density cholesterol level (LDL-C) of 3.24–5.44 mmol/L after a 4- to 10-week washout period. 654 patients were initially randomized in a double-blinded manner to receive the study drug, either 40 mg pravastatin or 80 mg atorvastatin. 502 patients had intravascular ultrasound (IVUS) examinations that could be evaluated both at baseline and after 18 months treatment. The target vessel for IVUS must not have undergone angioplasty or have a luminal narrowing of >50% throughout a target segment with a minimum length of 30 mm.

REVERSAL

The main outcome measure was percentage change in atheroma volume. A secondary outcome measure was change in percentage atheroma volume, a measure of absolute, not relative, change in atheroma volume.

Follow-up: 18 months

Results: Baseline LDL-C value (mean 3.89 mmol/L in both groups) was reduced to 2.85 mmol/L in the pravastatin group and 2.05 mmol/L in the atorvastatin group (p <0.001). C-reactive protein (CRP) decreased 5.2% in the pravastatin group and 36.4% with atorvastatin. There was a significantly lower reduction in progression of percentage change in atheroma volume (primary end point) in the atorvastatin group compared with pravastatin. No significant progression of atheroma burden occurred in the atorvastatin group, but it did in the pravastatin group compared to baseline. These changes may be related to reduction in LDL-C and CRP. There were no significant numbers of adverse drug reactions in either group.

Reference: Nissen SE, et al. (2004). *JAMA* 291:1071–1080.

RITA-2

Second Randomized Intervention Treatment of Angina

Purpose: To compare long-term consequences in 1018 patients with unstable angina randomized to PTCA vs. conservative therapy.

Follow-up: Median 7 years

Results: Death or MI occurred in 14.5% PTCA patients and in 12.3% medical patients, which was not significantly different. CABG and repeat arteriography were more common in the PTCA group. The PTCA group had improved exercise tolerance and anginal symptoms.

References: *Lancet* 1997; 350(9076):461–468; Henderson RA, et al. (2003). *J Am Coll Cardiol* 42:1161–1170.

SAFE T

Amiodarone versus sotalol for atrial fibrillation

Purpose: To evaluate the safety and efficacy of amiodarone compared with sotalol for restoration and maintenance of sinus rhythm among patients with atrial fibrillation. A total of 6582 patients were screened for the study, however, only 665 were enrolled.

Follow-up: Mean 12–54 months

Results: The primary end point of time to first recurrence of atrial fibrillation was longer in the amiodarone group (median 487 days, 48% by 1 year) than in either the sotalol group (median 74 days, 68% by 1 year, $p = 0.002$) or placebo group (median 6 days, 87% by 1 year, $p < 0.001$ for both amiodarone and sotalol comparisons). Spontaneous cardioversion in the first 28 days was similar in the amiodarone and sotalol groups, both of which were higher than the placebo group.

Reference: Singh BN, et al. (2005). N *Engl J Med* 352: 1861–1872.

Stenting and Angioplasty with Protection in Patients at High Risk for Endarterectomy (SAPPHIRE)

SAPPHIRE

Purpose: To compare stenting with protection vs. endarterectomy in patients with severe symptomatic or asymptomatic carotid artery stenosis. The rate of the composite end point of death, myocardial infarction, or stroke at 30 days and ipsilateral stroke or death from neurological causes within 31 days to 1 year was studied in 334 patients. Mean age of patients was 72 years.

Follow-up: 3 years

Results: Among patients with severe atherosclerotic carotid artery stenosis, treatment with stenting was noninferior compared to carotid endarterectomy (CEA) for the composite of death, stroke, or MI at 30 days plus ipsilateral stroke or death from neurological causes within 31 days to 1 year. The directionality of the individual end points at 1 year all favored stenting, none reached significance (death 7.4% vs. 13.5%, $p = 0.08$; MI 3.0% vs. 7.5%, $p = 0.07$; stroke 6.2% vs. 7.9%, $p = 0.60$). There was no significant difference in transient ischemic attack or major bleed between the 2 arms. However, the rate of cranial nerve injury was higher in the CEA arm (0% vs. 4.9%, $p < 0.01$). The trial was discontinued prematurely secondary to low enrollment. Long-term results of the trial through 3 years are pending.

Reference: Yadav JS, et al. (2004). *N Engl J Med* 351: 1493–1501.

Survival And Ventricular Enlargement Study

SAVE

Purpose: To evaluate the effect of captopril starting 3–16 days after MI in improving mortality and left ventricular function in 2231 patients with LVEF <40% but no overt heart failure.

Follow-up: Mean 42 months

Results: All-cause mortality risk was reduced in the captopril arm by 19%. Recurrent MI risk was reduced by 25% and death after recurrent MI by 32%. Patients in the captopril arm were less likely to require coronary revascularization but there was no difference in hospitalization rates compared to placebo. Symptoms of cough, dizziness, diarrhea, and taste alteration were more common in the captopril group.

Reference: Rutherford JD, et al. (1994). *Circulation* 90: 1731–1738.

SIRIUS

A randomized trial of a sirolimus-eluting stent versus a standard stent in patients at high risk of coronary restenosis

Purpose: To evaluate the effect of sirolimus drug-eluting stents vs. bare-metal stents on 1058 patients with de novo coronary artery stenosis.

Follow-up: 12 months

Results: At 9 months, clinical restenosis (target lesion revascularization) was 4.1% in the sirolimus limb and 16.6% in the control (*p* < 0.001); at 12 months values were 4.9% and 20%, respectively (*p* <0.001). There were no differences in death or MI rates. In high-risk subsets and in presence of diabetes, there was a reduction of 70%–80% clinical restenosis at 1 year. At 9 months, clinical restenosis (target lesion revascularization) was 4.1% in the sirolimus limb and 16.6% in the control (*p* < 0.001). At 12 months these values were 4.9% and 20%, respectively (*p* < 0.001). There were no differences in death or MI rates.

Reference: Holmes DR Jr, et al. (2004) *Circulation* 105: 634–640.

SOLVD

Studies Of Left Ventricular Dysfunction

Purpose: To evaluate the impact of enalapril on long-term survival in patients with LVEF ≤0.35 with or without a history of cardiac failure, and on LV function and volume, arrhythmias, and quality of life. Study design was randomized, double blind, placebo controlled. 4228 patients aged 21–80 years had no overt congestive cardiac failure, and 2568 patients had overt cardiac failure. Both groups were randomized to receive enalapril (starting at 2.5 mg twice daily, titrating to 10 mg twice daily) or placebo.

Follow-up: 3 years

Results: In the group without heart failure there was no statistically significant decrease in mortality, either all-cause or related to cardiovascular disease. There was, however, a 29% risk reduction in the combined incidence of death and development of overt cardiac failure. In the group with symptoms of heart failure, there was a 16% risk reduction in all-cause mortality. There was no change in quality of life in either group compared to placebo after 1 year, or in the incidence of ventricular arrhythmias. However, left ventricular end diastolic volumes and left ventricular mass increased in the placebo group but not in the enalapril-treated groups. Enalapril-treated patients lived 0.16 years longer than the placebo group, translating into a lifetime increase of 0.4 years over placebo. The enalapril groups had significantly fewer hospitalizations than the placebo group.

Reference: Glick H, et al. (1995). *J Card Fail* 1:371–380.

Scandinavian Simvastatin Survival Study

SSSS (4S)

Purpose: To evaluate the impact of 20 mg simvastatin in patients with total serum cholesterol 5.5–8 mmol/L (after 8 weeks of dietary therapy) on mortality and the incidence of major coronary artery disease. 4444 patients aged 35–69 years were in the study.

Follow-up: Median 5.4 years

Results: There was a 30% relative risk reduction in all-cause mortality, 42% reduction in coronary mortality, 34% reduction in coronary events, 32% reduction in cost of hospitalization, and 37% reduction in revascularization procedures in the simvastatin group. Simvastatin significantly reduced the risk of major coronary events in all quartiles of baseline total, LDL, and HDL cholesterol to a comparable degree in each quartile. There was one case of reversible myopathy that was the most serious drug-related adverse event.

Reference: Jönsson B, et al. (1996) *Eur Heart J* 17: 1001–1007.

Trials evaluating a slow-release paclitaxel-eluting stent (TAXUS) for coronary lesions

TAXUS

TAXUS 1: This trial was to evaluate the safety and feasibility of a TAXUS stent delivering paclitaxel locally to coronary plaques via a slow-release polymer coating, compared to a bare-metal control stent. 61 patients with de novo or restenotic lesions (≤12 mm) were randomized to receive a TAXUS stent or control stent that was non-drug eluting (diameters 3.0 or 3.5 mm). The primary end point, 30-day major adverse clinical event (MACE), rate was 0% in both groups. At 12 months, the MACE rate was 3% in the TAXUS group and 10% in the control. The restenosis rate measured by QCA was 0% in the TAXUS group vs. 10% in controls at 6 months. IVUS showed significant improvements in normalized neointimal hyperplasia in the TAXUS group compared to controls.

TAXUS 2: A comparison of slow-release (SR) and moderate-release (MR) paclitaxel-eluting stents with control bare-metal stents (BMS). All 536 patients had post-procedure and 6-month follow-up with IVUS. There was significant reduction in MACE rates, in-stent restenosis (ISR), and in-stent volume reduction with SR or MR stents compared to controls. There was no significant difference between the TAXUS groups.

TAXUS 3: 28 patients with ISR with lesions <30 mm in length and 50%–99% diameter stenosis in 3.0–3.5 mm vessels were treated with one or more TAXUS stents. 25 people completed the angiographic follow-up at 6 months. The MACE rate was 29% (8 patients). IVUS was recommended to ensure good stent deployment and complete coverage of target lesion.

TAXUS

TAXUS 4: This trial evaluated the safety and efficacy of slow-release polymer-based paclitaxel stents after implantation in de novo coronary lesions after 1 year. 1314 patients with de novo coronary lesions 10–28 mm length, diameter 2.5–3.75 mm, coverable by a single stent, were randomized to a TAXUS or bare metal (EXPRESS) stent. At 1 year, MACE rates and target vessel revascularization rates were lower in the TAXUS group. Rates of cardiac death, MI, and subacute thrombosis were not significantly different.

References: Grube E, et al. (2003). *Circulation* 107:38–42; Columbo A, et al. (2003) *Circulation* 108:788–794; Tanabe K, et al. (2003). *Circulation* 107:559–564; Stone GW, et al. (2004) *Circulation* 109:1942–1947.

TIMI 1

Efficacy of tPA (with IV heparin) was compared to streptokinase in achieving reperfusion in 290 patients presenting with acute STEMI <6 hours after symptom onset. All patients underwent baseline coronary angiography after randomization. Significantly higher rates of perfusion were found in the TPA arm. Patients with a patent artery at 90 minutes after starting reperfusing therapy had lower 6-month and 1-year mortality regardless of treatment group.

TIMI 2A

Patients with acute MI were given tPA within 4 hours of symptom onset and randomized to an immediate invasive (angiogram within 2 hours), delayed invasive (within 18–48 hours), and conservative (angiogram if ETT positive at 6 weeks or further ischemia) strategy. They were then given a predischarge angiogram and 6-week ETT, and followed up at 1 year. At 6 weeks there was no difference between the groups in death or reinfarction. Infarct-related artery patency at time of discharge was similar in all groups, with more complications in the invasive arms.

TIMI 2B

3339 patients with AMI were given tPA within 4 hours of symptom onset and randomized to an invasive strategy (angiogram within 18–48 hours) or a conservative strategy (angiogram if ETT positive at 6 weeks or further ischemia). Patients were also randomized to immediate IV followed by oral β-blockade, or deferred β-blockade. There was no difference in the composite end point of death or recurrent MI at 42 days between the invasive and conservative groups. But those in the invasive arm were twice as likely to need PTCA or CABG at 1 year. In the early β-blockade group, there was significantly lower reinfarction and recurrent ischemia at 6 weeks.

391 patients with unstable angina or NQWMI were given aspirin, IV heparin, β-blockers, nitrates and calcium antagonists, and then randomized to receive tPA or placebo after baseline angiography had excluded patients with left main stem disease or no coronary disease. They then underwent repeat angiography at 18–36 hours and were followed up at 6 weeks with an ETT. Baseline angiography showed 35% had apparent thrombus, and 30% had possible thrombus, with no difference in the degree of lesion improvement at angiography after randomization (25% tPA vs. 19% placebo).

TIMI 3A

1473 patients with unstable angina or NQWMI were treated with maximal medical therapy and randomized in a 2x2 factorial design to receive tPA or placebo, and to follow invasive or conservative strategies. There was no difference in composite end points of death, infarction, or ischemia in tPA and placebo groups, although the risk of MI, death, or cerebral bleeding was higher in the tPA group. Similarly, there was no difference between the conservative and invasive groups in the primary end points, although the invasive group required more readmission to the hospital for angina. The TIMI 3 registry showed that ST deviation was a prognostic indicator in unstable angina, whereas new T-wave inversion was not.

TIMI 3B

382 patients with AMI <6 hours were randomized to tPA, APSAC, or a combination of the two (at reduced dosage). Each underwent angiograms at 90 minutes, and at 18–36 hours. tPA was shown to have higher patency than APSAC or the combination, fewer unsatisfactory outcomes prior to discharge, and lower mortality at 1 year.

TIMI 4

Patients with AMI <6 hours were randomized to hirudin (a direct thrombin inhibitor) or unfractionated heparin, combined with aspirin and tPA, followed by angiography at 90 minutes and 18–36 hours. The hirudin arm had higher TIMI 3 flow rates and fewer re-occlusions.

TIMI 5

This study compared different doses of hirudin and unfractionated heparin in AMI patients in combination with streptokinase and aspirin. There was a lower incidence of death, recurrent MI, or new-onset CHF in the hirudin groups than in the heparin groups.

TIMI 6

Hirulog was used to treat 250 patients with unstable angina at a high and low dose. The incidence of death and MI was lower using higher doses of hirulog.

TIMI 7

This follow-up trial compared hirulog and heparin in a multicenter, double-blind, randomized study. The sponsor stopped it for business reasons after enrollment.

TIMI 8

TIMI 9A   This trial evaluated the safety and efficacy of hirudin compared to heparin as an adjunct to thrombolysis with tPA or streptokinase. As there were higher rates of bleeding than expected with hirudin, TIMI 9B was designed using lower hirudin doses.

TIMI 9B   This was similar to TIMI 9A but using lower doses of hirudin. No significant difference in death or reinfarction was seen between the hirudin and heparin groups.

TIMI 10A   This was a dose-ranging trial of TNK-tPA with aspirin and unfractionated heparin for treating acute STEMI.

TIMI 10B   Using TIMI 10A data, bolus doses of 30, 40, and 50 mg of TNK-tPA were chosen for comparison with accelerated tPA in conjunction with aspirin and IV heparin. A single bolus of TNK 40 mg achieved similar TIMI 3 flow to tPA at 90 minutes.

TIMI 11A   This dose-ranging trial for IV enoxaparin treated patients with unstable angina/NQWMI. Due to a higher than expected bleeding rate, the trial was reconfigured to look at a 1 mg/kg of enoxaparin to give bleeding rates similar to those in heparin plus placebo arm of TIMI 3B.

TIMI 11B   This was a comparison of enoxaparin and unfractionated heparin to treat unstable angina/NQWMI looking at the benefit of an extended courses of enoxaparin compared to a shorter course (8 vs. 43 days). Those randomized to unfractionated heparin continued on placebo. The enoxaparin group had reduced death, MI, and revascularization at both time points.

TIMI 12   This was a dose-ranging study for the gpIIb/IIIa inhibitor sibrafiban in patients 1–7 days after presenting with acute coronary syndrome. Results showed a dose-dependent rise in platelet inhibition.

TIMI 14   Abciximab was evaluated for treatment of STEMI, in combination with tPA, streptokinase, reteplase, or with no thrombolytic drug, compared to a group receiving tPA and heparin only. The combination of abciximab and half-dose tPA achieved the highest rates of reperfusion.

TIMI 15A   This dose-ranging study of the GpIIb/IIIa inhibitor Klerval (avail-able both orally and IV) for acute coronary syndrome showed a dose-dependent increase in platelet inhibition. The data were used in selecting the dose for the TIMI 15B trial.

TIMI 15B   This dose-ranging trial examined IV Klerval for 24–96 hours then oral Klerval for 4 weeks in the management of acute coronary syndromes (unstable angina, NSTEMI, STEMI), vs. placebo. Results showed potent predictable dose-related platelet inhibition with intravenous use, but moderate inhibition only with oral use.

(OPUS TIMI 16) Patients with acute coronary syndrome were randomized to two dosing strategies of oral orbofiban vs. placebo to evaluate the benefit of orbofiban in addition to standard therapy. No significant benefit was observed.

TIMI 16

(InTIME II) A multicenter trial of bolus lanoteplase vs. accelerated tPA was conducted for 15087 patients with STEMI. No significant difference was observed in mortality at 30 days between the two groups.

TIMI 17

(TACTICS TIMI-18) Treat angina with aggrastat and determine cost of therapy with an invasive or conservative strategy TIMI 18

TIMI 18

2220 patients with an unstable angina or NQWMI had baseline troponin measured and were given aspirin, heparin, and tirofiban. They were then randomized to an early invasive (angiogram in 4–48 hours) or early conservative strategy, and would proceed to PCI or CABG depending on their symptoms, treadmill testing, or other evidence of ischemia. They were followed up for 6 months. The combined primary end point of death, MI, and rehospitalization at 6 months was 19.4% in the conservative arm and 15.9% in the invasive arm. The reduction in patients who reached the primary end point was most marked in the 54% who were troponin positive (>0.01 ng/mL) and in patients who had an intermediate- and high-risk TIMI score. There was no significant difference in stroke, although major bleeding rate was higher in the invasive group. Hence there was benefit for "upstream" use of tirofiban in early intervention, using troponin levels and TIMI scores to guide potential usefulness of an early interventional approach.

Pravastatin or atorvastatin evaluation and infection therapy (PROVE IT)

TIMI 22

This study aimed to evaluate whether statins are effective in reducing events in patients with an acute coronary syndrome (ACS) and to see whether intensive lipid lowering of LDL-C (to an average 65 mg/dL) achieves greater reduction in clinical events than standard lowering (to an average 95 mg/dl). 4162 patients with an ACS within 10 days were given standard therapy and randomized to pravastatin 40 mg (standard therapy) or atorvastatin 80 mg (intensive therapy), as well as gatifloxacin vs. placebo in a 2×2 factorial manner. There was a mean 2-year follow-up after which the following primary end points were measured: death, MI, documented unstable angina requiring hospitalization, revascularization (>30 days after randomization), and stroke. The findings were that for the atorvastatin group, the risk of all-cause mortality or major cardiac events was reduced by 16% ($p = 0.005$). The benefits emerged at 30 days post-ACS and were maintained throughout follow-up and were consistent across all cardiovascular end points except stroke, and most clinical subgroups.

**TIMI 28
CLARITY**

The role of clopidogrel in early and sustained arterial patency after fibrinolysis for ST-segment elevation myocardial infarction

This trial evaluated treatment with clopidogrel compared with placebo among patients with ST elevation myocardial infarction (STEMI) treated with an initial medical management strategy. In patients with STEMI treated with an early medical management strategy, use of clopidogrel was associated with a reduction in the primary composite end point compared with placebo, driven by the reduction in infarct-artery occlusion. It should be noted that patients in the study were treated with an early medical management strategy and did not undergo coronary angiography for a median of 3.5 days. The risk of TIMI major bleeding did not differ significantly between the clopidogrel and placebo groups.

VANQWISH

Veterans Affairs Non-Q Wave Infarction Strategies in Hospital

Purpose: To compare the role of early invasive vs. conservative management strategies in patients with NQWMI with or without prior MI. The background of this study was that patients with a first NQWMI have a better prognosis than those with prior myocardial infarction who suffer another NQWMI. 920 patients were enrolled; 396 had had prior MI, 524 had not. These two groups were randomly assigned to an invasive strategy or conservative strategy, with subsequent invasive management if there was spontaneous or inducible ischemia within 72 hours of the NQWMI. The combined primary end point was death or nonfatal MI.

Follow-up: Mean 23 months

Results: Mortality did not differ significantly between the invasive and conservative strategy groups. Those with previous MI were identified as a high-risk subset of NQWMI patients who have similar outcomes regardless of the strategy used. But patients with a first infarct had better prognosis if managed conservatively, or with an ischemia-guided approach.

Reference: VANQWISH Trial Investigators (1998). *N Engl J Med* 338:1785–1792.

Vasodilator Heart FailureTrial II

V-HEFT II

Purpose: To compare the impact of enalapril with the combination of hydralazine plus isosorbide dinitrate in treating 804 patients with chronic congestive cardiac failure.

Follow-up: Mean 2.5 years

Results: The enalapril group had significantly lower mortality attributable mainly to a reduction in sudden cardiac death. Blood pressure reduction was greater in the enalapril group in the first 13 weeks. There was increased incidence of symptomatic hypotension and cough in the enalapril group, and increased headache in the hydralazine plus isosorbide dinitrate group.

Reference: Cohn JN, et al. (1991) *N Engl J Med* 325: 303–310.

West of Scotland Coronary Prevention Study

WOSCOPS

Purpose: A primary prevention study to evaluate the effect of 5 years of once-daily 40 mg pravastatin on the risk of MI, in 6595 men aged 45–64 years with LDL cholesterol 4–6 mmol/L and no history of MI, in a randomized, double-blind, placebo-controlled trial.

Follow-up: Mean 4.9 years

Results: Total cholesterol and LDL cholesterol were lowered by 20% and 26%, respectively, in the pravastatin group. There was a 31% relative risk reduction in the number of definite coronary events in the pravastatin group, and a 31% reduction in nonfatal MI, 33% reduction in death from coronary heart disease, and 32% reduction in death from all cardiovascular causes. All-cause mortality was reduced by 22% in the pravastatin group ($p = 0.051$).

Reference: The WOSCOPS Study Group (1996). *Eur Heart J* 17:163–164.

Special populations: women and elderly

Women and heart disease

Background

Cardiovascular disease in women is a health problem of epidemic proportions throughout the world. In the United States, cardiovascular disease (CVD) affects over 37 million American women, representing over one-third of the American female population, with coronary heart disease (CHD) affecting 5.9 million women.

By age 55, the prevalence of cardiovascular disease in women exceeds that in men. Cardiovascular disease accounts for 1 in 2.5 female deaths compared to 1 in 30 deaths attributable to breast cancer. Despite the high prevalence and mortality rate of cardiovascular disease, only 13% of women consider it to be their greatest health risk.

Although the past two to three decades have seen a decline in the overall mortality rate from CVD in men, the mortality rates for women have remained stable. In addition, when women do present with a new diagnosis of stable angina, they are less often referred for noninvasive or invasive studies and are less likely to undergo revascularization or given optimal secondary prevention medication even in the presence of confirmed obstructive coronary artery disease than are men.

Many studies have been done that highlight the discrepancies in the recognition and appropriate treatment of CHD between women and men and underscore the importance of appropriately identifying women who are at risk for CHD.

Diagnosis and prognosis

Exercise treadmill testing (ETT)

Women generally manifest CHD about 10 years later than men, present more commonly with atypical chest pain or dyspnea, and have a lower prevalence of luminal obstructive coronary disease by angiography. However, when women do present with obstructive coronary disease, they have higher morbidity and mortality rates than those of age-matched men.

It is therefore imperative to not only find effective primary and secondary prevention measures in women but also appropriately identify and risk stratify women with CHD. Historically, the noninvasive diagnostic workup in women has been underused, secondary to a lack of physician confidence in the accuracy of the test results.

While exercise stress testing is the most commonly used noninvasive diagnostic modality for detecting coronary artery disease in men, many studies have demonstrated a low sensitivity and specificity for exercise treadmill testing in women. In fact, women are 5 to 20 times more likely than men to have a false-positive exercise ECG.

Several mechanisms for the reduced specificity of exercise ECG testing in women have been proposed. These mechanisms include a lower prevalence of disease in women tested, lower achieved workload, the digoxin-like effect of estrogen, an inappropriate catecholamine response to exercise in women, a higher incidence of mitral valve prolapse, and different chest wall anatomy.

In addition, it is important to note that the standards for an abnormal exercise ECG test were developed in a male population.

Perfusion imaging and stress echocardiography in women

As a result of the high false-positive rate in exercise ECG testing in women, various imaging modalities have been evaluated in the diagnosis and risk stratification of CHD in women. Myocardial perfusion imaging has been shown to have a significantly higher sensitivity and specificity than that of ETT for detecting CAD in men.

Nevertheless, the small size of the left ventricle in women and breast artifact have led to some concerns regarding its utility in women. Studies evaluating the utility of myocardial perfusion imaging (MPI) in women with both Tc-99m sestamibi and Tl-201, however, have confirmed their value in diagnosing CAD in women. The use of gated SPECT imaging further increased the specificity of MPI findings in women.

Exercise echocardiography has also been shown to be an accurate modality to noninvasively diagnose CAD in men. There have, however, been conflicting reports regarding its utility in women, with specificities ranging from 46% to 93%.

In a study dedicated to evaluating the diagnostic accuracy of stress echocardiography compared to cardiac catheterization in 161 women, the sensitivity of exercise echocardiography for detecting CAD (>50% stenosis) was 80%, the specificity was 81%, the positive predictive value was 71%, and the negative predictive value was 87%.

Based on these studies, it is clear that exercise ECG is a less than ideal test for detecting CAD in women, with a very high false-positive rate, which in turn leads to many unnecessary invasive coronary angiograms. The addition of perfusion imaging or echocardiography to the exercise ECG provides an effective and cost-efficient way to diagnose women with suspected CAD without a high rate of false positives.

What is the prognostic utility of stress testing in women?

Both myocardial perfusion imaging and stress echocardiography have been evaluated for their roles in risk stratification of women with suspected CAD. It has been demonstrated that abnormal MPI is a more powerful predictor of future cardiac events in women than in men, with women

Table 16.1 Sensitivity and specificity of stress test modalities (for detecting stenoses >50%)

Test	Sensitivity	Specificity
ETT (men)	70%	77%
ETT (women)	61%	70%
Tl-201 MPI	75%	61.9%
Tc-99m MPI	71.9%	85.7%
Gated Tc-99m MPI	N/A	94.1%
Exercise ECHO	80%	81%

having a greater than twofold higher event rate than that of men with a similar scan result. The nuclear scan information added 17% and 37% additional prognostic information in men and women, respectively.

Exercise and dobutamine stress echocardiography have also been proven beneficial in risk stratifying both men and women with a relative risk of a cardiac event (nonfatal MI or cardiac death) in patients with an abnormal stress ECHO of 1.45.

Based on these studies, both exercise and pharmacological myocardial perfusion imaging and stress echocardiography are valuable tools in women for risk stratification. The choice of imaging modality will need to be based on each individual woman's risk factors, body habitus, and local expertise.

Hormone replacement therapy (HRT)

Proposed mechanism for estrogen's cardiovascular protection

The rates of coronary heart disease in postmenopausal women are two to three times greater than in premenopausal women of the same age. This is thought to be secondary to the cardioprotective effects of estrogen. In the basic science arena, researchers have demonstrated that estrogen has systemic effects as well as direct effects on the vasculature (see Box 16.1).

Data from observational trials—initial support for HRT

The role for estrogen replacement therapy (ERT) and hormone replacement therapy was initially supported by numerous observational epidemiological studies. A meta-analysis of these initial studies published from 1970 through the 1990s showed a significant reduction (35%–40%) in risk of CHD in women taking HRT.

Based on these observational data, the use of HRT/ERT in the primary and secondary prevention of CHD in women was the standard of care until 1998, when results from large, randomized controlled trials (RCTs) contradicted the findings of earlier observational studies.

Data from randomized controlled trials—increased risk with HRT in primary and secondary prevention

When HRT was evaluated in a large, randomized controlled study in postmenopausal women with known CHD (HERS trial), there was no difference in recurrent CHD events between the placebo group and the HRT

Box 16.1 Effects of estrogen

- Alteration in lipoprotein profile: decrease in total cholesterol, LDLc, and Lp(a); increase in HDLc and triglycerides
- Regulate expression of fibrinogen and ATIII and protein S
- Rapid effects on vasculature: vasodilation and increased nitric oxide (NO) synthesis
- Long-term effects on vasculature: alterations in gene expressions that decrease atherosclerosis, decrease vascular injury, decrease smooth muscle cell growth, and increase endothelial cell growth
- Proinflammatory: increase in C-reactive protein (CRP)

group. In fact, a post-hoc time trend analysis showed a 52% increase in CHD events during the first year of HRT use compared to placebo and a trend toward a decrease in CHD events in years 3 and 4. Further studies looking at the benefit of estrogen replacement therapy alone in the secondary prevention of CHD also did not show a benefit in reducing cardiac events.

Similarly, a large randomized controlled trial of HRT in the primary prevention of CHD in postmenopausal women (Women's Health Initiative) did not show a reduction in CHD events. In fact, there was a trend toward an increase in CHD events, with the greatest amount of risk occurring in the first year after randomization with a hazard ratio of 1.81 (95% CI 1.09–3.01).

Interestingly, a subgroup analysis of women stratified according to years since menopause revealed a nonsignificant trend toward a reduction in CHD in women less than 10 years since menopause (HR 0.89, 95% CI 0.5–1.7). When estrogen replacement alone was evaluated in the primary prevention of CHD, there was also no significant difference in CHD events between the active treatment arm and the placebo.

Possible future role for HRT in prevention of CHD

Regardless of the type of estrogen used, the method of hormone delivery or the combination of hormone replacement with estrogen and progestin, no significant benefit in CHD prevention was found in the aforementioned randomized trials. In the randomized trials, however, the average time between menopause and enrollment in the studies ranged from 16 years to over 20 years.

The initiation of hormone or estrogen therapy at this late stage may not truly represent physiological replacement and may contribute to lack of benefit in both primary and secondary prevention of CHD. The delay in HRT/ERT may have allowed subclinical atherosclerosis to develop and may have reduced the cardiovascular benefits of estrogen.

The trend toward a reduction in CHD events in the subgroup analysis in the Women's Health Initiative of women who began HRT/ERT within 10 years of menopause and results from a series of experiments in primates, which showed a benefit of ERT on atherogenesis progression only when started immediately post-oophorectomy, lend support to this theory.

These observations have kept the door open for a possible role of HRT in primary prevention in women at the inception of menopause and are the basis for the ongoing Kronos Early Estrogen Prevention Study (KEEPS). For now, however, there is no clear role of HRT or ERT for either primary or secondary prevention of CHD in postmenopausal women.

Dietary and vitamin supplements

Role of antioxidant vitamin supplements in women

As with the debate over HRT in the primary and secondary prevention of CHD in women, the role of antioxidant vitamins has been investigated over the past two decades. Like estrogen, vitamin E had a plausible biological basis for a postulated role in atherosclerosis prevention.

This theory was based on the hypothesis that oxidative modification of low-density lipoprotein (LDL) initiates atherosclerosis and on the idea that antioxidant vitamins, such as vitamin E, could inhibit lipid peroxidation, thereby preventing the development or progression of atherosclerosis and CHD.

Observational data from the Nurses Health Study and Iowa Women's Study initially supported this hypothesis. However, the positive benefit of vitamin E supplements noted in observational studies has not been consistently supported by subsequent randomized placebo-controlled clinical trials. The GISSI-Prevenzione trial, the Heart Protection Study (HPS), and the WAVE trial found no benefit of vitamin E in the secondary prevention of CHD events or in the angiographic progression of coronary atherosclerosis. The ability to apply these results to a female population, however, is limited because of the low proportion of women (19% in GISSI, 25% in HPS) in the majority of these trials.

Similarly, data for the role of vitamin E supplements in the primary prevention of CHD in women have also not been borne out in randomized placebo-controlled studies. In subgroup analyses of the HOPE and HOPE-TOO trials, there was no reduction in CHD events in women assigned to vitamin E supplementation.

However, a study dedicated to addressing this issue in women, the Women's Health Study, found a nonsignificant 7% reduction in major cardiovascular events (nonfatal MI, nonfatal stroke, cardiovascular death), and a significant reduction in major cardiovascular events in the subgroup of women aged 65 years or older, suggesting a possible role in the primary prevention of CHD events in this elderly subset of women. The use of vitamin E in this subgroup of women needs to be investigated further.

While data regarding the use of antioxidant vitamins, specifically vitamin E, in the primary and secondary prevention of CHD have been contradictory, the bulk of the data does not support the use of vitamin E in the prevention of CHD in women. At this point in time, vitamin E should not be recommended for the primary or secondary prevention of CHD in women.

Role of folic acid or vitamin B_6 in CHD prevention in women

Plasma homocysteine levels have been shown to be a strong, independent predictor of cardiovascular disease in both men and women. The correlation between homocysteine and CHD mortality ($r = 0.71$) suggests that homocysteine may play an important role in determining CHD mortality among different populations.

Several plausible mechanisms by which homocysteine could increase risk of CHD (direct toxicity to endothelial cells, increased coagulation, decreased endothelial reactivity, and stimulation of smooth muscle cell proliferation) have been previously elucidated.

Folate and vitamin B_6 are important cofactors in the metabolism of homocysteine, and changing the intake of folic acid and vitamin B_6 can modify homocysteine levels. Accordingly, studies have shown that low dietary intake of vitamin B_6 is also associated with increased risk of CHD.

Based on these observations, some investigators have hypothesized that lowering levels of homocysteine via folate and vitamin B_6 supplementation would translate into a reduction in cardiovascular events. Support for this hypothesis in women was initially offered from observations from the

Nurse's Health Study, which showed a relationship between folate and B_6 intake and incidence of CHD events.

The concern that the observed relation of homocysteine and vitamin B_6/folate to CHD risk may actually represent unrecognized confounders rather than a true causal relationship has led to the development of randomized clinical trials. Similar to the HRT and vitamin E story, randomized controlled studies evaluating the role of vitamin B_6 and folate in the secondary prevention of CHD have been negative (NORWIT trial).

The role of these vitamins in the primary prevention of CHD, however, is still a question. Until a randomized, clinical trial addresses this issue, the routine use of these supplements in primary prevention of CHD in women is not recommended.

Role of omega 3 fatty acid supplements

The observation that populations with a high intake of fish have a lower rate of cardiovascular disease initially led to the hypothesis that fish consumption may have a protective effect for atherosclerosis (Box 16.2).

Several prospective epidemiological studies in men have lent support to this hypothesis. Similar risk reductions were also observed in women in the Nurse's Health Study cohort. Although these epidemiological data are compelling, to date, there are no randomized controlled clinical trials to support the role of fish or fish oil in the primary prevention of CHD events in women.

Currently, the JELIS investigators are following 10,796 postmenopausal women and 4204 men who were free of CHD, in a trial of eicosapentaenoic acid (EPA), a component of fish oil, in addition to treatment with a statin in hyperlipidemic patients for 5 years. The primary end points in this trial are major coronary events (sudden cardiac death, fatal and nonfatal MI, unstable angina, and coronary revascularization).

The initial results of this trial, which were presented at the American Heart Association scientific session in 2005, revealed a 19% risk reduction in major cardiovascular events (RR 0.81, 95% CI 0.69–0.95) in the group treated with EPA plus statin therapy, compared to statin therapy alone, and a 24% risk reduction in unstable angina (RR 0.76, 95% CI 0.62–0.95).

In contrast to the dearth of data from randomized controlled trials on the role of fish oil in the primary prevention of CHD, there have been several observational trials and randomized controlled clinical trials showing

---

Box 16.2 Proposed biological mechanisms for omega 3 fatty acid CV protective effects

- Reduced susceptibility of the heart to ventricular arrhythmias
- Antithrombogenic properties
- Lowering of triglyceride levels
- Retardation of atherosclerotic plaque growth via reduced adhesion molecule expression
- Reduction in platelet derived growth factor
- Anti-inflammatory mediator
- Promotion of NO-induced endothelial relaxation

a benefit of fish oil on the secondary prevention of CHD events (GISSI-Prevenzione trial). The low number of female subjects participating in these trials, however, limits the applicability of the results to women.

Although the data are limited in women at this time, it is reasonable to recommend the use of n-3 omega fatty acids for the secondary prevention of CHD events in women who have recently had an MI. The recent results from the JELIS study also support the recommendation of adding fish oil to the treatment of hyperlipidemics in the primary prevention of CHD events.

Aspirin use in women

Aspirin for primary prevention in women

The role of aspirin in the secondary prevention of cardiovascular events is well established in both men and women. The role of aspirin in the primary prevention of cardiovascular disease in women, on the other hand, is not clear.

The Physician's Health Study, which was the first trial to uncover a significant 44% reduction in first MI with aspirin use only included men in its subject population. The data from the Hypertension Optimal Treatment Study (HOT) and the Primary Prevention Project, (each trial included about 50% women) present a less than convincing argument for the use of aspirin in the primary prevention of MI in women.

The Women's Health Study sought to finally answer this question in women. This study enrolled 39,876 women who were free of cardiovascular disease and had low-risk cardiovascular profiles. The investigators found a nonsignificant 9% risk reduction in major cardiovascular events, with no significant effect on fatal or nonfatal MI and with a concomitant increase in the rate of bleeding complications in those taking aspirin. Only in the subgroup of women over the age of 65 did they find a significant reduction in major cardiovascular events and in MI event rate.

Based on these data, there does not appear to be a clear role for aspirin in the primary prevention of cardiovascular disease in women in the low-risk female population. There may be a benefit in the elderly female population.

However, given the risk of bleeding complications, this needs to be further evaluated with a large-scale trial dedicated to answering this question. Although there is no clear role of aspirin use in the primary prevention of CHD events in women, this does not negate its use in women with established coronary artery disease, especially in the setting of acute myocardial infarction or post-angioplasty and stenting.

Cholesterol and inflammatory biomarkers of CHD in women

Optimal lipid levels in women for secondary prevention of CHD

The role of LDL cholesterol in the development of atherosclerosis has been well established. However, the best lipid parameter for predicting CHD events in women continues to be an issue of some debate. In a nested case–control study from the Nurse's Health Study cohort, the data suggest that measurements of both LDL and HDL are essential in the prediction of CHD events in women.

A similar contribution to the prediction model was seen when the ratio of total cholesterol to HDL was added (ROC increased to 0.72). This ratio reflects the proportion of atherogenic-to-antiatherogenic lipid fractions and appears to be a powerful tool for predicting CHD in postmenopausal women.

From these data it follows that lowering LDL cholesterol and raising HDL cholesterol should play a role in CHD prevention in women. Accordingly, the data from secondary prevention randomized controlled trials of statin therapy have shown reduced risks of CHD events in women placed on statin therapy.

The female subgroup analyses of the 4S trial, the CARE trial, and the PROVE-IT-TIMI22 trial have all shown significant reductions in major coronary events in women with known CAD who are placed on statins. Based on observational and clinical trial data, the goal LDL in women with a history of CHD or diabetes should be ≤70 mg/dL.

Role of CRP in predicting CHD risk in women

In addition to LDL and HDL cholesterol, recent data have shown that various markers of inflammation are also potent predictors of CHD events in women. Women in general have higher CRP levels than those in men, and black women have significantly higher CRP levels than white, Hispanic, or Asian women.

These higher CRP levels may provide insight into the pathogenesis of angina in women with nonobstructive coronary disease and further aid in assessing CHD risk in women.

Using the Women's Health Study cohort (27,939 women), both CRP and LDL were identified as strong, independent predictors of cardiovascular events, each measurement identifying different high-risk groups. Screening for both markers provided better information than either measurement alone. In fact, 77% of first cardiovascular events occurred in women with an LDL <160 mg/dL and 46% occurred in women with LDL <130 mg/dL. The addition of CRP measurements would have helped to identify at-risk women that were missed by the standards set by the National Cholesterol Education Program.

The JUPITER trial, a prospective, randomized controlled study of the use of rosuvastatin in the primary prevention of cardiovascular disease in patients with low LDL cholesterol levels (<130 mg/dL) and elevated CRP levels (≥ 2 mg/L), has recently confirmed these observational data. By targeting women with elevated CRP, even in the absence of significant LDL elevation, we will be able to identify more women who are at risk of CHD and be able to aggressively treat them with statin therapy.

The elderly and heart disease

Coronary heart disease (CHD)

Coronary heart disease is the leading cause of death in the United States in patients older than 65 years of age. Patients over the age of 65 account for greater than 50% of all myocardial infarctions, CABG procedures, and about 45% of all percutaneous coronary interventions.

As the life expectancy of Americans continues to increase, the population at risk for CHD and its complications will also increase. It is therefore imperative to pursue aggressive primary and secondary prevention measures in these patients to determine any unique interaction or considerations for this group and to establish standard preventive and therapeutic strategies in this growing segment of the American population.

Treatment of dyslipidemia in the elderly

Given that the absolute risk for CHD increases with age, the absolute numbers of people benefiting from cholesterol lowering is greater in the elderly patient population. As with a younger patient cohort, total cholesterol, low HDLc, and high LDLc have all been shown to be significant risk factors for CHD in the elderly.

Although it was previously thought that it would take several years to see a potential benefit from statin therapy on the course atherosclerosis, therefore limiting its use in an elderly population, it has now been shown that the clinical benefits of statins can be seen as early as 6 months and that they can improve endothelial dysfunction within 3 days of initiating therapy.

The secondary prevention trials of LDLc-lowering therapies have shown significant reductions in cardiac events in the studied populations. The applicability of these results, however, to an elderly patient population is somewhat limited secondary to the small number of elderly subjects in these studies.

In subgroup analyses of the studies that did include elderly patients, there does appear to be a similar benefit to lipid lowering in this cohort of elderly patients to that for younger patients (see Table 16.2). Similarly, the limited data available for the use of statins in the primary prevention of CHD in the elderly also supports its use in this group.

Currently, lipid-lowering therapy is markedly underused in the elderly. In the absence of other contraindications, lipid-lowering therapy should be initiated in the elderly following the same ATP III guidelines used to guide therapy in a younger patient population.

Treatment of hypertension in the elderly

Similar to dyslipidemia, hypertension (HTN) is a common problem in the elderly, with a prevalence of over 60% in patients over the age of 60 years. There is a large body of literature supporting the benefit of treating HTN in the elderly, including patients over the age of 80 years. In a meta-analysis of trials of treatment of isolated systolic HTN, it was found that only 19 patients over the age of 70 would need to be treated for 5 years in order to prevent one cardiovascular event.

When initiating antihypertensive therapy in the elderly, there may be several potential limiting factors, namely postural/postprandial hypotension and sluggish baroreceptor and sympathetic nervous system

Table 16.2 Lipid-lowering therapy in those over 65 years old

Study	No. of elderly subjects	Results
4S	1021 subjects >65 years old	34% lower all-cause mortality, 43% lower CHD mortality, 34% lower MACE, 41% lower revascularization procedures
CARE	1283 subjects between 65 and 75 years old	For every 1000 elderly patients treated, 225 CV hospitalizations and 207 CV events were prevented.
LIPID	3514 subjects between 65 and 75 years old	Absolute benefit was greater in the elderly compared to the younger patients (fewer patients needed to be treated to prevent a death, MI, or stroke).
HPS	20K patients age 40–80 years old	Similar reduction in CV events in patients above and below age 65
CARDS	N/A	38% reduction in first CV event in subjects older than 65 years

---

Box 16.3 Antihypertensive therapy in the elderly

- First line: thiazide diuretics
- Second line: ACE inhibitor/ARB or long-acting dihydropyridine calcium channel blocker (i.e., amlodipine)
- β-Blockers should not be used as primary therapy for hypertension in the elderly in the absence of another specific indication (i.e., prior MI or CHF)

---

responsiveness, as well as impaired cerebral autoregulation, which necessitates cautious initiation of therapy to prevent or minimize ischemic and orthostatic side effects (see Box 16.3).

Therefore, when starting antihypertensive therapy, lower initial doses should be used (about one-half the dose used in younger patients).

Valvular heart disease in the elderly

Aortic stenosis

Calcific or degenerative aortic valve disease is the most common valvular abnormality seen in the elderly. The prevalence of at least moderate aortic stenosis (AVA <1.2 cm^2) in patients aged 75–85 years old was 5% in the Helsinki Aging Study.

Currently, the recommendations for aortic valve placement in aortic stenosis are the same as in the younger patient population, namely development of symptoms, severe AS in patients undergoing CABG or other valve surgery, or severe AS with LVEF <50%.

However, when considering aortic valve replacement in the elderly, it is important to note that elderly patients typically have poorer preoperative status than that of younger patients, leading to higher in-hospital mortality, ranging between 5% and 18% in various studies with age being a very important determinant of outcome.

Elderly patients also have more nonfatal complications and longer perioperative hospitalizations than a younger patient cohort. However, if the elderly patient survives the perioperative period, the patient typically does very well with good long-term survival and significant improvement in symptoms (similar survival to the general population of age-matched subjects). Therefore, more and more elderly patients are being considered for aortic valve surgery as surgical and supportive techniques continue to improve.

In addition, for patients who are considered too high a risk for surgical correction, percutaneous aortic valve replacement techniques are currently being developed in Europe and South America and may eventually be a viable alternative therapy in the elderly patient population.

Aortic regurgitation

Aortic regurgitation is less common in the elderly than calcific aortic stenosis or mitral regurgitation and is most often associated with aortic stenosis or dilation of the ascending aorta from long-standing hypertension.

Although prophylactic aortic valve surgery is usually recommended for asymptomatic patients with severe aortic insufficiency (AI) and evidence of LV dysfunction, in the elderly (especially patients over the age of 80), it is recommended that aortic valve surgery be reserved for those patients with symptoms and severe AI, given the increased risk of operative and long-term mortality with increasing age.

Mitral regurgitation

Mitral regurgitation (MR) is the second most common indication for valve surgery in the elderly, accounting for 30%–35% of cases. Myxomatous degeneration of the valve and ischemic heart disease are the two most common etiologies of mitral regurgitation in this patient population.

Similar to aortic regurgitation, it is preferable to refer patients over the age of 80 for mitral valve surgery only if they are symptomatic, as the 30-day mortality in patients over the age of 80 is >10% with mitral valve replacement.

The outcome after surgery varies on the basis of patient age, comorbidites, and disease severity and is improved with mitral valve repair compared to replacement. In addition, it has been shown that functional MR secondary to ischemia may improve significantly with CABG alone, thereby simplifying any potential procedure in this higher-risk patient population.

Mitral stenosis

Mitral stenosis remains a disease primarily of younger patients, with rheumatic heart disease being the most common etiology. In elderly patients the most common cause of mitral stenosis is impingement on the mitral valve by mitral annular calcification.

The preferred surgical treatment for mitral stenosis is mitral commissurotomy. However, this is often not possible in the elderly, necessitating mitral valve replacement.

The ideal treatment for those elderly patients with favorable valvular morphology is percutaneous valvotomy. However, the number of elderly patients who have valvular morphology amenable to this technique is quite limited.

Index

Framingham risk scoring system for women

Age

Years	Points
30–34	–9
35–39	–4
40–44	0
45–49	3
50–54	6
55–59	7
60–64	8
65–69	8
70–74	8

Diabetes

	Points
No	0
Yes	4

Smoker

	Points
No	0
Yes	2

LDL-C (mg/dL)

	Points
<100	–3
100–129	0
130–159	0
160–190	1
>190	2

HDL-C (mg/dL)

	Points
<35	5
35–44	2
45–49	1
50–54	0
>60	–2

SBP (mmHg) / DBP (mmHg)

SBP (mmHg)	< 80	80–84	85–89	90–99	≥100
<120	–3	0	0	2	3
120–129	0	0	0	2	3
130–139	0	0	0	2	3
140–159	2	2	2	2	3
≥160	3	3	3	3	3

Coronary heart disease risk

Total points	10 yr risk (%)
< –2	1
–2	2
0	2
1	2
2	3
3	3
4	4
5	5
6	6
7	7
8	8
9	9
10	11
11	13
12	15
13	17
14	10
15	24
16	27
17	32

Reprinted with permission from Wilson, PW, et al. Prediction of coronary heart disease using risk factor categories. *Circulation* 1998; 97:1837–1847.

Common Exercise Stress Protocols

Stage	Duration (min)	Bruce			Modified Bruce		
		Grade (%)	Speed (mph)	METS	Grade (%)	Speed (mph)	METS
1	3	10	1.7	5	0	1.7	1.7
2	3	12	2.5	7	5	1.7	2.8
3	3	14	3.4	10	10	1.7	5.4
4	3	16	4.2	13	12	2.5	7
5	3	18	5.0	16	14	3.4	10
6	3	20	5.5	19	16	4.2	13
7	3	22	6.0	22	18	5.0	17

ECG Localization of myocardial infarction

Anterior	ST elevation and/or Q waves in V1–V4/V5.
Anteroseptal	ST elevation and/or Q waves in V1–V3.
Anterolateral	ST elevation and/or Q waves in V1–V6 and I and aVL.
Lateral	ST elevation and/or Q waves in V5–V6 and T wave inversion/ST elevation/Q waves in I and aVL.
Inferolateral	ST elevation and/or Q waves in II, III, aVF and V5–V6 (sometimes I and aVL).
Inferior	ST elevation and/or Q waves in II, III and aVF.
Inferoseptal	ST elevation and/or Q waves in II, III, aVF, V1–V3.
True posterior	Tall R waves in V1–V2 with ST depression in V1–V3. T waves remain upright in V1–V2. This can be confirmed with an esophageal lead if available (method similar to an NG tube). Usually occurs in conjunction with an inferior or lateral infarct.
RV infarction	ST segment elevation in the right precordial leads (V3R–V4R). Usually found in conjunction with inferior infarction. This may only be present in the early hours of infarction.

JNC 7 Blood pressure classification

Category	SBP (mmHg)	DBP (mmHg)
Normal BP	<120 AND	<80
Pre-hypertension	120–139 OR	80–89
Stage 1 Hypertension	140–159 OR	90–99
Stage 2 Hypertension	≥160 OR	≥100

Reprinted with permission from Chobanian AV, et al. *Hypertension* 2003; 42(6): 1206–1252.